Women in Medicine

In telling the history of women in medicine, the pioneers (especially the turbulent ones) are rightly remembered and celebrated in books, articles, memorials, awards, names of buildings, and organizations – even in stone statues and memorials. In contrast, the generation who began the transition from minority status to the current numerical equity is seldom memorialized, yet without the efforts of these few determined women in what was unambiguously a male profession, the achievements of these pioneers could easily have withered.

This book is written to celebrate the unique generation of women who entered medicine between the Second World War and the early 1970s – determined women who just wanted to be doctors but ended up fundamentally changing the profession. Utilizing oral histories from 37 women who became physicians between 1948 and 1975, these women tell their stories in their own words and provide a valid picture of their experiences throughout their careers that has much resonance for those entering or practicing medicine today.

Women in Medicine: Stories from the Girls in White will be of interest to all health professionals or those considering entering health professions, particularly women, and their advisers and supporters, to medical educators, and to medical historians seeking to understand the progress of women in medicine and other professions since the end of WWII.

W0234857

Women in Medicine
Stories from the Girls in White

Anne Walling

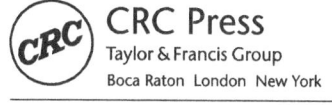

CRC Press
Taylor & Francis Group
Boca Raton London New York

CRC Press is an imprint of the
Taylor & Francis Group, an **informa** business

Designed cover image: University of Kansas Medical Center Archives, Kansas City, Kansas.

First edition published 2025
by CRC Press
2385 NW Executive Center Drive, Suite 320, Boca Raton FL 33431

and by CRC Press
4 Park Square, Milton Park, Abingdon, Oxon, OX14 4RN

CRC Press is an imprint of Taylor & Francis Group, LLC

© 2025 Anne Walling

ISBN: 978-1-032-88759-3 (hbk)
ISBN: 978-1-032-87319-0 (pbk)
ISBN: 978-1-003-53956-8 (ebk)

DOI: 10.1201/9781003539568

Typeset in Times LT Std
by Apex CoVantage, LLC

Contents

Acknowledgments

This project would not have been possible without my diligent and thoughtful co-investigators, Kari Nilsen, PhD, and Morgan Gillam, MD. We were assisted by several individuals associated with the University of Kansas School of Medicine, including our advisory board of Kim Templeton, MD; Grace Shih, MD; Barbara Lukert, MD; Susan Pingleton, MD; and Robert Daugherty, MD, as well as Jordann Snow and the staff of the Medical Alumni Association. Special thanks to Christopher Crenner, MD, and Alex Welborn of the Department of History and Philosophy of Medicine for their support and generous access to archival material. Developing the book owes much to the encouragement and expertise of Tim Butzen, MLIS, and Jo Koster, PhD. Above all, we are deeply grateful to the wonderful women who shared their life experiences in medicine and made the interviews so enjoyable and thought-provoking.

Acknowledgments

Author

Anne Walling, MB, ChB, FFPHM, is a Scottish physician who has lived in the United States since 1980. She is a 1971 graduate of the University of St. Andrews School of Medicine and a fellow of the Faculty of Public Health Medicine of the Royal College of Physicians. Since joining the University of Kansas School of Medicine in 1981, Dr. Walling has been a practicing family physician with academic roles, including clerkship director and vice-chair of the Department of Family and Community Medicine, vice-chair of the Department of Public Health and Preventive Medicine, and director of the standardized patient program. Becoming the first associate dean for faculty affairs and professional development in 1998, she supervised reorganization of the promotion and tenure system, bylaws revisions, and faculty development. She has been deeply involved in medical education and received major teaching awards at the departmental, school, and university level. After focusing on the Wichita campus in 2002, Dr. Walling was responsible for faculty affairs and professional development, taught in geriatrics and family medicine clerkships, and provided care to frail elderly patients. Moving to Emerita status in 2017 has enabled Dr. Walling to continue coaching faculty members in career development and scholarship, as well as pursue her interests in issues for senior female physicians.

Dr. Walling has been an associate editor for *American Family Physician* since 1989 and is a reviewer for several major journals. She has published 145 peer-reviewed articles, over 25 book chapters, and several monographs. Dr. Walling's first book, *Academic Promotion for Clinicians*, was published in 2018, and a second edition is scheduled for publication in 2025. The motivation to tell the stories of *The Girls in White* came from conversations with the few senior women colleagues in the medical community but does owe something to having been forced to read "Boys in White" for a medical sociology course in 1968 and wanting to give voice to the women who were excluded from that study as being irrelevant to the "man's work" of medicine!

Interview Guide for the Alumnae Oral History Project

What motivated you to think about becoming a physician?
Did you have any role models or mentors?
Tell me more about your background.
What did your family think/do about you becoming a physician?
What happened in high school to encourage or discourage your career choice?
What was college like? What college experiences encouraged or discouraged your career choice?
Did you train for or work in another career before medicine?
Tell me about the admissions process.
• Was there a quota for women?
• Who conducted the interview?
• What were you asked?
What was medical school like for you?
• How did you finance your training?
• How were you treated by faculty, interns/residents, nurses, patients, classmates?
• Did you have any role models or mentors?
How did you select your specialty?
Tell me about getting an intern or residency position.
What was being an intern/resident like for you?
• How were you treated by faculty, fellow interns/residents, nurses, patients, others?
• Did you have any role models or mentors?
Overall, what do you think about your medical education?
Tell me about working as a physician.
How did you manage professional responsibilities with your personal and family life?
Did you ever feel burned out or want to quit?
Did you ever work part-time or take any significant time away from medicine?
Overall, what do you think about your career?
• What were the best aspects? The worst aspects?
• How would things have been different if you were male?
• If you had a "do-over," what would you do differently?
What advice do you have for women thinking of entering medicine now or in training?
What do you think about the *#MeToo* movement? Did you or your friends encounter sexual harassment?

1

Introduction: Capturing the Stories

We need to write our own history before someone else writes it for us!

In the summer of 1934, a 10-year-old girl watched as a seriously injured boy was carried into her father's rural medical office. It was harvesttime in Kansas, time for the local boys to shoot the terrified rabbits flushed out by the advancing combines. In the dust, excitement, and confusion, one of the boys took shotgun blasts to his abdomen and thighs. The girl's father was delivering a baby at a remote farm and could not be reached. Her mother, a nurse, did what she could to staunch the profuse bleeding and triage his wounds, but the boy had to be put in the back of a truck and driven over unpaved roads to Wichita. *I thought right then, if Mother had been a doctor, we could have treated him here and not sent him off. I realized being a nurse would be inadequate. I absolutely decided right then to become a doctor and stuck to it!*

From this vivid Depression-era recollection of an emergency on a hot Kansas after-noon, we set out to gather the stories of women who became physicians when medicine was an unusual, and often extremely difficult, career choice. We were interested in what motivated them to make this controversial choice of profession, how they navigated medical training and professional life, and what factors had supported and nurtured their development – as well as all the items and events that discouraged or impeded their progress. Above all, we wanted to hear firsthand accounts of becoming and living as a physician when the profession was overwhelmingly male and doctors were always assumed to be men.

The project originated in enjoying the war stories of senior colleagues. We realized that as these ladies retired or became frail, their stories would be lost. The stimulus to action was the contrast between their robust anecdotes and the common perceptions that all older female physicians had battled career-long, unrelenting misogyny and mistreatment. Our senior colleagues were perplexed and frustrated by such interpre-tations of their experiences. While they readily acknowledged the many challeng-ing, inappropriate, and unfair situations they had faced, they were unwilling to have their histories reinterpreted as completely negative. They vigorously resisted being regarded as victims or survivors but were more uncomfortable being cast as hero-ines by their students and junior colleagues. As one put it: *I keep getting told, "You were so BRAVE to go to medical school – you were HEROIC!" Everyone likes being praised and put on a pedestal, but I don't know what to say. I don't want to burst their bubbles. Of course, it was tough and plenty of bad things happened, but it was not all bad and we managed to have a lot of fun along the way. We need to write our own history before someone else writes it for us!*

DOI: 10.1201/9781003539568-1

The Only Woman in the Room Study

In 2018, the Medical Society of Sedgwick County invited older female members living in the Wichita area to share their stories. The findings were published in "The Only Woman in the Room" (OWR) – a title suggested by a retired surgeon, but a sentiment shared by all 23 participants of the sudy.[1]

The OWR study provided a vivid and positive picture of young women navigating medical education in the 1960s and early 1970s. The overall tone of the discussions was upbeat, but participants did not shy away from describing their adverse experiences. The wide-ranging discussions and personal anecdotes included frank accounts of discrimination, mistreatment, and diverse negative experiences occurring from high school to retirement. Participants attributed much of what now would be considered gender-based discrimination and mistreatment to the accepted attitudes and treatment of women at that time. *It was the '60s – that stuff went on everywhere. It was just the way it was. We knew what we were getting into.* They focused on overcoming challenges, learning, growing in their profession, and finding joy in being able to *make a difference, be useful, help people*, rather than dwelling on negative aspects of their training and careers. Only one expressed enduring bitterness over incidents during her training and practice. Overall, the participants expressed great satisfaction and a sense of fulfillment from their careers and enthusiastically endorsed medicine as *a wonderful career for women.*

From the masses of information in the notes and transcripts, the key themes were the tenacity, resilience, and humor of these feisty ladies – as well as the surprising diversity of their personal and professional experiences. The discussions generated many anecdotes and personal stories but limited the number of recollections and opportunities for in-depth discussion of shared experiences. In addition, the groups immediately established an upbeat and collegial atmosphere that may have inhibited sharing sensitive or distressing experiences. The OWR project provided a fascinating picture, mainly of the trainee experiences during the 1960s and the 1970s. A larger study was needed to flesh out the picture of becoming a female physician in the 1960s and the 1970s and the professional experiences of women in medicine over the following decades.

The Alumnae Project

In 2019, we partnered with the University of Kansas Medical Alumni Association to seek information from women who attended the University of Kansas School of Medicine (KUSM) prior to the influx of women that began in the mid-1970s. By 1975, women finally represented about 25% of medical school matriculants, having more than doubled in five years.[1] The OWR discussions revealed marked differences in the experiences and attitudes of the women who entered medical school after 1975. Although they were still a minority, once women represented one quarter of the class, they were no longer so unusual, isolated, or invisible.

We decided on an oral history format using guided interviews – a technique designed to "complement and enrich the written record of significant events and improve understanding of crucial periods by drawing on the recollections of participants or witnesses."[2] This approach has been used to document the careers and insights of several distinguished female physicians, most graduating prior to the 1970s.[3-8] Our goal was a wider representation of women entering medicine prior to 1975. We designed the interview guide based on our OWR experience, an updated literature review,[8-17] the best practice recommendations of the Oral History Association, and input from our advisory board, comprised of alumnae (classes of 1960 and 1972), an alumnus (class of 1958), senior female faculty members, and alumni association representatives. A question was included about sexual harassment because of contemporary attention to the problem and concerns that it could have been downplayed or avoided during the group OWR discussions.

The medical alumni association used newsletters and personal contacts to invite alumnae from the class of 1975 and earlier to participate. We were able to complete interviews with 37 of the 49 women who volunteered to share their stories. Nine could not be contacted despite repeated efforts. Three withdrew because of poor health. Our oldest participant graduated in 1948 and was 96 years of age. Some ladies were frail but struggled determinedly to participate; others were so active that we had difficulty finding time in their busy schedules to complete an interview. Since ours was an approved university study, we provided participants with detailed information, including arrangements to ensure confidentiality of information, and obtained signed consent forms prior to each interview.

During the winter of 2020–2021, we interviewed alumnae living from the east coast of Maine to the west coast of Maui. The COVID-19 pandemic proved an unexpected benefit, as it necessitated the use of interactive communication services that captured the body language, facial expressions, and conversational nuances of participants and recorded interviews for reference. Each interview began with an invitation for the alumna to tell her story, starting with family background and why she had been attracted to medicine. Participants were encouraged to describe their lives in their own words, with the interviewer only using prompt questions as necessary to ensure all areas of interest were addressed. The tone was friendly and conversational. Most interviews were completed within 60 minutes; some lasted over two hours, and a few required two sessions. Within two days of the interview, each participant received her transcript, along with a note expressing thanks and requesting any additional information, corrections, or clarifications. This feedback was incorporated into the final written record of each interview. We are enormously grateful to the many family members, friends, and caretakers who assisted often frail or technologically challenged participants to master the mysteries of remote interactive interviews. We have also been moved by the feedback from several family members that the project prompted mothers and grandmothers to tell long-forgotten stories about *being a girl who went into medicine*.

The interviews were conducted by a retired physician who spent her career at KUSM but had trained in the United Kingdom, graduating in 1971. To analyze the data, she was joined by a fourth-year KUSM student and a PhD psychologist with expertise in qualitative research and women's issues, including aging, employment, and retirement. This team used thematic analysis to identify and interpret patterns of meaning across the masses of qualitative data in the interviewer's field notes, interview transcripts, and recordings.[18] The three investigators each independently analyzed the recordings, then worked together to reach consensus on the principal themes expressed by interviewees and to identify illustrative quotations. Alumnae quotations are provided in italics throughout this book. The very different backgrounds and perspectives of the three evaluators generated rich discussions in reaching consensus. When necessary, investigators returned to the recoded interviews for verification of information.

The 37 interviewees described diverse pathways to medicine and a rich plethora of experiences during training and throughout their long professional lives. They served thousands of patients through 13 different medical specialties and practiced in a wide range of environments, from rural Appalachian clinics to prestigious cancer research institutes. Over the years, they practiced medicine in 16 different states plus several countries overseas. Ten (27%) had predominantly academic careers, and others taught medical students and other health professionals in their practices. Three retrained in a second specialty after some time in practice. While their stories are those of women mostly from one area of the country who entered medicine through one institution, their experiences are likely to resonate with other contemporary female physicians, certainly those attending similar medical schools in the central United States. We hope our experience will encourage other medical schools and professional organizations to gather oral histories of this generation of women. In particular, we hope the stories of women from minority groups will be sought and recorded, as only one of our volunteers was non-White.

REFERENCES

1. Walling A, Nilsen K, Templeton KJ. The only woman in the room: oral histories of senior women physicians in a Midwestern City. Womens Health Rep (New Rochelle). 2020 Aug 24;1(1):279–86.
2. Davis C, Back K, MacLean K. Oral history: from tape to type. Chicago: American Library Association;1977.
3. Morantz RM, Pomerleau CS, Fenichel CH. In her own words. Westport (CT): Greenwood Press;1982.
4. East C, Bridges D. Women physicians at Baylor University Medical Center. BUMC Proceed. 2004;17:304–17.
5. Center for the History of Medicine at Countway Library. Oral histories. The Women in Medicine Legacy Foundation [cited August 2024]. Available from: https://www.wimlf.org/oral-histories
6. Women in white: women physicians oral history. University of Kentucky Libraries. Louie B Nunn Center for Oral History Project [cited August 2024]. Available from: https://kentuckyoralhistory.org/ark:/16417/xt77d7959s9f
7. Women in Duke Health [cited August 2024]. Available from: https://exhibits.mclibrary.duke.edu/duke-women/
8. Detweiler S, Cartwright L. Women physician pioneers of the 1960s: their lives and profession over a half century. San Francisco (CA): University of California Medical Humanities Press;2022.

9. Walsh MR. Doctors wanted: no women need apply: sexual barriers in the medical profession 1835–1975. New Haven and London: Yale University Press;1977.
10. Morantz-Sanchez R. Sympathy & science: women physicians in American medicine. New York (NY): Oxford University Press;1985.
11. More ES. Restoring the balance: women physicians and the profession of medicine 1985–1995. Cambridge (MA): Harvard University Press;1999.
12. Campbell MA. Why would a girl go into medicine? Old Westbury (NY): Feminist Press;1975.
13. Lopate C. Women in medicine. Baltimore (MD): Johns Hopkins Press;1968.
14. Matthews MR. The training and practice of women physicians: a case study. J Med Educ. 1970;45:1016–24.
15. Williams PA. Women in medicine: some themes and variations. J Med Educ. 1971;46:584–91.
16. Boulis A, Jacobs J. The changing face of medicine: women doctors and the evolution of heath care in America. Ithaca (NY): Cornell University Press;2008.
17. Dubé WF. Woman students in U.S. medical schools: past and present trends. J Med Educ. 1973;48(2):186–9.
18. Clarke V, Braun V, Terry G, Hayfield N. Thematic analysis. In: Liamputtong P, editor. Handbook of research methods in health and social sciences. Singapore: Springer;2019.

2

Women in Medicine: Does the History Matter Now?

"Remembering what it took to get us here will, I hope, help to ensure the equal success of future generations of physicians independent of their sex."[1]

A rich history underlies the continuing efforts to enhance the careers of women in medicine. The experiences of women who entered medicine between the end of World War II and the early 1970s are especially important as they lived the transition from long-established minority status to numerical gender equity and, we hope, established the secure foundation for continuing progress. By 2023, over half of medical students, 48% of residents and fellows, and 38% of active physicians were women, and their representation and influence in the profession continue to grow.[2,3] Unfortunately, rising numbers do not guarantee equality. There is ample evidence that women's salaries continue to lag behind those of their male colleagues, and that they remain underrepresented in several specialties and in leadership positions.[2] More than 50 years since the first large numbers of women entered medical school, these issues seem unlikely to self-correct, as ever-larger cohorts of female physicians advance in their careers and achieve critical mass in many areas of the profession. Women in medicine continue to be disadvantaged despite policies, regulations, and the efforts of diverse initiatives, services, and programs to support their careers.[2,4]

Further progress depends on addressing complex structural and cultural factors in the profession and its institutions. The focus of women's issues in medicine has gradually shifted from increasing numbers and facilitating the careers of individuals to addressing fundamental organizational and cultural factors that impede women from achieving their full potentials.[2,4–7] Addressing such issues requires understanding the history behind many of the ingrained misconceptions and recurring challenges for women in the profession. Topics such as women's perceived suitability for medicine and concerns about their sexuality, stamina, productivity, and ability to manage both family and professional roles have deep roots and remarkable tenacity. They repeatedly re-emerge in different guises or with new variations on the underlying themes, but they never completely disappear from considerations of women's careers in medicine. The language may change, but ingrained issues can intervene unexpectedly to sabotage women's progress or the credibility of female leaders. History teaches that continued progress is neither inevitable nor achieved solely on the basis of merit, equality of numbers, or justice. Current hard-won and well-deserved gains must not be taken for granted; they can be reversed, stalled, or perverted. This has happened in the past on more than one occasion.[8]

DOI: 10.1201/9781003539568-2

The story of women in US medicine is one of successive advances and setbacks rather than sustained progress. The current generation is not the first to claim a breakthrough for women in US medicine. New dawns have been confidently proclaimed at least three times – once in the late 19th century, and again in the later periods of each world war – only to be eclipsed by subsequent events.[8] The generation of women covered by our interviews has the unique distinction of establishing a presence in the profession that has endured and grown rather than peaked then ebbed under the pressures of backlash and multiple challenges. They were not another temporary wave of female entrants but the transition to a new normal in the profession.

The New Century: A Bright Future

By the end of the 19th century, women were established in American medicine and seemed poised for sustained progress. In 1900, 7,387 women were registered physicians. This was a 60% increase in a decade but only represented 5.6% of physicians.[8]

Women were making gains in many aspects of the profession. By the 1890s, women could apply to 19 medical schools exclusively for women as well as compete for places at several co-educational institutions. In 1893, women accounted for 37% of medical students at Boston University, and 31% at the Kansas Medical College. Co-educational medical schools in states including Colorado, Oregon, Iowa, and Massachusetts reported 20% or more of their enrolled students were women.[8] The expanding opportunities led to questioning the need for women-only medical schools, as the larger co-educational institutions had the potential to provide more resources and opportunities for female students and faculty members. In 1899, a women's medical school closed, having "fulfilled its purpose, and medical education may hereafter be obtained by women in New York in the same classes, under the same faculty, with the same clinical opportunities as men."[8] By 1910, only two medical colleges for women remained. Even the pioneering Dr. Emily Blackwell concluded that women's medical colleges had provided an essential but temporary service that was now obsolete, having "held open the doors for women until broader gates had swung open for their admission."[8]

This rosy picture failed to recognize that several institutions refused to admit women and the widespread use of quotas to limit the number of female students. The doors of medical schools had not been flung wide to welcome women; rather, they had been pried open by sustained moral, political, social, and other pressures. Some schools only accepted women in return for bribes of large endowments.[8] Women faced many impediments to entering the profession. Aspiring female physicians encountered discouragement, dismissal, ridicule, or insult. Medicine was widely considered unnatural for women, or at least unfeminine. Being regarded as unfeminine has been a recurring theme for female physicians but now may be less flagrantly expressed than in 1867: "We hope never to see the day when the female character shall be so completely unsexed as to fit it for the disgusting duties which imperatively devolve upon one who would obtain proficiency in the healing arts."[9]

Aspiring female physicians could, and still do, also encounter barriers erected in the guise of concern for their physical and emotional welfare. A popular book, *Sex in Education: Or, A Fair Chance for the Girls*, warned in 1873 that "excessive education" damaged women's health and stunted their development. The resulting "monstrous brains and puny bodies made over-educated women unfit for their most important roles as wives and mothers."[10] Despite considerable evidence to the contrary, including an 1881 survey of 430 female physicians demonstrating that they enjoyed better health than their peers, it was widely believed that women lacked the physical and emotional stamina required for medical school and practice.[8] Admitting women to medical school would destroy their health and waste resources that could have been used to train robust male physicians. The waste of resources or poor investment is another recurring theme – usually twinned with the denial of opportunities to deserving men.

Female medical students at the turn of the century were generally older than their male counterparts, had often been employed (many as teachers), and were mostly dependent on family or their own resources for financial support. They often encountered hostility from faculty and fellow students and had to navigate institutional obstacles, such as being barred from participating in certain procedures or areas of hospitals, denied membership in honor societies, and refused access to financial support.[8,11] Nevertheless, women performed well. In 1902, women gained 60% of the graduation honors at Tufts, although representing only 26% of the class.[8,11] Academic success caused consternation among male classmates and faculty members, contributing to a backlash against women. When the first woman graduated from the University of Michigan in 1871, she achieved the highest honors but was "hooted and showered with abusive notes."[8]

Once qualified, women faced multiple challenges. Nevertheless, by the end of the 19th century, many female physicians were well established, and several had large and lucrative practices.[8] Female physician were slowly overcoming the expectations that they would limit their practices to the health of women and children and were undertaking an increasing variety of specialties, including surgery.[8,11-13] They were also countering the notions that women might not be fully committed to medicine and be willing to be tolerated only as amusing, demure, and decorative adjuncts to the profession, such as the "dilettante female physician" who treated her practice as a part-time hobby rather than a serious profession.[8] These "beauteous damsels who flitted about the tables of medical society meetings like joys forever"[8] may have allayed the fears of their male colleagues about professional competition but did little to enhance the image of women as intelligent and competent physicians. The dilettantes may have been more fanciful than real. An 1881 survey showed that over 90% of female graduates were professionally active, but the idea that women are less committed to medicine than their male colleagues has been another recurring problem. Commitment to medicine has repeatedly been linked to remaining single. Marriage raises the thorny issue of reconciling family and professional responsibilities – perhaps the most serious and enduring external challenge and internal concern for female physicians. As early as the 1881 survey, over 40% of respondents reported being married. This was higher than for other college-educated women, demonstrating over 140 years ago that medicine was compatible with marriage and motherhood. Overall, despite the many diverse challenges, the women of American medicine made significant gains during the latter years of the 19th century and entered the 20th century on a wave of optimism, confident that the momentum of the previous decade would be sustained.[8]

Backlash and Retreat

At first, this optimism seemed justified. The 1910 Flexner Report that revolutionized US medical education concluded that women faced few, if any, barriers in medical school admission:

> "Medical education is now, in the United States and Canada, open to women upon practically the same terms as men. . . . No woman desiring an education in medicine is under any disability in finding a school to which she may gain admittance. Her choice is free and varied. She will find schools of every grade accessible."[14]

Nevertheless, it was already evident that progress had stalled. In 1910, the number of female physicians peaked at 9,015 (6% of the total), a number that would not be equaled until the 1950s.[8,11] The early 1900s saw nationwide declines in the numbers of female medical students, even in institutions that had previously reported high percentages of female students. At Tufts University in 1900, women accounted for 42% of graduates in medicine; by 1908, they represented fewer than 10% of medical students. Institutions in Kansas, Colorado, Oregon, Iowa, Massachusetts, and other states that had previously reported 20–30% female medical students reported rates of 4–6% by 1908.[8] Over a relatively short period, several schools began to refuse women students; others imposed quotas and/or made successful application difficult or nearly impossible. Northwestern University abruptly closed its women's medical school in 1902 without notice to faculty or students. The results of these institutional changes were dramatic, effectively choking off the pipeline for women in medicine. In 1910, the entire United States had 907 female medical students (4.0% of the total), and only 116 women graduated in medicine (2.6% of the total). By 1915, the number of students had dropped to 592, and a mere 92 women graduated in medicine. At the lowest point in 1912, women represented only 2.3% of US medical students.[11]

Why women faded from medicine in the early 20th century remains unclear. Flexner attributed the dramatic reduction in the number of women physicians and their loss of influence in the profession to "decreasing inclination of women to enter medicine, possibly augmented by the lack of any strong demand for women physicians."[14] Historians point to multiple social, educational, financial, institutional, personal, and other factors acting synergistically to make medicine a difficult and unappealing career for women, discourage their admission to medical training, and impede their success in the profession. Some authors also suggest that female physicians and their supporters contributed to the decline by relaxing their crusading efforts too soon in the belief that the future was assured.[8]

A major factor was backlash against the success of female physicians. In the early 1900s, America had a physician surplus. Competition for patients and fees was intense and could be unscrupulous, fueled by popular publications, such as *Dollars to Doctors; or, Diplomacy and Prosperity in Medical Practice* (1903) and *Large Fees and How to Get Them: A Book for the Private Use of Physicians* (1911). Although the profession was hardly "overcrowded to the starving point with a flood of hungry graduates poured into it each Spring," as the *Journal of the American Medical Association* (JAMA) wailed in 1898,[15] many physicians faced financial uncertainty, exacerbated by the annual entry of "swarms of young men and young women to the profession."[16] The rising availability of female physicians was of particular concern as practices (and income) could be impacted if female patients were to prefer female physicians.

An influx of women into medicine threatened both incomes and prestige. In addition to attracting patients away from their male colleagues, female physicians were believed to be less motivated by financial rewards. This might lower fees for all physicians. Prestige was enhanced by income but was contingent upon medicine remaining a resolutely male profession. A few token women might be tolerated as long as they knew their place and conformed to the expectations of their male colleagues. A noticeable presence of women risked the profession being considered as "women's work," and thus of lower prestige.[8,13,17] An increasing presence of women plus the oversupply of physicians was a formula for disruption, decreased income, increased competition, and lowered prestige.[8,13,17,18] "Meddlesome females are crowding into medicine, taking the bread out of our mouths, and turning the divine order of things completely topsy-turvy."[18]

These very practical considerations played out against major upheavals in both medicine and society concerning the roles of women. Medicine was perceived as natural for women when it focused on alleviating suffering, soothing and nurturing patients, and other humanitarian activities. As science, rationality, and efficiency became dominant in American medicine, women's attributes, interests, and talents were increasingly seen as inappropriate for robust scientifically based medicine. The duties of a physician became increasingly incompatible with the acceptable activities of a respectable woman.[8,13,17] Those women who felt a vocation to care for the sick were encouraged to divert their energies into becoming nurses – regarded as the handmaidens of supervising physicians. "Nurses are docile, submissive and keep their proper place; let a woman study medicine and she thinks her opinion is as good as a man!"[18] The "sympathy versus science" argument that women are inherently more suited to the softer aspects of medicine than to its hard science may explain much of the dramatic reduction in women entering medicine.[13] The 1910 Flexner Report established modern medical education grounded firmly in the sciences and dominated by teaching hospitals and institutions.[14] This report consolidated many "masculine" attributes of medicine and led to the closure of many inferior medical schools, but the decline in women's entry to the profession was already well underway and cannot be attributed to Flexner's reforms. Women had established a record of academic achievement even in the most scientific and competitive schools; they were more likely to gain than lose by the elimination of inferior medical colleges and the elevation of the intellectual and ethical standards of the profession.[8]

The retrenchment of women in medicine reflected a wave of antifeminism in the early 20th century. Focus on the duty of young women to become wives and mothers almost excluded any consideration of medicine as a career. Such an unfeminine career was openly opposed even by the AMA.[8,11,13] "The girl's vocation in the world is to be a wife and mother, to be the mistress, caretaker and manager of her home."[19] Societal pressures were brought to bear on families and others to whom a woman might turn for financial and other support of her career ambitions. Obtaining the necessary preparation in science was possible but increasingly discouraged, even at the most academic women's colleges.[20] Studies in home economics became well established as an alternative to hard sciences to prepare "college women to make cheery efficient homes."[8] Pursuing a career in science or medicine was associated with more radical views – perhaps even the dangerous and unladylike Women's Suffrage movement! Female physicians were overwhelmingly supportive of Women's Suffrage, and about half identified as Suffrage leaders.[8] Those few women who entered medicine in the early years of the 20th century were robust and determined. Compared to later graduates, they reported significantly less concern about the disapproval of others, combining practice with marriage and children, or doubts about their motivation, health, stamina, or intellectual abilities. None reported concerns about being considered unfeminine or emotionally unstable.[21]

1915: Optimism and Opportunities

By 1915, supporters of women in US medicine had rallied. In that year, the AMA admitted its first female members, and the American Medical Women's Association (AMWA) was formed. As 1915 saw the lowest recorded number of female medical students (592) and graduates (92), there was much to be done.[10]

The onset of World War I presented opportunities for women due to the combination of reduced availability of male applicants to medical schools plus increasing demand for physicians. Thirteen of the exclusionary medical schools began accepting women.[8] Those women who were admitted still had to navigate a hostile environment and were made very aware that their presence was only tolerated because of the shortage of male applicants. "If enough men applied, she would be 'thrown out.'"[11]

The shortage of male physicians also presented opportunities for women to prove their worth. The war brought a temporary increase in the availability of internship positions for women. Female physicians also stepped up to fill the gaps in civilian care left by enlisted physicians. Many volunteered for military service but were rejected. Over 50 women served as contract surgeons in military hospitals in Europe through a collaboration of AMWA, the Suffrage Association, and the Red Cross.[8,11] These women had no military commissions, status, or benefits but provided impressive services. A 1915 *JAMA* commentary concluded that because of wartime,

> "excellent service, it will be impossible for conservatism any longer to deny all opportunity to women. After the War, there will be a readjustment accompanied by more or less friction: . . . women physicians may undoubtedly look

forward in the end to a fair field, from which old prejudices have been to a considerable degree eliminated by the pressure of necessity. It will be interesting to see what use they make of their enlarged opportunities."[22]

Interwar Years: Faltering Momentum and Elusive Promise

The gains of WWI may have been exaggerated, and the expectations of new and deserved opportunities over-optimistic. Hopes for advancement of women in US medicine following the war quickly dissipated. Old prejudices showed no difficulty in resurrecting themselves, and new challenges arose.[8,11,17] Following the wartime influx, the number of female US medical students reached 818 by 1920 but represented only 5.8% of medical students.[11] Women represented 4–5% of US medical students and graduates until 1946, reflecting the general quota of up to 5% per class.[8] The number of female students first reached over 1,000 (1,056, 4.7%) in 1933. As late as 1934, 28% of US medical schools had never graduated a woman.[11]

The interwar years saw great social, political, and financial upheavals. For female physicians, they were "decades of faltering momentum and elusive promise."[17] Women continued to face the well-established challenges in obtaining medical education and advancing in the profession, but with the rise of specialization in medicine, issues concerning postgraduate training assumed greater significance.[8,11,13]

Difficulties for women in obtaining postgraduate training had been noted in the 1910 Flexner Report.[14] Flexner recommended that "internal privileges must be granted to women graduates on the same terms as men" as a condition of the elimination of women's medical colleges in favor of co-educational institutions. Nevertheless, women had always experienced considerable difficulty in obtaining any postgraduate training, except in a few female-oriented institutions. The extreme shortage of physicians during WWI had opened internships at some institutions, but many of these closed to women as soon as the war ended. Typical comments were to "not consider a woman unless it is impossible to get a desirable man."[13] Institutions used a variety of justifications – if any were offered – such as lack of accommodation for female physicians, patient resistance to being treated by a woman, causing distractions or not fitting in with the working environment, resistance from nurses, and the ever-present danger of disruption of work due to female ailments or even pregnancy. In 1921, only 40 (8.3%) of the 482 hospitals offering approved internships accepted women.[8] These hospitals were clustered in certain cities, forcing women to compete for positions that might be distant from family and support systems, while their male classmates were recruited by a plethora of institutions. The situation only improved slowly. In 1934 (the year our oldest participant crystalized her intent to become a physician), 43% of US hospitals had never employed a female physician.[11] Although an increasing number of states required completion of an approved internship for licensure, by 1938, only 185 internships were available nationwide for the 237 female graduates, whereas 6,154 internships competed for the attention of their 4,844 male classmates.[8]

The interwar years were challenging for practicing female physicians. They often struggled with issues that had little or no impact on their male colleagues. In addition to usually being supported by a wife and free from many domestic and family responsibilities, male physicians could assume that essentials such as obtaining hospital privileges or licensure would be managed easily. Men could also count on support from their colleagues for patient referrals or consultations, coverage for absences, and inclusion in professional and social events. Female physicians were often marginalized and ignored. As one stated in 1929, "Men do not want women in their institutions and organizations except as subordinates and auxiliaries. As assistants, technicians, nurses, and stenographers, they are greatly appreciated and most indispensable. As competitors for equal recognition men simply tolerate us under compulsion."[23]

Finances proved particularly challenging for women in the interwar period, both in terms of sustaining income and in obtaining financial support from banks, financial institutions, and hospitals or practice groups. Typical contemporary comments include how "Women have to work harder, do more, and seldom are equally paid. A woman must be about 50% superior in the quality of her work to receive the same consideration as a medical man."[13] The income of female physicians was impacted by patient choices as well as by discrimination from colleagues and institutions. During the interwar years, female patients became more willing to consult male physicians, while a growing disapproval of feminism led to discomfort with female physicians – the net effect decreased the availability of the traditional pool of female patients.[8] Financial challenges and social disapproval were even greater for married female physicians, especially those with children. In the 1920s, only 7–8% of married women were employed outside the home, and 26 states had laws prohibiting the employment of married women.[24] Even within the profession, the possibility (or wisdom) of combining a career with marriage and motherhood was debated. Some of the most vigorous attacks came from female physicians who had dedicated their lives to medicine and expressed outrage at the disgraceful prospect of a woman attempting to succeed in both medicine and marriage/motherhood.[13] A 1932 graduate dismissed her married colleagues, stating, "The modern quest for fulfillment seems crazy to me."[11] If tolerated, married female physicians were expected to seek positions with less responsibility and/or ones more accommodating of disruptions, such as laboratory work, public health, or salaried positions.[8] A 1928 publication concluded that "having children is almost an insurmountable barrier to a career."[17]

Driven by the need for professional survival, many female physicians turned away from their traditionally liberal positions, but others persisted in promoting public health and social programs, especially for women and children.[17] Such programs received a significant boost from the Sheppard–Towner Act of 1921 that established the US Children's Bureau and a national program of prenatal and child health centers.[17] These programs and those of the later New Deal provided opportunities for female physicians, but they exacerbated the schism between public and private practice, further marginalizing female physicians and enhancing the perception that women physicians should be limited to practicing public health or pediatrics.[13,17]

World War II

As the United States entered the 1940s, the status of women in US medicine had reached a low point in both numbers and prestige. "For women born in the early 20th century, medicine as a career was unlikely in the extreme; it took an unusually strong-minded woman."[25] Female physicians appeared to have little energy or incentive to break out of their predominantly passive roles.

> "Women physicians who came of age after 1930 were trained in a medical world almost totally bereft of female-run institutions, female support systems, or a traditionally female point of view. Young women physicians learned to accept the prevailing values of the profession without wielding any real power within it."[17]

They eyed the onset of war with mixed feelings – would it offer new opportunities for women to enter medicine and finally prove their worth? More importantly, would ground gained and promises given during wartime be maintained into the following peace – or would women step up, provide essential service, and be relegated to submissive roles as soon as the old order could be re-established? Amid this uncertainty, our first interviewees entered medical school in the 1940s.

The number of female medical students increased only modestly from 1,145 (5.4%) in 1940 to 1,352 (5.6%) in 1945.[11] Despite the wartime demand for physicians and the diversion of young men into military and war-related occupations, several factors inhibited an influx of women into medicine. First was the substantial social pressure (plus the attraction of unprecedented earnings) for women to put personal ambitions on hold and devote themselves to the war effort. Over six million women joined the workforce, presumably including some who might otherwise have considered medical careers.[24] Secondly, medical schools moved to reduce the number of female students or refuse them admission for the duration of the war "for patriotic motives," presumably to use all available places to prepare male physicians for military service.[8] Finally, male students could access substantial financial support – in some years, up to 80% had all their expenses covered from military sources.[8] Nevertheless, the percentage of women admitted each year increased during the war to a high of 14.4% of freshmen in 1945. By 1947, the United States had over 2,000 female medical students, reaching an unprecedented 9.5% of all students in 1948. Similarly, the number of female graduates peaked at 612 (12.1%) in 1949.[11] The war years also saw unprecedented gains in the availability of internships for women. In 1941, only 105 hospitals accepted female interns; by 1942, this had escalated to 463.

Female physicians contributed to the war effort in multiple ways, including stepping in to serve civilian populations in the absence of physicians called to military service. As during WWI, the American Medical Women's Association (AMWA) led efforts to directly involve female physicians in the military, registering over 2,000 to serve in the American Women's Hospital Service and advocating for women to be commissioned in the Army and Navy Medical Corps. This was finally achieved in 1943 – nurses had been commissioned since 1920.[8,11]

Female physicians anticipated the postwar era with optimism. A *New York Times* article validated this positive outlook, echoing the sentiments of the 1915 *JAMA* article: "Women doctors who took the place of men and worked long hours have come into their own. They have arrived, they are wanted, and their position is at last secure."[8]

A commentary in the *AMWA Journal* took things even further, stating that wartime achievements would ensure "an undeniable right to consideration for entrance into the country's finest medical schools and acceptance for training in the foremost hospitals in the land."[8] Unfortunately, signs of a backlash were already evident in the postwar resurgence of the "cult of domesticity" as the ideal role for American women.[26] In a 1942 speech, the NIH director anticipated appropriate roles for women physicians as limited to general practice, maternal and childcare, psychiatry, public health, research, and teaching medical students.[17] Even more troubling is the 1946 advertisement in the *New York Herald Tribune* proclaiming, "Doctors Wanted: no women need apply."[8]

The Great Withdrawal[27]

Progress for women in medicine stalled, then declined, during the 1950s and early 1960s. The number of female medical students fell below 2,000 (1,806) in 1950 and did not recover until reaching 2,081 in 1963. Throughout the decade, the percentage of female medical students stagnated around 5.5%.[11] Again, the reasons are debatable but clearly reflect the synergistic impact of movements within medicine and society. The widespread use of quotas and frank antipathy from medical school leaders demonstrated the pervasive opposition to the admission of women to medical school. "We do keep women out, when we can. We don't want them here – and they don't want them elsewhere either, whether or not they'll admit it."[8] Those women who achieved admission entered a decidedly male world and hostile environment in which "many students and a significant number of faculty resent women and openly show their attitude."[28] Several articles documented "the special problems of women medical students" during this period.[28] In addition to overt institutional and other discrimination and mistreatment documented in the national literature, the class yearbooks of our early participants convey the atmosphere of pervasive immature misogyny through which they navigated the multiple personal and professional challenges medical school posed for women.

Things were not much better in practice. As during the interwar years, female physicians during the 1950s and 1960s clustered in a few specialties (notably pediatrics and psychiatry), tended to prefer salaried positions, and generally assumed low profiles.[8,11] Accounts from leading medical women of that time describe professional isolation and lack of support as they were buffeted by recurrent political, social, economic, and other problems. "Every step of the way is a way I had to work out myself," one said.[25] Male colleagues could be overtly hostile. In a 1949 survey, hospital chiefs of staff characterized their female colleagues as "emotionally unstable, always defensive, and talk too much. If married and childless, she is frustrated: if she raises a family, she is neglecting her practice."[11] Similarly, a 1953 national survey of 1925–1940 graduates generated comments such as: "Women were created to be wives: I dislike female doctors of either sex: and I prefer a third-rate man to a first-rate woman."[29] This survey's conclusion that female physicians were less productive than their male colleagues had a persisting negative impact on the progress of women in medicine. As in a later study of 1931–1956 graduates published in 1969, the authors concluded that female physicians were about 30% less productive than their male colleagues in terms of hours practiced and numbers of patients.[29,30] The "waste of training women physicians" was correlated with family size, reporting that 86% of single women worked full-time compared to 40% of those with three or more children.[30]

A related attack on training women targeted the higher dropout rates among female medical students. Although these were clearly attributable to non-academic issues, especially financial stress and family responsibilities, the only proposed solution was to limit the number of women admitted.[11,31,32] Little attention was given to addressing the unique personal and financial disadvantages of female medical students. Multiple subsequent studies countered the "low productivity" arguments and demonstrated the volume and quality of the work of female physicians.[8,11,21,33] Nevertheless, beliefs that women were twice as likely to drop out of training and only 60% as productive as their male colleagues in practice haunted the admissions interviews and career progress of our interviewees and of their contemporaries. Several recalled battling assumptions – *She's going to leave or ask for time off to have babies* – when applying for positions.

The setbacks for women in medicine during the 1950s and 1960s cannot be entirely blamed on attitudes and actions within the profession. As in the 1920s and 1930s, the postwar rise in male chauvinism and the emphasis on domesticity isolated female physicians from societal support. Cultural expectations acted synergistically with pressures within the profession to exacerbate the challenges for female physicians, especially in reconciling the responsibilities of both families and careers. Societal concepts of appropriate female roles and behavior reverted from the wartime enthusiasm for participation in the workforce – "there's practically no limit to the types of jobs women can do"[24] – to the primacy of excelling as a wife and mother. Women in the professions were regarded as abnormal, if not deviant. Contemporary books and movies portrayed any successful professional or businesswoman as coming to a miserable end, alone, despised, and bitter.[24,26] The "great withdrawal"[27] of women did not only impact medicine; its effects were also seen in reduced interest in science-related courses from high school girls and college women, encouraged by shifts in academic counseling and other pressures toward home economics and other female-appropriate topics.[8,11,27] Girls were not only socialized away from medicine and the professions but also encouraged to doubt or downplay their abilities in order to avoid being considered arrogant, pushy, or unfeminine.[8,11,27] Certainly, our interviewees, most of whom grew up during this era, are among "the few who persist and become physicians must be exceptionally motivated."[11]

New Dawn – Again

The 1960s and 1970s brought great political and social upheavals. Young women were especially impacted by movements such as those supporting civil rights, women's liberation, and other causes, including opposition to the Vietnam War. Everything changed: Demure dirndls gave way to miniskirts (or even hot pants), music was revolutionized, and issues such as sexuality – even contraception – were suddenly discussed openly. Amid the turmoil, young people perceived new possibilities and career opportunities. In particular, young women felt emboldened, if not entitled, to enter the professions.[24] They either encountered less societal disapproval and/or felt better equipped to achieve their career ambitions, despite criticism and discouragement.

The number of female medical students and their representation in the student body grew slowly during the 1960s from 1,710 (6.7%) in 1959–1960 to 3,390 (9.0%) in 1969–1970. Numbers began to escalate about 1971–1972, and by 1980, the 16,141 women represented 25.3% of all US medical students.[34]

Much of this dramatic increase is attributable to external social and political forces.[8,11,13,17,34,35] Medical schools were reluctant to receive an influx of women – and woefully unprepared. A 1973 survey of female students at 41 US medical schools reported pervasive and multifaceted discrimination and mistreatment of women at all levels of the institutions as an "unremitting recital of Bad Things" – with little motivation for change perceived at any institution.[36] Change, however, was underway. In 1970, discrimination in admissions was the subject of congressional hearings and a class action complaint filed against all US medical schools by the Women's Equity Action League.[8] This was quickly followed by an Association of American Medical Colleges (AAMC) resolution on equal opportunity for women and calls for individual schools to promptly initiate programs and practices to improve opportunities and foster a more supportive environment for women.[34] Regulatory and financial considerations may have been stronger motivations to improve the status of women in medical schools than the aspirations and exhortations of professional organizations. The Civil Rights Act (1964), Title IX of the Educational Amendments of 1972, and other legislation and federal regulations tied funding to institutional progress in opportunities for minority groups, including women.[34] Other funding sources followed the federal lead. Attention to discrimination and the experience of minority students became necessary for institutions to access essential core funding, including several types of grants and contracts, and for student eligibility for loan programs.

Despite these pressures, women in medicine still found themselves in an alien and often uncomfortable environment. Appropriate female roles and behaviors had not been clarified, and their accustomed behaviors could be counterproductive.[13,17,26,28,37–39]

> "Women who enter the domain of medicine, which has been male-defined, are likely to find that their presence is jarring and upsetting to others. First, women are unexpected and therefore feared as unpredictable. Second, their personal 'female' characteristics and qualities (which may be stereotypically imputed or actually theirs) are incongruent with those expected and valued for a physician."[37]

Medical schools were slow to adapt to the growing presence of women – by 1993, only half had offices or committees on women's issues.[17] By 1978, a comprehensive study concluded that

> "Affirmative action policies to increase the number of women in medical training institutions are indispensable for ultimate change, but are impotent at present to correct the effects of a discriminatory environment. Numbers alone will not undo the norms and values we have observed; these will

remain until we change the relation of male roles to the family, and crucial features of the structure and organization of professional work."[37]

Recognizing the powerful influence of culture (both within the profession and in society at large), some writers in the 1970s and since have worried about another antifeminist backlash and a repeat of the three historical great withdrawals from medicine and other professions in the early 20th century, the interwar years, and the 1950s.[8,24,38] Despite these concerns, the numbers of women in medicine have continued to grow, and progress continues to advance their status within the profession, especially in academic leadership.[2] While the gender revolution does not appear to have stalled as feared,[8,38] ample evidence can be found for continuing challenges and inequities for women in medicine.[2] The old stereotypes and beliefs may have gone underground, but they could easily reappear to challenge the appropriate participation of women and other minorities in medicine. Among these stereotypes are the prevailing perceptions of the women who entered medicine in the post-WWII era as victims, buffeted by hostile systems, and frustrated in their professional aspirations. One interviewee described a student's *righteous indignation on my behalf about my mistreatment!* It is tempting to interpret history as completely negative, but even in the study claiming women's experiences as "an unremitting recital of bad things," closer examination of the data and narratives from participants shows a much more nuanced picture.[36] Similarly, most oral histories, biographies, essays, and other writings from female physicians of the period do not convey an unrelentingly bleak experience. Without minimizing the many unfair, cruel, discriminatory, and difficult aspects of their lives and careers, the literature and surveys suggest older female physicians regard themselves as satisfied and successful – not downtrodden victims.[25,39] The literature is, however, limited to those few individuals who have provided information on their lives. Our interviews with 37 alumnae who graduated between 1948 and 1975 are also limited by this selection bias, but do provide a vivid picture of this period from women who lived the progression from under 5% to over 25% of the class. These ladies were not the first who got a foot in the door – that had been done more than a century previously – but they were the ones who kept the door open and demonstrated the sustained competence, dedication, and tenacity that gradually blunted criticism, tempered discrimination, and built (often reluctant) acceptance that women could be successful in medicine. They steadily wore down stereotypes and provided younger women with the realization and confidence that *women could be physicians!* Their efforts laid the foundation for (we hope) the enduring transformation of medicine into a profession in which all individuals can achieve their full potential unhampered by discrimination based on gender or any other personal characteristic. We have much to learn from their experiences.

REFERENCES

1. Wood M. Women in medicine: then and now. Anesth Analg. 2015 May;120(5):963–5.
2. Lautenberger DM, Dandar VM. The state of women in academic medicine 2023–2024: progressing towards equity. Washington (DC): AAMC;2024.
3. Association of American Medical Colleges (AAMC). U.S. physician workforce data dashboard 2022 [cited May 2024]. Available from: https://www.aamc.org/data-reports/report/us-physician-workforce-data-dashboard

4. Ellinas EH, Kaljo K, Patitucci TN, Novalija J, Byars-Winston A, Fouad NA. No room to 'lean in': a qualitative study on gendered barriers to promotion and leadership. J Womens Health (Larchmt). 2019 Mar;28(3):393–402.

5. Winkel AF, Telzak B, Shaw J, Hollond C, Magro J, Nicholson J, et al. The role of gender in careers in medicine: a systematic review and thematic synthesis of qualitative literature. J Gen Intern Med. 2021 Aug;36(8):2392–9.

6. Vassie C, Smith S, Leedham-Green K. Factors impacting on retention, success and equitable participation in clinical academic careers: a scoping review and meta-thematic synthesis. BMJ Open. 2020 Mar 25;10(3):e033480.

7. Helitzer DL, Newbill SL, Cardinali G, Morahan PS, Chang S, Magrane D. Changing the culture of academic medicine: critical mass or critical actors? J Womens Health (Larchmt). 2017 May;26(5):540–8.

8. Walsh MR. Doctors wanted: no women need apply: sexual barriers in the medical profession 1835–1975. New Haven and London: Yale University Press;1977.

9. Friesen SR, Hudson RP. The Kansas School of Medicine eyewitness reflections on its formative years. Kansas City: University of Kansas School of Medicine;1996.

10. Clarke EH. Sex in education; or, a fair chance for the girls. Boston (MA);1873.

11. Lopate C. Women in medicine. Baltimore (MD): Johns Hopkins Press;1968.

12. Pope EF, Call EL, Pope CA. The practice of medicine by women in the United States. Boston (MA);1881.

13. Morantz-Sanchez R, Sympathy & science: women physicians in American medicine. New York (NY): Oxford University Press;1985.

14. Flexner A. Medical education in the United States and Canada. Carnegie Foundation for the Advancement of Teaching. Bulletin No. 4;1910.

15. Anon. Our prospects as a profession. JAMA. 1898;31(16):932–3 [cited May 2024]. Available from: https://archive.org/details/pub_jama

16. Anon. An overcrowded profession. Boston Med Surg J. 1884;111:90 [cited January 26, 2022].

17. More ES. Restoring the balance: women physicians and the profession of medicine 1985–1995. Cambridge (MA): Harvard University Press;1999.

18. Fogy T. A doctor in distress (letter to editor). Woman's J (Boston). 1884 Jan 5; XV(1):6–7 [cited May 2024]. Available from: https://iiif.lib.harvard.edu/manifests/view/drs:48880300$1i

19. Public-school instruction in cooking. JAMA. 1899;XXXII(21):1183 [cited January 1, 2022].

20. Wein R. Women's colleges and domesticity, 1875–1918. Hist Educ Q. 1974;14(1):31–47.

21. Williams PA. Women in medicine: some themes and variations. J Med Educ. 1971;46:584–91.

22. Anon. Women physicians and the war. JAMA. 1915;65(21):1823.

23. Philbrick I. Women, let us be loyal to women. Med Womens J. 1929;36:39–42.

24. Douglas SJ. Where the girls are: growing up female with the mass media. New York (NY): Times Books;1994.

25. Morantz RM, Pomerleau CS, Fenichel CH. In her own words: oral histories of women physicians. Westport (CT); Old Westbury (NY): Greenwood Press;1982.

26. Friedan B. The feminine mystique. New York (NY): Norton;1963.

27. Bernard J. Academic women. University Park (PA): Pennsylvania State University Press;1964.

28. Bowers JZ. Special problems of women medical students. J Med Educ. 1968;43:532–7.

29. Dykman RA, Stalnaker JM. Survey of women physicians graduating from medical school 1925–1940. J Med Educ. 1957 Mar;32(3 Part 2):3–38.

30. Powers L, Parmelle RD, Wiesenfelder H. Practice patterns of women and men physicians. J Med Educ. 1969 Jun;44(6):481–91.
31. Johnson DG, Hutchins EB. Doctor or dropout? A study of medical student attrition. J Med Educ. 1966;41(12):1107–203.
32. Hutchins EB. Minorities, manpower and medicine. Division of Education, AAMC Technical Report No. S-663;1966.
33. Shapiro CS, Stibler BJ, Zelkovic AA, Mausner JS. Careers of women physicians: a survey of women graduates from seven medical schools, 1945–1951. J Med Educ. 1968 Oct;43(10):1033–40.
34. Braslow JB, Heins M. Women in medical education: a decade of change. N Engl J Med. 1981 May 7;304(19):1129–35.
35. Boulis A, Jacobs J. The changing face of medicine: women doctors and the evolution of heath care in America. Ithaca (NY): Cornell University Press;2008.
36. Campbell MA. Why would a girl go into medicine? Old Westbury (NY): Feminist Press;1975.
37. Bourne PG, Wikler NJ. Commitment and the cultural mandate: women in medicine. Soc Probl. 1978;25(4):430–40.
38. England P. The gender revolution: uneven and stalled. Gend Soc. 2010;24:149–66.
39. Detweiler S, Cartwright L. Women physician pioneers of the 1960s: their lives and profession over a half century. San Francisco (CA): University of California Medical Humanities Press;2022.

3

Motivation: Why Would a Girl Go into Medicine?

"There is little wonder that so few women are attracted to careers as doctors when all of society's cues are negative."[1]

The findings of a 1973 study of women in US medical schools were so discouraging that the report was plaintively titled "Why Would a Girl Go into Medicine?"[2] Even if she survived the rigors of medical training, a woman was faced with building her life and career in a society where female physicians were uncommon and often demeaned or patronizingly tolerated as eccentric. Hopefully, a distinguished physician was exaggerating in 1971 when she described the popular image of a medical woman as

> "a horse-faced, flat chested female in supphose who sublimates her sex starvation in a passionate embrace of the *New England Journal of Medicine* and cyclic AMP. It takes considerable determination for a young girl to ignore this threat to her image as a desirable woman and only a pitifully small number of women risk it. It's enough to make a cat cry!"[3]

Even the possibility of such an image speaks volumes about public perceptions of female physicians during the decades when our interviewees were deciding on their medical careers.

Young women growing up in the 1950s and 1960s faced sustained societal pressures steering them toward marriage, motherhood, and domesticity.[1,4–11] Study of "masculine" topics, such as science or mathematics, was both overtly and more subtly discouraged. Any consideration of entering prestigious professions such as law or medicine was generally regarded as inappropriate, foolish, or arrogant, indicating hubris that was certain to end in a well-deserved downfall.[4] Even our interviewees from the most supportive environments encountered expectations that they would follow more "normal" career paths for girls.

In those days, women were not encouraged to be doctors. It was just not even discussed – there was no idea of women going into medicine.

We were expected to be a secretary, teacher, or a librarian. I couldn't be a secretary – my typing skills were too bad.

Official recruiting materials for medicine were not encouraging. The AMA cautioned prospective medical students that the profession was "not for the weak or easily discouraged," citing long hours, arduous work, truncated family and personal life, rigorous intellectual demands, and personality requirements including "intelligence, scientific curiosity, self-discipline, physical and emotional strength, interest in people and objectivity."[12] Other resources for potential applicants added requirements of "compassion, good judgement, insight, equanimity, and pleasing personal appearance."[13] The desired personal appearance for female applicants was not specified. The few materials for women projected a superwoman image of an attractive young woman joyfully and effortless excelling as wife, mother, socialite, cook, and physician – all while beautifully groomed and smartly dressed, including high heels![14] Given the well-documented insecurity of young women about their intellectual abilities and appearance, plus the ever-prevalent impostor syndrome, the superwoman approach may have been even more discouraging to young women than the potential rigors of the profession.[1,4,5,15,16]

A woman needed strong motivation, resolute determination, or even a spiritual vocation – perhaps all three – to become a physician in the decades following WWII.[1-11,17,18] For young women of that time, medicine was a challenging and controversial career choice with life-changing consequences. We were, therefore, surprised that several of our interviewees struggled to articulate why they had made this crucial decision. Few cited a single motivation, and even fewer could describe a "light bulb" moment when the decision was suddenly clear. For most, medicine was a long-standing consideration influenced by various positive and negative factors, people, and experiences. Some described a sustained, almost gravitational pull by different synergistic forces, whereas others described an interest that ebbed and flowed. Even the majority of those who entered medicine relatively late and/or had pursued other interests or careers acknowledged an underlying and often suppressed long-term interest in medicine: *I just kept coming back to medicine.*

Motivation had to withstand diverse challenges, rebuffs, and practical problems. Multiple different references were made to medicine being *inappropriate for girls* and to self-doubt about *being good enough* to be accepted into medical school and succeed as a physician. All our interviewees spoke about medicine with respect and humility, almost reverence. Even those who were determined to be physicians from an early age recognized that a career in medicine was an ambitious aspiration. Many had initially considered it out of reach and expressed surprise that their younger selves had the courage or audacity to apply.

I wasn't sure I could reach for it. Cost was a major barrier. Plus, medicine was an elite thing.

I thought it was a pipe dream. I never thought I would be able to be a doctor.

Timing of the Decision to become a Physician

About half of the interviewees felt committed to medicine from a very young age. Some described feeling vocationally called or predestined to become physicians; others just unquestioningly accepted that medicine was what they wanted to do.

I always felt it was a calling.

I can't explain it – it was just something I always wanted to do.

I always wanted to be a physician from about 3 years of age.

I was definitely sure by age 7.

I always wanted to be a doctor. Remember talking about it from the age of 7.

Many clearly recalled being committed to the career during elementary school and making this decision known to family, teachers, and classmates, with mixed reactions, as described in the next chapter.

I told my fourth-grade teacher, "I am going to be a doctor."

At age 12, I wrote in my journal about being a child psychiatrist – it never crossed my mind to be a nurse.

In fourth grade, I have exquisite memories of being in hospital for about a month. That solidified my interest in medicine, but I knew I had to do well in school and my chances of getting into medical school were slim.

Only four identified the decision being made during high school. One interviewee cited the influence of a future medical professions club, and two linked the decision to career-oriented projects. Interestingly, neither project anticipated girls becoming physicians.

I came full circle from thinking about nurse anesthesia for my high school project to becoming an anesthesiologist.

Did a career project on med tech and got to visit KUMC labs and spoke with people there – it looked interesting.

The final participant who decided in high school identified her decision moment when a career counselor was scathingly dismissive of her ever being accepted into medical school.

I just thought, "I'm not wavering from medicine. I'll show YOU!"

Most early deciders remained fixed in their determination to become physicians. A few considered alternative careers, returning to medicine after finding other professions unsatisfying and/or overcoming the discouragement and obstacles placed in their way. Most interviewees made final decisions during college, often toward the end of their undergraduate studies. Seventeen made late changes from graduate studies in science to commit to medicine. For most, this was a final recognition of wanting to do medicine and/or at last gaining the confidence to apply to medical school. Some described the realization that girls *could* apply to medical school. Several commented they had been over-awed by the premed students but suddenly realized they were *just as smart* as their male classmates. Others reported that frustration about the limited career options in pure science pushed them toward a final decision for medicine.

I enjoyed science in college, and the place was loaded with premeds, so I thought,

"Why not me?"

I decided I was as smart as the male premeds in college.

I was planning on graduate work in psychology, but some of the psychology majors were weird and scared me.

The plan was a PhD in medical genetics, but I was stuck in a lab, experimenting on rats. I wanted to work with people, to help people.

I was struggling with my independent study project in sociology when I met an LPN who worked in the emergency department. I was immediately fascinated by the work.

One interviewee only seriously considered medicine after a pre-graduation aptitude test. *I loved science and wanted to be a theoretician but didn't think I was smart enough to go to Princeton to be paid to think. And I didn't want to teach or work in industry. They offered aptitude testing, and I tested out for medicine, so I thought I should give it a go.* Another very late decider was accepted by both medical and veterinary schools and claimed that finances determined her choice to become a physician. *I asked vet school about jobs and loans. I couldn't get loans, and the only job was cleaning out kennels for 50 cents an hour. Medicine offered me a job right away doing surveys and had loans available. They were much more welcoming. Better than cleaning out dog poop!*

Seven interviewees had careers before entering medicine. Three taught sciences at the high school level, one was a medical technician, and the others had unconventional premedical careers. One served in the Peace Corps, doing community development overseas, then worked in a medical research laboratory; one was a nun; and the third entered medicine after graduate studies in Anglo-Saxon and medieval languages and working in several environments, including a politician's office and a psychotherapy training program.

Motivating Factors

Each of our participants described her personal path to medicine, but common motivational themes emerged across the group. (See Table 3.1 for factors and additional illustrative quotations.) Most reported being influenced by several factors and described a gradual but not always linear process, even if the initial idea of medicine or the final decision to apply was precipitated by a critical "light bulb" moment.

Role Models

More than half of the group reported being motivated by a role model. Role models were particularly important for those who had medical family members, but about

TABLE 3.1

Motivating Factors in the Decision to become a Physician

Factor	Number Reporting (%)	Illustrative Quotations
Inspiring role model (physician, nurse, pharmacist, lab technician, veterinarian, pharmacist, physical therapist)	22 (60%)	• *My father took great pleasure in his work.* • *I was so proud of my father.* • *Dad talked a lot about patients and their emotional needs. I thought that was very interesting and decided about age 12 to become a psychiatrist.* • *My grandfather died when I was 8, but he was definitely an influence. I have vivid memories of spending time in his office. We played at writing prescriptions and grinding up medicines in pestle and mortar. He had an X-ray machine, and I used to put my hand in it to see my bones! We had no idea it was dangerous; I was just fascinated.*
Love of science	17 (46%)	• *I fell in love with medicine and science when I got my polio immunization aged 15 – I thought, "WOW, that's really neat!"* • *I found science very interesting and was pretty good at math and chemistry. LOVED bacteriology.* • *LOVED science and math – they were fun!*
Helping people	17 (46%)	• *I initially thought about aeronautical engineering, but I always enjoyed people.* • *I though how great to be able to bring comfort and consolation to people.* • *I always felt it was a calling.*
Illness experience	12 (32%)	• *At age 7, I had severe pneumonia and was hospitalized. Several other family members had serious illnesses when I was a youngster, so I had very favorable impressions of doctors and nurses from a very young age.* • *My sister was born with congenital abnormalities so was in and out of hospitals and had multiple surgeries – got me interested in medicine.* • *I was certainly influenced by my parents having to deal with health problems.*
Books	10 (27%)	• *I read all the* Nurse Sue Barton *books and loved them. Patients liked and needed Sue Barton: I wanted to be liked and needed.* • *My father was always looking at his medical books from being a Navy Corpsman during WWII. I was fascinated by them.* • *At one stage in junior high school, cafeteria was closed, so I ate lunch every day in Father's office. I read his medical books.*

(Continued)

TABLE 3.1 (*Continued*)

Motivating Factors in the Decision to become a Physician

Factor	Number Reporting (%)	Illustrative Quotations
Volunteer or work experience (lab assistant, nurse aide, candy striper, PT assistant)	7 (19%)	• *My mother let me fill in for her working in an internist's office as a medical technologist. She taught me how to do blood counts, blood sugars, etc. I was not very adept – probably a bit over my head as a high school student.* • *I was working in the hospital lab during the summer. The pathologist let me look at slides, took an interest in me.* • *A friend persuaded me to go with her for a summer job at a camp for handicapped children. I spent two summers working with handicapped kids at the camp and was so impressed about what physical therapy could do.*

Note: Participants could identify more than one factor.

one-third of our group had no personal connection with a health professional. Most role models were physicians, usually general practitioners, but also nurses, veterinarians, pharmacists, laboratory technicians, and physical therapists. Only four participants mentioned female role models prior to college. Some mentioned multiple influential individuals who sparked or encouraged their interest. The common factor was a committed professional who relished doing worthwhile work and enthusiastically shared their experience.

My family doctor knew about my interest. Even as a child, whenever I was there, he and his staff would show me things.

My pediatrician had a great deal of influence on me; medicine felt possible because she was there.

When I was 4, a wonderful old female physician came out to my grandmother's farm after we had drunk bichloride of mercury. I was so impressed!

A female ENT surgeon gave a talk to a club at school. I was amazed she was allowed to do surgery.

Eight (36%) of the 22 interviewees who identified an inspiring professional role model named a parent: seven were physician fathers, and one mother was a nurse who specialized in the care of cancer patients.

My mother was a patient advocate. She would get frustrated when doctors did not prescribe enough pain medications for her patients.

Several ladies identified influential grandparents, uncles, other relatives, or close family friends, almost all of whom were physicians. They shared an ability to communicate enthusiasm about care of patients and to convey the love of medicine to a receptive young woman.

My father was doing something he enjoyed every day – and getting paid for it seemed like a great idea!

My uncle LOVED practicing medicine.

These young women were not under any illusions about the demands of practice or the nature of the work. In some cases, the degree of exposure to medicine even at very young ages was astonishing. One woman described accompanying her father on house calls and Sunday hospital rounds after church services, all dressed up in her Sunday best.

I would "advise" him on the treatment of his patients. The patients loved it, and the nurses spoilt me!

My father was a rural family doctor. Patients were always coming to the house with injuries and all kinds of things.

When I was about 6, I asked my dad about the difference between girls and boys, so he had me watch a circumcision. I watched a cesarean section when I was about 9 years old!

Although not specifically medical role models, five participants reflected on being influenced by the frustrated medical ambitions of a relative.

Father started medical school but had a serious illness in first year, then family financial problems caused him to switch to chemistry.

Much later, my mother revealed she had wanted to study medicine, but during the Depression, the priority was to educate the boys in the family.

Love of Science

Although they grew up during a period when science was not always perceived as appropriate for girls, almost all interviewees were interested in science from an early age, and about half cited love of science as a primary motivation for medicine. Several participants also volunteered love of mathematics, including the challenges of advanced calculus. Many still spoke about science and related topics with energy and delight. Several enthusiastically discussed current advances in sciences and were excited and optimistic about current and potential developments in science and medicine.

My grandfather gave me a science set in junior high – much against my mother's wishes – and I was hooked!

Always liked science – at age 10, I wrote a paper about wanting to become a physicist.

I always loved biology and worked hard to get good grades.

I LOVED math and science. I aced three calculus courses, loved equations and everything like that.

Not all science and math came easily. In particular, chemistry and calculus caused great concern for a few ladies trying to acquire competitive credentials for medical school. Some vividly recalled their distress that poor grades in any subject could sabotage admission to medical school or undermine their self-confidence to make the application. Sometimes they succeeded through sheer determination.

I got a C in inorganic chemistry and was devastated – then I found it wasn't required for medical school at that time!

Desire to Help Others

Interest in people and desire to help others permeated all interviews, especially in the sections addressing participants' time in practice and identification of the best aspects of their careers. Just under half of interviewees identified helping others as a motivation to become a physician, but we had the strong impression that this was a driving force for all participants. Perhaps participants believed "helping others" was self-evident and did not need to be mentioned, or maybe older Midwestern ladies did not want to reveal the zeal of their youthful selves early in the interview.

Commitment to helping others as a motivation was expressed in several ways, ranging from non-specific aspirations *to be useful* up to sincere spiritual vocation and dedication to the welfare of others. Three ladies mentioned aspiration to participate in medical missionary work. All three remained active volunteers for overseas missions throughout their careers.

I always wanted to help people. I decided that medicine was something I wanted to do to REALLY help people.

At age 12, the church was visited by missionaries from India, where the women could not be treated by men. I asked myself why women could be doctors in other countries.

I wanted to find something useful in the mission field.

Illness Experiences

In several cases, both the interactions with role models and the desire to serve others were interwoven with experience of personal or family illness. As a teenager, one lady was called upon to care for three young children while her older sister underwent treatment for thyroid cancer. Her brother-in-law was a medical student. Despite the pressures on the family, *he came back every evening and explained how wonderful it was to be a doctor.*

Twelve (32%) participants identified illness experiences as leading motivational factors in their decision to become physicians. In most cases, impressions of health professionals were positive, even inspirational. These experiences often occurred at a young age, and many were dramatic. At that time, conditions such as pneumonia or appendicitis could be life-threatening, especially for those living in rural areas.

When I was 6, my mother had appendicitis and peritonitis. She was hospitalized over 30 miles away for six weeks. Once she got home, our family doctor visited the farm every Saturday evening. He brought reassurance, helped the family relax and have confidence in her recovery.

I had a major illness in fourth grade, a ruptured appendix. The hospital stay was about a month and solidified my interest in medicine.

Several women recalled polio epidemics during the 1950s, with everyone living in fear, *waiting for the next child to be struck down.*

My brother had polio when he was 4. We saw lots of doctors and experienced lots of health care.

A few illness experiences were negative or distressing, providing a paradoxical motivation to enter medicine *to do things better.* One woman linked her subsequent career in obstetrics to poor care during the birth of her first child and the dramatic contrast with the good experience of her second delivery: *I didn't know care could make such a difference!*

My decision was solidified helping take care of my grandparents when they passed away and when my father died during my college sophomore year. I thought there should be a way to provide better care.

Medically Related Books

Ten (27%) interviewees identified books read during their pre-teen and teenage years as motivation for medical careers. These were described as adjuncts to developing interest in medicine rather than primary motivational forces. One specified that she had sought out the books *after* beginning to think seriously about a career in one of the health professions and the stories turned her away from nursing and toward medicine. The three types of books mentioned were novels, medical texts, and biographies.

Several participants referenced popular books for girls in which nurses were heroines. The seven *Nurse Sue Barton* books were written between 1936 and 1952 and follow Sue's adventures from student nurse to nursing superintendent and head of a nursing school – a position she unfortunately leaves because of pressures to support her physician husband and their children. The period stereotypes continue when she has to return to work to support her family during her husband's illness, but the conclusion implies she will be content to return to the roles of wife and mother on his recovery. The *Nurse Cherry Ames* series combines the promotion of nursing as a career with a mystery/adventure format, making the heroine as much a special agent as a nurse. The 27 novels, written between 1943 and 1968, document the adventures of an apparently never-aging nurse who has a remarkable ability to change locations and roles within nursing (27 times in 25 years) while solving mysteries and capturing criminals who have eluded all other attempts to bring them to justice – rather like Nancy Drew in a white cap, or a non-violent solo Charlie's Angel.

Although the interviewees had enjoyed these stories as girls, the impact was more likely to diminish than nurture consideration of a nursing career. Whatever their merits, the *Nurse Sue Barton* and *Nurse Cherry Ames* books were very popular among girls in the decades following WWII and were almost unique in having female heroines at a time when other literature, television shows, movies, and other sources of information about medicine were dominated by masculine stereotypes.[1,4,5]

When I was very young, I read all the Nurse Nancy *books – and decided I didn't want to be a nurse.*

I read all the Nurse Cherry Ames *books. I loved the books, but it never crossed my mind to be a nurse.*

Even at very young ages, some participants had morbid fascination for medical textbooks, especially those with gruesome illustrations.

I read all my grandfather's books, looking at pictures of malformed children and that sort of thing. He died when I was 8, so this was very young.

I loved snow days. We could go to Dad's office and read his books – mainly looked at the pictures.

Three individuals mentioned being influenced by medical biographies: a history of Marie Curie, a book about pioneer female physicians, and a biography of a male medical missionary.

Volunteer or Work Experience

Seven (19%) interviewees identified volunteer or work experience as important in their decisions to enter medicine. For some, work experience was pivotal in deciding to become a physician; for others, the experience reinforced a growing commitment to medicine. The majority were summer or part-time jobs related to medicine during high school or college. Three identified working in research labs as a primary motivation.

My first summer job at about 16 was in the hospital lab. The chief technologist assigned me to microbiology, and I loved it. We did mouse pregnancy tests, and I had to sacrifice the mice! The pathologist was very helpful. I thought what he was doing was very interesting. I vividly remember watching an autopsy on a pregnant woman. Probably why I became a pathologist.

I spent the summer helping my uncle, who was an old-fashioned rural GP. He did surgery and all his own stuff. I thought, "Oh, yes. This is what I want to do."

In college, I worked in a lab and volunteered in ER – got to do things.

In at least three cases, negative work experiences only strengthened the resolve to enter medicine.

I worked as a nurse's aide in college, decided I should do medicine.

I volunteered as a candy striper in high school, but when I applied to the same hospital for a summer research job between my sophomore and junior year of college, I was told, "We do not accept women; we do not think women should be doctors." I thought, "I'll show you!"

I had a summer job as a waitress during high school. When some customers found out I wanted to become a physician, they were rude and dismissed the idea. "You can't do THAT. Girls don't go to med school." I think it just made me more determined.

In addition, five of our interviewees commented that early experiences caring for sick animals influenced their interest in medicine, and each struggled with the choice between human and veterinary medicine.

I loved caring for sick calves in the basement of the house. I could always tell which ones were going to do well and which ones weren't. I assumed I couldn't be a vet because I was a girl.

I was accustomed to dealing with one emergency after another with farm animals and finding ways to fix problems.

I told my grandfather I wanted to be a veterinarian, but he said I wouldn't be strong enough.

My uncle was a vet, and I helped with veterinary medicine all the time.

I loved caring for animals and was accepted into both vet and med school – getting into med school was easier!

Summary: So Why *Would* a Girl Go into Medicine?

"A woman's decision to enter medical school is statistically unusual and therefore occupationally innovative."[18]

We were particularly interested in our participants' motivations to enter medicine because of the overwhelmingly negative and pessimistic tone of writings about women in medicine in the decades following WWII. From the perspective of the 2020s, when more than half of medical students and one-third of practicing physicians are women, we constantly had to remind ourselves that the interviewees were describing events and decisions that unfolded in a different era. The majority of our participants grew up in the 1950s and 1960s, when the literature indicates that even intelligent women were expected to be decorative adjuncts to husbands or male bosses and women were encouraged or expected to include home economics in their college courses, as "college women make cheery, efficient homes!"[5] A flippant comment attributed to a college career counselor of that time may be uncomfortably close to an accurate reflection of the prevailing attitudes when our participants were considering their career options: "Yes, my dear, medicine can be a VERY rewarding career. Why not plan to MARRY a doctor?"[5]

Our interviewees referred to pressures to follow more conventional or "suitable" careers, but none of their experiences approached the degree of negativity, even hostility, that is conveyed in the literature about women attempting to enter the professions in the 1950s, 1960s, and 1970s. They are, of course, a select group whose experiences may not represent those of the majority of women at that time. Not only did they all graduate from the same medical school and share many demographic characteristics; they also successfully completed careers in medicine and felt comfortable recounting events and feelings from more than 50 years previous. Experiences may have been forgotten, reprocessed to fit different narratives, or omitted from our discussions because they were judged inappropriate or too personal, but nevertheless, we were impressed by the open and thoughtful responses of our participants and have no reason to doubt the accuracy of their input. Consistency within interviews and across the group, along with the similarities to the results reported by other studies, supports the validity of the information.

A possible explanation for the discrepancies between the literature and the recollection of our interviewees is that young women in the Midwest may have experienced different societal pressures or encountered different issues in seeking medical careers than those in other regions of the country. We found little contemporary information about the motivation of women entering medicine – perhaps because women represented only about 5–9% of medical students at that time and there was little societal interest in increasing the availability of women physicians.[1,5] As best as we can tell, the only available information comes from three surveys conducted in the late 1960s, the oral histories mentioned earlier, biographical accounts, and some unpublished work cited in books about women in medicine.[1,5,17–24,25]

These sources all cite interest in science and a desire to help others as principal factors in women's motivation toward becoming physicians. They also highlighted the importance of relationships with role models and experience of illness. Only one survey mentioned the influence of books or movies about medical careers.[5] Our respondents differed from those of other studies in the rare mentions of desire for independence or the prestige of the profession as strong motivational factors.[5,17,18]

In contrast to their male colleagues, prestige and financial success were not leading motivations in any of the literature on female medical students. Our interviewees only referred to status and prestige in terms of family attitudes toward medicine, usually describing concerns that medicine was regarded as *elite* and concerns about fitting in with classmates from wealthier, more upper-class families. Money was only mentioned in the context of struggles to finance college and/or medical school.

While the question from 1974 of "Why would a girl go into medicine?"[2] may never be conclusively answered, our interviewees add to the scanty knowledge available about the motivations of women who graduated prior to 1975. Their recollections are those of women who succeeded in medicine and willingly volunteered to reflect on their motivations for decisions made more than a half-century ago. They reported the interplay of societal pressures and stereotypes with the influence of family members, friends, teachers, career counselors, and others in a complex process that enhanced or discouraged their personal aspirations to enter medicine but cited the same major factors as other sources.

Our interviewees rarely identified a single motivation leading them to medicine, but the combination of interest in science and a desire to help others appears to be essential and universal. *I wanted to do something with science, but to help people too, so that equaled being a doctor.* In the end, the best answer to the question "Why would a girl go into medicine?"[2] may be that of our participant who paused for some time before answering: *It was just something I had to do.*

REFERENCES

1. Walsh MR. 'Doctors wanted: no women need apply': sexual barriers in the medical profession 1835–1975. New Haven (CT): Yale University Press;1977.
2. Campbell MA. Why would a girl go into medicine? Medical education in the US: a guide for women. Old Westbury (NY): Feminist Press;1974.
3. Ramey E. An interview with Dr. Estelle Ramey. Perspect Biol Med. 1971;14(3): 424–31.
4. Douglas SJ. Where the girls are: growing up female with the mass media. New York (NY): Times Books, Random House;1994.
5. Lopate C. Women in medicine. Baltimore (MD): Johns Hopkins Press;1968.
6. Morantz RM, Pomerleau CS, Fenichel CH. In her own words: oral histories of women physicians. Westport (CT): Greenwood Press;1982.
7. Bowers JZ. Special problems of women medical students. J Med Educ. 1968;43: 532–7.
8. Morantz-Sanchez R, Sympathy & science: women physicians in American medicine. New York (NY): Oxford University Press;1985.
9. More ES. Restoring the balance: women physicians and the profession of medicine 1985–1995. Cambridge (MA): Harvard University Press;1999.
10. Mattfield JA, Van Allen CG, editors. Women and the scientific professions. Cambridge (MA): MIT Press;1965.
11. Bourne PG, Wiker NJ. Commitment and the cultural mandate: women in medicine. Soc Probl. 1978;25:430–40.
12. American Medical Association. Horizons unlimited. Dearborn (IL): AMA;1966.
13. Kalb WS. Your future as a physician. New York (NY): Richard Rosen Press;1963.
14. American Medical Women's Association. Medicine as a career for women. New York (NY): AMWA;1965.

15. Weir WD. Honors and the liberal arts college. In: Cohen JW, editor. The superior student. New York (NY): McGraw-Hill;1966.

16. Bernard J. Academic women. New York (NY): Meridian;1966.

17. Williams PC. Women in medicine: some themes and variations. J Med Educ. 1971;46:584–91.

18. Cartwright LK. Conscious factors entering into decisions of women to study medicine. J Soc Iss. 1972;28:201–15.

19. East C, Bridges D. Women physicians at Baylor University Medical Center. BUMC Proceed. 2004;17:304–17.

20. Center for the History of Medicine at Countway Library. Oral histories. The Women in Medicine Legacy Foundation [cited January 17, 2022]. Available from: https://www.wimlf.org/oral-histories

21. Women in white: women physicians oral history. University of Kentucky Libraries. Louie B Nunn Center for Oral History Project. Available from: https://kentuckyoralhistory.org/ark:/16417/xt77d7959s9f

22. Women in Duke medicine: an oral history exhibit. Available from: http://digital dukemed.mc.duke.edu/med_women/interviews.html

23. Martin T. When the personal is political; five women doctors look back. Lincoln (NE): iUniverse;2008.

24. Chin EL, editor. This side of doctoring; reflections from women in medicine. New York (NY): Oxford University Press;2003.

25. Detweiler S, Cartwright L. Women physician pioneers of the 1960s: their lives and profession over a half century. San Francisco (CA): University of California Medical Humanities Press;2022.

4

Family Background and Early Life

"The Kansas medical students are a homogeneous body: they are young, white, male, Protestant, small-town natives . . . provincial."[1]

Over 80% of our 37 interviewees described themselves as being raised in Kansas. One interviewee was brought up in California, but both of her parents were University of Kansas School of Medicine (KUSM) graduates, and she had strong family ties to the state. One was raised in New England but married a Kansan. The remaining out-of-staters came from Texas, Montana, California, and Connecticut to attend college or graduate school in Kansas. For two, the attraction was to experience small college environments – plus exercise youthful independence. *I wanted a small college and had friends in Missouri, so I transferred to a college in that state. I liked the Midwest, so I applied to KUSM as my first choice.* An interviewee from New England bluntly stated: *I wanted to get away, attended a small religious college in Kansas and LOVED it.*

The preponderance of in-state residents is still typical of state-supported medical schools. States have a long history of relating funding to the expectation that graduates will establish practice in the state.[2] As for our matriculants of 1944–72, current Kansas residents are more likely to apply to KUSM than to other medical schools and are more likely to be admitted. Non-residents are at a disadvantage, unless they can demonstrate close family ties to the state or some compelling reason for admission.[1,3] Some of the in-state applicants' preference for KUSM can be attributed to tradition or familiarity with the state and its institutions. Many have family links to KUSM and/or have attended in-state colleges and universities. In-state applicants are also likely to know KUSM alumni, as a large percentage of the state's physicians have always been KUSM graduates. Financially, in-state applicants have strong incentives to attend KUSM. Nationwide, state-supported colleges and universities typically have large differences in tuition, sometimes charging almost double for out-of-state students. In addition, multiple scholarships, loan programs, and other incentives are available to encourage Kansans to receive their medical education and establish practice in the state. For most young Kansans considering the choice of medical school, the combination of personal and financial factors counters any temptations to seek newer pastures.[1,3,4] For at least a century, KUSM has been the normal route for a Kansan seeking to become a physician. For our interviewees and their modern counterparts, it would be considered very unusual and financially wasteful for a Kansas girl to apply anywhere else.

DOI: 10.1201/9781003539568-4

Communities of Origin

Our participants came from communities of various sizes and types, ranging from farms and tiny rural settlements to large cities and college towns. About half of our interviewees were raised in cities with populations of 100,000 or more, predominantly the state's two largest metropolitan areas of Wichita and Kansas City. During the 1950s and 1960s, when the majority of our participants were growing up, these were boom towns with rapidly expanding industries and growing populations. The other interviewees were raised in smaller towns or on farms. The largest town had about 40,000 inhabitants. Three towns had under 1,000 population – the smallest had approximately 200 inhabitants when our interviewee lived there. Several interviewees were raised in frontier areas, that is, counties with six or fewer persons per square mile. One woman described growing up on an isolated farm in northwest Kansas, 15 miles from the nearest town – itself a settlement of only 400 people!

In visualizing the environments in which our interviewees grew up, it is important to realize that communities have changed substantially over the intervening half-century or more. Wichita has tripled in population since the early life of most of our interviewees, and several nearby communities have grown even more rapidly. The rural community in which our opening story took place had about 700 inhabitants at that time and was considered a self-sufficient rural town some distance from Wichita – over mostly unpaved roads through farmland. The town currently has over 7,000 inhabitants and is within easy commuting distance of the city. Most of the intervening distance is now taken up with housing subdivisions rather than wheatfields, but rabbits and shotguns are still common in the area. Conversely, many more remote communities have lost population, and some are one-third to one-half smaller than in the 1950s and 1960s.

Participants raised in small towns or on farms did not consider themselves disadvantaged. Small communities could be very supportive of ambitious young people who, in turn, felt a sense of obligation to do well and repay the confidence of the community. It was a *very supportive small town. I had lots of affirmation and support. I always knew I had to do well in school.* Within an urban setting, an African American participant used almost exactly the same terms to describe being *encouraged and affirmed by everyone in my community.* The interviewees who were raised on farms were especially likely to credit their upbringing with developing tenacity, work ethic, sense of responsibility, and other valuable attributes that helped them succeed in medical school and throughout their careers. *I had been brought up on a farm. If something needed done, you did it and moved on to the next thing. If you're raised on a farm, you're trained to work. I had experienced lots of hard and nasty things on farm and learned to work through things: to do your best and wait for things to improve.*

Sometimes, a farm or small-town upbringing provided mixed motivations, both inspiration to help others and aspiration to escape to wider pastures.

I was accustomed to dealing with one emergency or another with the animals. Decided that medicine was something I wanted to do, to really help people, but I also wanted to get off the farm!

I had deep-rooted feelings of wanting to be away from the small town and to achieve.

Families of Origin

Parental Education and Occupation

About half of our participants reported that one or both parents had attended college. Mothers were just as likely to be college graduates as fathers, but maternal and paternal degrees and occupations were very different (Table 4.1). Mothers had sometimes made many compromises and sacrifices to obtain a college education. Their determination that their daughters would be well-educated resonated throughout the interviews.

Education was very important to my mother: She was the eldest of five siblings, neither of her parents had a college degree, and they were living in a little town in western Kansas. The only way they would help her financially was if she went to teachers college, a two-year program, so she did that initially even though she was not keen on teaching. She and my dad married after the war, and both attended college. My dad got a degree in civil engineering, and my mother got her BS in home economics, with hope of becoming a buyer for department stores. She became pregnant with me in the last semester of her junior year, unplanned. Completing her degree was so important to her that she sent me to my grandmother in western Kansas for the last semester of her senior year. I rejoined my family after my mom graduated. My dad felt she should stay home with me, but she did do some accounting work at home for a while. I think one of her fears was that my career would get derailed if I had children, a message my sisters received as well. I was the only one to have children, but I kept working!

One participant found out later in life that her mother had wanted to be a nurse but was discouraged by her family. Another discovered that financial problems had prevented her mother from becoming a physician.

Mother revealed that she had wanted to study medicine but was prevented by the financial priority to educate the son in the family. Mother studied chemistry and did very well.

For fathers, the most common occupation was farmer, followed by physician (five general practitioners/family physicians and one obstetrician/gynecologist). Most fathers were professionals, white-collar or skilled workers, but three were described by their daughters as unskilled workers. Three fathers had aspired to become physicians but were prevented from entering medicine due to health or financial reasons.

My father was a businessman, but I found out later that he had wanted to go to medical school but was prevented/discouraged because of rheumatic heart disease. He was told he could not handle the rigors of medical school.

Father intended to become a physician, but serious illness (pneumonia) in the first year plus financial problems caused him to switch to chemistry.

Father was a medical corpsman during the war. I think he wanted medicine, but the training was too long, and he was married and had a family to support. But he kept his books and was always looking at them. I think he always wished he had gone to medical school.

Mothers were more difficult to classify by occupation. Although 40% (14/35) were described as homemakers, this included nine farmers' wives – a full-time occupation in itself. In addition, we documented maternal occupation as described while the interviewee was growing up. Several mothers listed as homemakers in Table 4.1

TABLE 4.1

Parental Occupation and Education Level

Occupation	Father	Mother
Farmer	9 (24%)	
Physician	6 (16%)	1
Businessman/Businesswoman	5 (14%)	1
Teacher	3	8 (22%)
Accountant	2	
Laborer	3	1
Salesperson	2	
Banker	1	
Engineer	1	
Industrial chemist	1	1
Lawyer	1	
Linotype operator	1	
Homemaker		14 (38%)
Nurse		4 (11%)
Administrative assistant		2
Mathematician		1
Medical technologist		1
Pharmacist		1
Not recorded	2	2
College Degree	**Father**	**Mother**
Yes	20 (54%)	20 (54%)
No	15 (41%)	15 (41%)
Not recorded	2	2

Notes: 1. "Farmer" includes one beekeeper and two who also held other jobs (teaching, factory work).
2. "Physicians" comprised five family physicians and one obstetrician.
3. "Teacher" includes one university professor.
4. "Homemaker" includes nine co-farmers.

entered the workforce at a later stage. Their daughters spoke with great pride of their mothers' accomplishments, including establishing their own businesses and being continual sources of inspiration and support.

Mother did a degree in accounting and had a successful career in real estate, then in developing technology for the visually impaired. She remained active and engaged into her 90s.

After raising five children, she returned to college and got involved in starting the women's studies department.

My mother attended high school throughout WWII and was only 18 when they married, 19 when she had her first child. Mostly, she was a stay-at-home mother, but later, as my younger siblings grew, she did have a 20-plus-year career as an administrative assistant. She is very bright, and I always thought she would have been a wonderful nurse had she had the opportunity. My generation was the first to attend college and higher education.

Among mothers employed while their daughters were growing up, the most common occupation was teaching, followed by nursing. Most of the other employed mothers were in one of the professions (Table 4.1). The only physician mother died when her daughter was an infant. None of our participants grew up in a family with a close female physician relative, but one interviewee recounted with pride that, in the 1890s, her great-grandmother and great-great-aunt had been among the first physicians to qualify in osteopathic medicine. Several had grandfathers, uncles, and other male relatives who were physicians.

Living History: Children of the Depression – The Greatest Generation

The impact of historical events was obvious as our ladies described their families of origin. Some shared family histories of recent immigration, others of homesteading around the time of the Civil War. Several of those raised in cities retained strong ties to rural areas, such as grandparents still living on family farms. Most of our participants grew up in the 1950s and 1960s and described their parents as *children of the Depression – frugal and ambitious for their children.* We heard of family farms destroyed in the Dust Bowl, businesses and jobs lost during the Depression, family relocations and disruptions, and the struggles of their parents and grandparents to survive the financial recession of the 1930s. Several interviewees described how their parents' education had been impacted by financial hardship.

My parents had to help with the farm growing up – they never finished high school.

Mother had two years of college but left to help the family financially during the Depression.

Mother's family was impacted financially by the Depression, unable to send the daughters to college – just the son.

Both my parents were first-generation immigrants from Eastern Europe and suc-
ceeded by pursuing whatever education was available.

The other defining event for many families was WWII. For the majority of our participants, born during or just after the war, their parents were members of the "Greatest
Generation," or "GI Generation," born between 1901 and 1927. They are characterized as shaped by the Great Depression and by their experiences during WWII.[5]
The parents of some participants met because of the wartime requirements for military service or war-related employment, especially in aircraft manufacturing. Some
ladies described families moving and making adaptations to the war and its many
social upheavals. The war had multiple impacts, especially on the mothers of our
participants. War-related disruptions to mothers' education or career plans were
often credited with explaining their passion for education and determination for their
daughters to be successful.

Regarding my parents' education and occupations, I expect it was rather typical
for Depression era and WWII people. My father dropped out of high school and
joined the Civilian Conservation Corps. Shortly after Pearl Harbor, he enlisted in
the Navy and served on a ship in the South Pacific for nearly four full years. On
a leave in early 1945 while his ship was being repaired from a bomb attack, he
took the train back to KC and married my mother, the girl next door. They had a
month together before he shipped out again, but during that time, my older brother
was conceived. So when Dad returned after the war, he had a family to support.
He worked at a dairy during the day and attended printing school at night. He
became a linotype operator, which was the bulk of his career, although he changed
capably with the times as computer printing came along. He worked at various
newspapers and magazines. Many years later, he obtained his GED. He was very
bright and mostly self-taught by reading a lot. He used to read poetry to us at
bedtime. He was a compulsive stickler for spelling, grammar, and punctuation. It
was a sad day for him when newspapers got rid of proofreaders, and he groaned or
cursed when he saw errors in the papers or magazines! My mother attended high
school throughout WWII and was only 18 when they married, 19 when she had
her first child. Mostly, she was a stay-at-home mother, but later, as my younger
siblings grew, she did have a 20-plus-year career as an administrative assistant.
She is also very bright, and I always thought she would have been a wonderful
nurse had she had the opportunity. My generation was the first to attend college
and higher education.

My mother graduated from junior college in her hometown, then moved in with rela-
tives in Wichita to attend Wichita State. Everyone was excited about the war and
doing their part, so she dropped out of school and went to work in one of the airplane
factories. A real Rosie the Riveter! She met my father when he also came to Wichita
to live with family and work in the aircraft factories. He soon left for the South Seas
in the Army, they were engaged by mail, he came home fall of 1945, they married
in October 1945, [and] I was born December 1946. Mother never did get back to
school, but she was a great help in writing, spelling, grammar, and inspiring interest
in literature and music.

My mother was offered a scholarship to the Julliard School of Music in New York but did not attend as her family could not afford the tuition. She studied voice in Maryland and sang in an operetta with James Arness before her father's government job in Washington, DC, was transferred to Kansas City due to decentralizing government offices during WWII. She graduated with a degree in home economics from KU, where she met my father, a medical student. She worked for a short time and sang semi-professionally for weddings, funerals, church, and social events. After moving to a smaller town when he went into practice, she was the youth choir director at church. I think she always felt she had sacrificed a singing career for my father's career. Common situation for women of that generation. My sister was born a year after their marriage, and my mother raised four children – all college graduates. I have memories of her singing opera while she did housework.

The war provided opportunities as well as hardships. For at least four participants, the GI Bill enabled their fathers to attend college and establish financial support for their families. *My grandparents were immigrants, coal miners. My father was an Air Force navigator in WWII, then studied engineering. He was first in the family to attend college.* One of these fathers was a naval medical corpsman. Although he did not become a physician, his interest in medicine and his medical books were instrumental in his daughter's choice of profession. Interestingly, one participant's mother also used WWII to obtain professional qualifications. *She became a naval officer. Studied and received degree as a medical technologist.*

Although the parents and families of our interviewees were shaped by the Depression and WWII, they were also influenced by the multiple social, political, economic, and other influences of the 1950s, 1960s, and 1970s. When most of our interviewees were growing up, families enjoyed the prosperity of the postwar boom, followed by the alternating challenges and opportunities of the cycles of boom and bust that Kansas experienced, depending on the fortunes of major employers (especially aircraft manufacturers) and commodity prices associated with agriculture, oil, and natural gas. The attitudes of families toward women in medicine were not immune to the powerful movements that shook US society during these decades. At times, supporting a daughter who aspired to become a physician required going against convention and challenging norms – as at the height of the cult of domesticity in the 1950s. At the peak of the feminist movement in the late 1960s, such support could have been regarded as very worthy – or on the contrary, depending on the micro-environments of families, neighborhoods, and social communities (especially those based on ethnicity or religious affiliation). As families navigated the diverse challenges, opportunities, and issues thrown up by some of the most tumultuous years in US history, attitudes and concepts of what was appropriate or normal for young women changed. The one constant that shines through in the narratives of our participants is family support for their daughters to achieve as much as possible – even when parents may have inwardly thought her aspirations were too ambitious.

Family Attitudes – Above All, Get an Education

With rare exceptions, our respondents described being brought up in stable, supportive families. Only one experienced significant family disruption in her teens; another reported parental divorce around the same age. One mother died when the interviewee was an infant. In addition, one mother and one father died prior to the interviewee leaving home for college, and another father died when the participant was a college sophomore. The majority of our interviewees described their families as *typical* or *pretty ordinary*, even *very middle-class*. In describing their parents and families of origin, the alumnae consistently stressed the importance of education, strong work ethic, and frugality. These characteristics frequently acted synergistically.

My parents were very frugal. I think they thought paying for medical school was the best investment ever! Both my parents valued education and were pleased with my decision to go to medical school and proud when I graduated. They supported me financially throughout college and medical school. They taught me to live frugally, as they did. As it turned out, medical school was an excellent investment.

The value placed on education was explicitly mentioned by 30 (81%) respondents and alluded to by others. Education appeared to be a core value for all families. With only two possible exceptions, all participants were raised in families in which education was prized and children were expected to *aim high and work hard*. As described earlier, this priority was often driven by the experiences of parents, especially mothers, who had been denied or failed to fulfill their own academic aspirations.

Mother encouraged anything we wanted to do. All four children attended college.

My parents placed a very high value on education. All three of us girls were honor students. They were supportive of what we wanted to do, as long as we did it well.

Several participants who were raised on farms described an iconic picture.

My parents were very hardworking children of farmers during the Dust Bowl and Depression. They had been denied a high school education because they needed to work. They both saved and made education a high priority. All four children attended college.

Neither of my parents graduated high school, but they were extremely supportive of education. Wonderful parents, hard workers. We knew from the beginning that we were definitely going to graduate high school and go on. They were super supportive that we follow our dreams.

My parents did not attend college, but Father was very intelligent, curious, and successful in his business. There was a VERY high priority on education for daughters. Extreme value on education – all of their daughters were expected to go to college.

In most families, daughters were expected to strive to excel academically, and only one participant (the daughter of immigrants from Eastern Europe) echoed the experience of the previous generation in being expected to defer to her brother's academic needs. *My family were neither here nor there. I think they were proud of my academic achievements and very happy I became a doctor but never, ever encouraged me to keep doing more scholarly things. The priority, family's first responsibility, was to educate my brother.*

Some parents cited education as a means to enable their daughters to be self-sufficient and independent. Surprisingly, this message was conveyed more explicitly by fathers than mothers. *Father was a real caretaker. He insisted his daughters do well in school and be able to take care of yourself: "Even if you get married, you can't depend on a man to take care of you!"*

Father was very supportive of women getting education to support themselves. Mother, not so much. She was a bit stressed out about it. Thought I should find a husband.

Family Attitudes to Interviewee becoming a Physician: "You Want to Do MEDICINE?"

While almost all families were unequivocally supportive of education, attitudes about their daughters entering medicine were much more mixed. For some families, the news came as a complete surprise.

I think their heads were whipped around.

Most participants who had been secretive about their aspirations were concerned that they would fail to be accepted into medical school and avoided telling families until they had secured an interview. Others were concerned about family disapproval.

When I first mentioned it during college, my mother and sister were not encouraging, so I finished as med tech and didn't tell anyone about medicine. When I applied, I told them after my interview at Christmas. I think they were delighted when I got in.

In high school, I told my cousin I wanted to be a doctor. He laughed and made fun of me, so I didn't tell anyone else until I had passed the MCAT.

One participant did not inform her parents until the last minute because her father had a poor opinion of health professionals due to the family being treated rudely following a farming accident many years previously. *I had to tell my parents in order to get the car to drive to Kansas City when I got the notice about the interview. Parents were really surprised. I should have told them earlier but didn't want to burden them or give them the chance to dissuade me. My family was very stoic, non-demonstrative. I found out later they felt pretty good about it.*

For other families, the decision to apply to medical school did not come as a surprise. In fact, several interviewees credited their parents with the original idea – or with encouragement to aim for medicine instead of more female-oriented careers.

Everyone assumed it was my father who pushed for medicine, but it was my mother. She said, "You can't be a nurse – you have got to be a doctor." My parents encouraged me all the way. They said, "Of course women can be physicians."

My father said, "You have to decide if you want to be the one taking the bedpan or ordering the bedpan." He encouraged me to aim for medicine and told me, "You are intelligent enough to compete."

My father encouraged and supported me financially. He specifically discouraged the alternative consideration of becoming a med tech.

Initially, it was my dad's suggestion. I had been thinking of becoming a teacher, but Dad encouraged to set my goals higher. The idea took root and stuck. Mother was always very for it. Very supportive. I think she had a better idea of what I was getting into.

Father thought medicine would be good for me.

I wanted to be a vet, but my grandfather said I was not strong enough. Then I thought I should be a nurse, but Dad said, "Don't be a nurse."

About one-third of interviewees described immediate unqualified support and enthusiasm for their medical aspirations from both parents and other family members.

My family thought it was great.

I had nothing BUT encouragement from my family.

My parents were pleased and proud. Couldn't have done it without them.

I think they were thrilled. Neither had more than high school but they recognized the value of an education.

Both parents were enthusiastic about my career. Mother maybe more so because she had been denied opportunities because of growing up in the Depression. My parents were relieved when I chose medical school over vet school – there were even fewer women in vet school!

In other families, one or both parents were initially uncertain but came round to supporting their daughter's aspirations to become a physician.

Father was a bit iffy at first, but once he got used to the idea, he was supportive, proud, very proud.

Father was thrilled. Mother, not so much. She had mixed feelings about it.

In seventh grade, I asked Father what he thought about women doing medicine. He replied, "Not a good idea," and raised the issue of "taking the place of a man." He did not realize at that time that I was thinking of becoming a physician. Later, my parents were supportive.

Father went along with the idea. Mother explained her initial hesitancy based on her own experience of not being able to become a physician.

Father thought being a schoolteacher was ideal for women as she could be available for her children and have a satisfying career. Mother worried medicine would be too much for me. I think they were proud, happy I was doing what I wanted to do.

One mother came round reluctantly to support her daughter entering medical school, but only conditionally. *Mother said, "Fine, but get a teaching certificate first."*

Some participants attributed their parents' initial negative reactions to feeling caught out by their own emphasis on education and setting ambitious goals. These interviewees perceived that their parents were shocked, almost stunned, that their daughters had taken them at their word and aimed as high as academically possible.

They always encouraged us to aim high and achieve what we set out to do . . . but I don't think they expected me to aim quite that high!

My grandmother and aunts, all my family, had SUCH a high opinion of doctors. This made me uncomfortable, but I thought, "I can do this."

There was no prohibition to pursuing a career at any level. However, there was also no particular enthusiasm for an extraordinary education.

For at least one family, the concerns were social more than academic, as medical students were perceived to come from more affluent and influential families.

They were very supportive but dubious about my getting in, as they perceived "influence" was needed to succeed in admissions process, and country/farm people with no college experience or contacts were at a disadvantage. Mother worried I would not fit in with kids from rich and important families.

Several parents, especially mothers, offered qualified support or were conflicted about their daughter's career choice based on concerns about the difficulties facing a girl in medical school and the implications of a career in medicine on marriage and family life. As described in a previous chapter, these families were living in the post-WWII era of the "Great Retreat" from feminism and the national fervor for the "cult of domesticity."[6–8] Parents could face significant disapproval and criticism from friends, families, and others for supporting an errant daughter who wanted to become a physician.

Mother was supportive, but worried. She cautioned about hard work and a hard life that could be sad. Also, the need to make sacrifices.

My family were supportive of my going into medicine, but Mother may have worried about having children and all that.

Mother was cautious: "Well, you know that's a hard row to hoe." I think she was afraid for me, that I would find it difficult. Not academically, but other aspects of it. Father didn't say much, but he was proud of me and supportive.

Father really encouraged. Mother was more about getting married and having a family – but she acquiesced.

One mother's fears were not revealed for over 20 years. *Mother didn't say much at that time, but at the open house for my new private practice in 1984, she told a friend that she was proud of me but didn't really want me to go to medical school as she had seen my father's struggles in practice and did not want me to go through the same. She was also concerned about my being a woman in medicine, and if I would be accepted.*

The other major concern for many families was the financial cost of medical school. Almost all our interviewees described cost as an issue during family discussions about applying for medical school or in making decisions about which school to attend. *Of course, money was a concern.*

For approximately half of the group, families could not contribute and/or were concerned about a daughter taking on substantial debt. They simply did not have sufficient resources to support their daughters through three to four years of medical studies. None of our participants mentioned outright refusal to contribute to medical training from parents who could afford the expense. Nevertheless, four of our interviewees were explicitly told that parents would help support their daughter's college education, but not any additional studies. *They told me they would be able to help support through college, but for med school, you're on your own.*

Money was tight, but my parents paid for books and tuition in college. I did two years JUCO and two years KU. The family didn't have the money for med school. Knew I had to pay my own way, so I only applied to KU.

Although the post-WWII decades were generally prosperous for families living in the region, only one of our interviewees came from a wealthy family. Most families worked hard and were very careful with money. The interviewees who were financially supported by families were very grateful for this support and appreciated what the funding meant for their parents. One father even took on an additional part-time job to help finance his daughter's medical education. Very few families paid all the expenses associated with medical school; most interviewees understood that they were expected to make efforts to support themselves through loans, scholarships, or part-time work. They were certainly required to live frugally and not squander money on non-necessities and frivolities. Most interviewees described the family attitude toward financial support as a parental investment or expression of confidence in their daughter's future. Some spoke of family traditions of supporting education and a responsibility to *pay it forward*.

My parents did not believe in loans for college. They paid my tuition for medical school as well. It was $400 per semester and only a three-year program, so very inexpensive!

Couldn't have done it without them. My parents were very frugal. I think they thought paying for medical school was the best investment ever!

With so many issues and concerns influencing family attitudes, some families had substantial discussions and divided opinions on their female relative going into medicine.

Father was not crazy about my going into medicine. Didn't see medicine as a place for any daughter of his, but he was supportive. His family thought it was terrible. My mother's family were happy.

I discovered my father sent a "round-robin" letter to family members to seek opinions on me doing medicine. He expressed "many a slip between ambition and reality." The general consensus was that medicine was an unrealistic pipe dream for me.

Mother did not make a lot of comment. Only one relative was a physician, but he did not encourage me at all. He did not believe I had a chance to be admitted to medical school.

Only three participants recalled overt discouragement or disapproval from their families.

Everyone thought it was silly. I think they thought it sounded good but were not sure it would pan out.

Mother said, "Oh no, you'll have to wade through all that blood and gore, hear strong language, meet people you would rather not know."

My family were discouraging. The general attitude was, women should not be doctors: Find a nice husband, get married, have children. My siblings married as soon as they graduated from college.

Six interviewees were married when they entered medical school. These were older matriculants, five of whom had careers before medicine. Three had young children – including one with a 3-week-old baby. One husband was a senior medical student, and another an intern. Both were credited with encouraging their wives to become physicians, supporting them financially, and being very helpful with practical items and *insider information.*

For the interview, my husband was a third-year medical student, so I was able to talk with medical students and prepare. Going into med school, I felt fairly well prepared as I was a bit older than other students and my husband was a medical student, then a resident. . . . I had room and board covered!

My husband warned me there would be very few women in the class and I would be the only married one – we lived on his magnificent resident's salary!

One interviewee was married to a law student, and another to a lawyer. The latter interviewee was unsure about applying to medical school as she was older, had a

3-year-old child, and was pregnant. She had repeatedly *taken detours* working in various jobs and credited her husband with pushing her final decision to apply to medical school. *He told me, "You go, or I'll never be able to look you in the face."*

The husbands of the other married matriculants were a teacher and clergyman, respectively. All husbands supported their wives financially during medical school. In two cases, this was described as a staggered career arrangement, that is, the wives worked to support the husband during college and graduate studies in the expectation that she would resume studies once the family was more secure financially. *I taught school to put my husband through school, then grad school.*

Summary and Reflections

Almost all our interviewees grew up in Kansas and were raised in a wide range of environments, from isolated farms to large cities. Although the literature states that female medical students of that time predominantly came from urban areas,[7-10] about one-third (12/37) of our group was raised in communities of less than 10,000, and about a quarter (9/37) on farms.

The group also differed from contemporary literature in several aspects of family background. Studies indicate that medical students of that time predominantly came from upper-income families, and that female students came from even more financially secure backgrounds than their male classmates.[7-11] In contrast, most of our participants came from middle-class or modest backgrounds. Only one described an affluent upbringing, and money was a serious concern for several families.

Family income is closely related to parental occupation. Publications in 1968 and 1971 reported over 80% of the fathers of female physicians were in professional or white-collar occupations.[8-12] In contrast, only 62% of the fathers of our group were in such occupations. The discrepancy could be due to differences in classifications of occupations, especially farmers, or to changes over time. Our group included 1974 and 1975 graduates, part of the rapid expansion of medical school matriculants and influx of minorities, including women and those from different social backgrounds.[12] Compared to other studies of female medical students of the era, our group reported a higher percentage of at least one college-educated parent (57% vs. 35%), but a lower percentage of physician fathers (16% vs. 20%).[8-12] The mothers of our participants were just as likely to be college graduates as the fathers, resonating with the importance in the literature of maternal education and role modeling.[8,13]

Maternal education may explain the differences in family support reported by our interviewees and that reported in the literature. A 1968 review reported 19% of mothers being *against* a daughter's decision to enter and only 31% being *strongly in favor.*[8] Our group reported that even those mothers who had concerns or were initially opposed came around by the time the decision was final. Similarly, our group recalled almost all fathers being strongly supportive, as opposed to the 55% reported in the national study.[8] No parents remained strongly opposed once the daughter had committed to medicine. Again, our group included those who matriculated in the 1970s, later than those in the national study, so social attitudes could have changed. In addition, our participants could have recall bias and/or presented a more positive picture of family support. Nevertheless, the information from our interviewees is consistent with the strong family themes of valuing education, hard work, and self-reliance featured in the literature. Similar family values are reported in personal narratives of women entering other medical schools in widely different parts of the country during the same time period as our participants.[9,14–17] These narratives also describe the strong influence on family attitudes and resources of national events, especially the Depression and WWII.[14–17]

Regardless of the size or type of community in which they were raised, our participants described coming from stable, loving (if sometimes somewhat undemonstrative and stoic) families that valued education and encouraged their children to aim high and work hard to achieve their goals. Sometimes they were taken aback by their daughters' ambitions, and several were unable to fully support her financially, but most did what they could and were proud of *my daughter, the doctor.*

REFERENCES

1. Becker HS, Greer B, Hughes EC, Strauss AL. Boys in white. Chicago (IL): University of Chicago Press;1961.
2. Nowacek G, Sachs L. Demographic variables in medical school admission. Acad Med. 1990 Mar;65(3):140–4.
3. Friesen SR, Hudson RP. The Kansas School of Medicine eyewitness reflections on its formative years. Kansas City: University of Kansas School of Medicine;1996.
4. Major RH. An account of the University of Kansas School of Medicine. Kansas City: University of Kansas;1968.
5. Brokaw T. The greatest generation. New York (NY): Random House;1998.
6. Bernard J. Academic women. University Park (PA): Pennsylvania State University Press;1964.
7. Walsh MR. Doctors wanted: no women need apply: sexual barriers in the medical profession 1835–1975. New Haven (CT): Yale University Press;1977.
8. Lopate C. Women in medicine. Baltimore (MD): Johns Hopkins Press;1968.
9. Williams PA. Women in medicine: some themes and variations. J Med Educ. 1971;46:584–91.
10. Cartwright LK. The personality and family background of a sample of women medical students at the University of California. J Am Med Womens Assoc (1972). 1972 May;27(5):260–6.
11. Jolly P. Diversity of US medical students by parental income. AAMC Anal Brief. 2008;8(1).
12. Hall FR, Mikesell C, Cranston P, Julian E, Elam C. Longitudinal trends in the applicant pool for U.S. medical schools, 1974–1999. Acad Med. 2001 Aug;76(8):829–34.
13. Sewell WH, Shah VP. Parents' education and children's educational aspirations and achievements. Am Sociol Rev. 1968 Apr 1:191–209.
14. Morantz RM, Pomerleau CS, Fenichel CH. In her own words: oral histories of women physicians. Westport (CT): Greenwood Press;1982.

15. Chin EL, editor. This side of doctoring: reflections from women in medicine. New York (NY): Oxford University Press;2003.
16. Martin T. When the personal was political; five women doctors look back. New York (NY): iUniverse;2008.
17. Detweiler S, Cartwright L. Women physician pioneers of the 1960s: their lives and profession over a half century. San Francisco (CA): University of California Medical Humanities Press;2022.

5

The Road to Medicine: School Experiences

"Female education produces monstrous brains and puny bodies; abnormally active cerebration and abnormally weak digestion; flowing thought and constipated bowels."[1]

The oldest of our interviewees graduated from high school as the United States approached WWII, the youngest in the summer of love in 1968. For the majority, their education began in the post-WWII era that idealized domesticity and traditional roles for women as wives and mothers.[2-4] Their high school and college experiences occurred in institutions attempting to adapt to dramatic events and changing societal norms and expectations. The Cold War, the Civil Rights movement, the feminist revival, and the Vietnam War – plus associated counter-movements and backlashes – buffeted the education of Americans growing up during this period. For the high school curricula of our group, the Cold War was the most profound external influence, especially the launching of Sputnik in October 1957.[3-5] This was a watershed event for US education, leading to massive investment in programs to train scientists and engineers. Nearly 90% of our interviewees experienced high school during the immediate aftermath of the Sputnik launch and the pivot to science education.

Current readers may have difficulty appreciating the shock and near-panic resulting from the Sputnik launch. The public perceived that the United States had lost, or was perilously close to losing, the Cold War. Dire consequences, including thermonuclear annihilation, were imminently predicted.[3,4] The blame for the "cosmic humiliation" by the USSR was placed squarely on the failure of the US educational system to prepare adequate numbers of appropriately trained engineers and scientists.[2-6]

"The vital problem facing the nation, and the free world as a whole, is the fact that Russia is training scientists and technological personnel at a pace four times that of our own and that, unless something is done about it as a large-scale, national effort, Russia will definitely surpass us in the near future, with consequences too tragic to contemplate."[5]

The immediate reaction to Sputnik was a frantic race to train a large scientific workforce.

"It is no exaggeration to say that America's progress in many fields of endeavor in the years ahead – in fact, the very survival of our free country – may depend in large part upon the education we provide for our young people now."[6]

DOI: 10.1201/9781003539568-5

The language of the National Defense Education Act and other legislation enabling massive federal investment in scientific education was gender-neutral, but the clamor for training more scientists and engineers was not followed by a groundswell of support for women entering the workforce, including the scientific and technical professions. The United States was deeply conflicted over the appropriate role for women in addressing the national crisis of the Cold War.[3,4] Even prior to Sputnik, several reports had challenged the "wasted manpower resource" of low female employment.[6-9] Several experts called for more education of women in the sciences and their greater participation in the scientific community, specifically in the defense industry. Unfortunately, the rhetoric was not matched with practical recommendations, beyond optimistic aspirations about how maternal employment and family responsibilities could be handled by "Trousered Mothers and Dishwashing Dads."[6-12]

A 1957 report asserted that women working outside the home no longer encountered criticism and disapproval.

> "The attitudes of society which affect the participation of women in paid employment are deeply rooted and resist change, but they are far from immutable. They have altered sufficiently to make it easier for married, as well as for single, women to work outside the home without feeling that they are violating social conventions."[8]

The report offered no evidence to support this somewhat-tentative claim.

Despite the national emergency and initiatives to train more scientists and engineers, no concerted attempt was undertaken to attract young women into science-based careers. The images of the "bachelor girls of science" of the late 1950s seemed unlikely to inspire girls to enter scientific and technical professions or to contribute meaningfully to triumphing in the Cold War.[13] Female scientists (presumed to be single) were depicted as "well-groomed, intelligent girls with character" who required the help of their male colleagues or acted as their assistants.[13] This contrasts sharply with the bold, competent Rosie the Riveter, the image presented to avidly recruit women for the national emergency of the previous generation.[3] Imagery was a powerful force in the polarizing debate of the late 1950s and 1960s about women in the workforce. The contribution of Russian women to their nation's scientific success was portrayed as achieved at the cost of defeminizing women and destroying the nuclear family.[3,4,14-16] In contrast, the US ultra-feminine housewife and mother was portrayed as essential to the survival of the American way of life.[4] Female devotion to domesticity was weaponized by President Nixon in his 1959 Kitchen Debates with Khrushchev when he claimed that "American families, complete with working husbands and housewives who raised children *and* washed the family's clothes in electric washing machines, were superior to Soviet families, for they embodied the spirit of American liberty and freedom of choice."[4] A "normal" family and a vigilant mother became the "front line" of defense against treason. Any deviation from the model was linked to Communism and sedition.[11] Young women in high school during the 1950s and early 1960s, including most our interviewees, received highly conflicting messages about appropriate roles – should they save the American way of life by dedicating themselves to science and winning the technological race against the USSR, or could they better defeat the forces of evil by devotion to family and domestic duties?[3]

Size and Type of School (K–12)

The majority of our participants attended public schools in urban/suburban areas or small towns in Kansas. Their high schools included the largest in the state, with several hundred graduates every year, but the group also included women who were educated in very small schools.

I was in a class of 8 throughout from first grade to graduation.

There were 18 students – 10 girls and 8 boys – in my graduating class.

One participant described attending an iconic tiny schoolhouse out on the prairie.

I attended a two-roomed school with about eight grades, where the older taught the younger children. I was the only child in my class for four of the eight years. The school burned down and was replaced with a one-roomed schoolhouse.

The consolidation of rural school districts during the 1950s largely eliminated the one-roomed rural schoolhouse but resulted in *massive busing* to collect all the children from isolated farms and settlements to attend a single school serving a large but sparsely populated area. One participant provided a vivid picture of the school bus picking up children from multiple farms and small communities to take them to the school in the largest town – population 400! The bus was based with the family who lived farthest from the school. *Sometimes one of the older boys drove the bus, even on unpaved roads in the winter, to take the rest of us to school and back. It was 15 miles from our farm to the school.*

Schools in small communities could be lacking in resources and not accustomed to students, especially girls, with high academic aspirations. *I was the first from my high school to go to KU and the first to go to medical school. High school had very little influence on my career decisions. The school had few resources. No chemistry lab and science classes were a joke.*

Conversely, other small communities and schools actively encouraged academic aspirations. *It was a very supportive small town. The education system picked out and recognized the potential of people who were good at math and science and had special in-class groups. I had lots of affirmation and support. I always knew I had to do well in school.*

Four participants were educated predominantly in private all-girls' schools. Two of the private schools were Catholic institutions, one a boarding school. Two participants described being transferred from public schools because their parents were dissatisfied with the quality of the education provided. One woman recalled her mother's vigorous interactions with the principal of the public junior high school – very embarrassing for a teenager!

Mother was VERY invested in her children's education. After a confrontation with the headmaster of the junior high school about the sixth-grade curriculum, she transferred me to a private girls' school. She also told the headmaster he didn't speak English correctly! The new place was a rigorous girls' school, VERY good in science. Some unusual female teachers, but GREAT teachers. I LOVED science but had a terrible time with math.

I started in public schools but got a HORRIBLE education. When my grandparents realized I didn't know my alphabet, they moved me to small private girls' school with 4–12 pupils per class. I got a very good education – a bit light on math and physics.

All four who attended private schools believed they were well educated. The two Catholic school graduates also commented on character development and the absence of distraction from male classmates.

The convent was a fabulous education. I learned discipline, delayed gratification, other good stuff – helped in medicine!

The school had very high standards and provided a comprehensive education. Well-rounded curriculum. Required sciences and math, as well as arts, foreign languages, and humanities. Advantage to be able to focus on school without worrying on competing with a boy you might want to date – and act dumb. Encouraged girls to fulfill their dreams.

High Achievers

Whatever the educational environment, our participants were good students and high achievers. They described determination to excel academically in high school and to achieve excellent grades. Several were valedictorians. This determination was not described in terms of dutiful daughters striving to please family members, or on personal ambition to attain future wealth and prestige. Almost all our participants conveyed innate enthusiasm and love for education. Some expressed pure joy in learning.

I always LOVED school, wanted to keep learning for years and spend a long time in school.

Worked hard and got good grades.

My goal was to do well in school.

As described in the previous chapter, academic achievements were encouraged, or even expected, by most of their families. Several interviewees also described supportive schools in which advanced education for girls was a norm and college aspirations were expected.

Most of the women I associated with in high school were going to college with plans for a professional career (teachers, writers, med tech). No other friends were planning on medicine, but no one thought I was crazy. I just assumed that I could do it and didn't even think there might be barriers. Two guys in my high school class of 465 became physicians.

I was very good at science and especially math. Really enjoyed math. Was in Future Medical Careers club in high school. Did very well in high school and achieved good grades. Friends were all girls who intended to go to college. No issues over girls succeeding in math/science.

Many participants volunteered that they encountered no opposition to girls studying sciences and several credited science and/or math teachers as instrumental in their academic successes.

Always encouraged to do well – no issues over girls doing medicine or sciences.

Encountered no negatives in high school about girls in science.

Never had anyone tell me, "You can't do that because you're a girl."

Only one participant recounted discrimination in high school science studies because of her gender. The experience made her even more determined to succeed, despite her mother's enigmatic comment. After over 50 years, she remains angry over the injustice and underlying assumptions.

In my senior year, I was given an A– in physics despite grades qualifying for an A and male classmates with similar grades getting As. I was told the grade was an A– "because you are a girl." My mother commented, "You are making progress. I was given a B despite earning an A 'because girls don't understand science'."

Only a few of the oldest participants described striving to succeed in high school against assumptions about appropriate studies or encountering low academic expectations for girls.

Did courses like physics and chemistry – not into home economics. We were expected to get married and be taken care of.

Not a lot of people went to college from my town in those days.

At least four individuals recounted being socially isolated during high school but attributed this to shyness or *nerdiness*. None linked being isolated or lonely to being ostracized by classmates because of academic ambitions or success.

I wasn't very outgoing; my goal was to do well in school.

I wasn't popular like a cheerleader or something.

High school was not wonderful. Felt socially inept.

Didn't have much of a social life – put all my energy into school and music.

Inspiring Teachers and Other Influences

About half or our interviewees specifically mentioned inspirational teachers. These were found in all types of schools, from huge urban high schools to small rural school-houses, and could be male or female. Even in the smallest rural school, one enthusiastic and innovative teacher could make a huge difference.

One teacher taught all the sciences – he was very enterprising and early adopter of electronics (in the early 1960s!). He had students build an organ as a project.

We had two inspiring/encouraging female teachers (spinster sisters) at our tiny school. One converted a closet into a library and encouraged reading. About sixth grade, I read a book about women physicians. This was the 1950s. It inspired me to become a physician, but I didn't think it was possible.

Outstanding teachers were predominantly in science and/or math. As described in a previous chapter, interest in science was a primary factor in the motivation to become a physician. Some participants described teachers who inspired their original interest in the sciences or helped them overcome initial difficulties in mastering the material; more commonly, the key teacher recognized and encouraged a developing enthusiasm for science and related subjects. Some women spoke passionately about their love of these subjects in high school.

I had a wonderful teacher in math and chemistry. He took the time and trouble to recognize when I didn't understand and to present things in different ways till the light bulbs came on!

LOVED math and sciences. Aced three calculus courses, loved equations, etc. WONDERFUL female math teacher.

Found science very interesting. Pretty good at math and chemistry. Male science teacher was a positive influence. Even in small school, several outstanding teachers really helped me learn.

I LOVED science and math. Encouraged especially by male chemistry teacher.

Always encouraged in sciences. Encouraged by outstanding male science teacher.

Both male and female teachers were remembered as influential in our participants' love of science, academic success, and decision to aspire to medicine. In addition to stimulating learning, they fostered confidence in their pupils, and some were credited with giving the interviewee the *final push* to aim for medicine.

A positive influence was the course in human physiology. The teacher (male) had actually been to med school but decided to become a teacher. I was fascinated by how the body worked. I also took the first AP class in biology offered in Kansas.

I had a couple of very encouraging teachers (male in science and female in history). I was hesitating/unsure "would like to go to medical school . . . but." These teachers told me to "go for it."

Despite the many reports of a supportive high school environment and inspirational teachers, at least two participants described keeping quiet about medical aspirations, for fear of being thought inappropriately ambitious

In high school, I didn't tell anyone about medicine.

Did not disclose my medical ambitions in high school, in case they laughed at me.

Another woman was ridiculed by teachers for her early decision to become a psychiatrist – a specialty about which she still speaks with enthusiasm after 50 years' experience!

About the age of 12, decided I wanted to be a psychiatrist. The teachers laughed, said psychiatrists were all crazy.

Surprisingly, only two interviewees mentioned career counselors when describing their high school experiences. Both recalled negative interactions, and the interviewees were scornful of the advice – which they both ignored. One counselor discouraged focusing on science with a rather strange metaphor. The second expressed doubts that made our interviewee even more determined to become a physician.

My high school counselor tried to discourage me from taking so many science classes. He said, "I like bananas, but you shouldn't eat too many." I suppose he meant too much of a thing is bad for you – anyway I ignored that bit of advice, and it was one of the smartest choices I made.

The high school counselor was dismissive of me going into medicine. Said, "Don't apply, consider something else." My reaction was, "Sign me up." I'll show YOU. I did not waver from my intent to do medicine.

Summary and Reflection

About one-third of the group initially reported that high school experiences had little or no influence on the decision to enter medicine. The remainder reported generally positive influences, but with less impact than other factors, such as family, mentors, role models, or college studies. In retrospect, we believe participants may have underestimated the role of high school experiences in shaping their career decisions.

After reading the contemporary literature, we were surprised that our participants rarely mentioned academic discrimination, especially in girls studying science. Studies conducted in the 1960s, when most of our ladies were in high school, demonstrated a significant waning of academic ambition among girls during high school.[17,18] The erosion of interest was particularly striking for girls considering medicine. In the reported studies, half of the eleventh-grade boys intending to be physicians retained that intent one year later, compared to only 18% of the girls. Conversely, most of our interviewees described their studies in science and/or math with enthusiasm, and several mentioned encouraging teachers. About one-third of the way through the project, we began to ask specifically about opposition or resistance to girls studying science in high school. Neither the open-ended approach ("Tell me about high school. Did anything happen to encourage or discourage you to become a doctor?") nor direct questioning about their experiences in studying science ("Did you run into any issues over the girls' studying science?") unearthed evidence of widespread discouragement of girls studying science. The only mentions of being discouraged from science or *pressured to do something more appropriate for a girl* were in our oldest participant, who attended high school in the 1940s and 1950s.

Several factors could account for the apparent discrepancy between the experiences reported by our group and those of national studies. The most likely is the preponderance of graduates from the 1970s. Being discouraged from science features less prominently in descriptions of their education by women in this group compared to earlier cohorts.[19] In addition, our interviewees could have selectively recalled positive experiences and been unable or unwilling to share negative or discouraging influences. Importantly, our interviewees are a select group of survivors and high achievers. As discussed in the previous chapter, they mostly enjoyed the support of strong families and appeared to have thrived in school, regardless of the size or type of school attended. As described in Chapter 3, about half of our interviewees reported serious interest or even firm commitment to medicine early in life. They managed to retain or even solidify this early interest during high school and to achieve the academic credentials to advance to the next stage in the process of becoming a physician: excelling in college.

REFERENCES

1. Clarke EH. Sex in education; or, a fair chance for the girls. Boston (MA);1873.
2. Miller DT, Nowak M, The fifties: the way we really were. Garden City (NY): Doubleday & Company;1977.
3. Douglas SJ. Where the girls are: growing up female with the mass media. New York (NY): Times Books;1994.
4. Pabst ES. Cold war insecurity as women's opportunity: Sputnik, the National Defense Education Act of 1958, and shifting gender roles in Eisenhower's America [Unpublished Honors Thesis]. Boston College, Department of History. 2005 April. Available from: http://hdl.handle.net/2345/403
5. Laurence WT. Science in review: Soviet success in rocketry draws attention to need for more students in the sciences. New York Times. 1957 Oct 13:191.

6. National Defense Education Act, 20 U.S.C. §§ 401–602. 1958 US House of Representatives. 85th Congress Committee on Education and Labor National Defense Education Act 1958 National Defense Education Act I US House of Representatives: History, Art & Archives.

7. Howes RF, editor. Women in the defense decade: report of a national conference of persons representing schools, colleges, universities, government agencies, and selected national organizations, New York City, 1951 Sep 27–28. Washington (DC): American Council on Education;1952.

8. National Manpower Council. Womanpower. New York (NY): Columbia University Press;1957.

9. Conference on the Present Status and Prospective Trends of Research on the Education of Women. The education of women: signs for the future. Washington (DC): American Council on Education;1959.

10. Clowse B. Brainpower for the cold war: the sputnik crisis and national defense education act of 1958. Westport (CT): Greenwood Press;1981.

11. Coontz S. The way we never were: American families and the nostalgia trap. New York (NY): Basic Books;1992.

12. Barclay D. Trousered mothers and dishwashing dads. New York Times. 1957 Apr 28;SM257–9.

13. M.I.T.'s bachelor girls of science. New York Times. 1958 Apr 27:SM84–5.

14. Samuels G. Why Russian women work like men. New York Times. 1958 Nov 2:22–5.

15. Turk C. They do a man sized job: the Olgas and Tanyas trade femininity for muscle power on farm, in factory. Chicago Daily Tribune. 1958 Aug 10:F30.

16. Meyerowitz J, editor. Not June Cleaver: women and gender in postwar America, 1945–1960. Philadelphia: Temple University Press;1994.

17. Walsh MR. Doctors wanted: no women need apply: sexual barriers in the medical profession 1835–1975. New Haven and London: Yale University Press;1977.

18. Lopate C. Women in medicine. Baltimore (MD): Johns Hopkins Press;1968.

19. Detweiler S, Cartwright L. Women physician pioneers of the 1960s: their lives and profession over a half century. San Francisco (CA): University of California Medical Humanities Press;2022.

6

College Girls

"Premed is a waste of time for girls: you need to do Home Ec."

(College Counselor 1965)

The college years of our interviewees spanned the turbulent decades from 1941 to 1971. In her first year, our oldest participant saw male classmates depart for military duties and the campus fill with individuals attempting accelerated degrees in subjects essential to the WWII war effort. She and her sorority sisters were caught up in campaigns to collect scrap metal and other war-related volunteer activities. In contrast, some of the graduates from the late 1960s and early 1970s were active in antiwar protests that disrupted campuses and divided communities. Our interviewees attended college against the backdrop of WWII, the Cold War, Civil Rights movement, Women's Liberation, the Vietnam War, and other upheavals that rocked American society and had profound impact on the challenges and opportunities for aspiring female physicians.[1]

Our oldest participant was criticized in 1942 for not returning home from college to work in the aircraft factories. During WWII, Wichita became a major aircraft manufacturing center, drawing in huge numbers of workers. Similarly, the area around Lawrence, the home of the University of Kansas (KU), experienced an influx of thousands of workers for munitions plants and military installations. The 1948 medical class yearbook describes heady times in Lawrence during the early 1940s:

> "Everyone had plenty of money, everyone had jobs, carousing at racetracks
> and nightclubs reached an all-time peak, and American were drinking more
> whiskey than had ever been drunk before as the breath of victory rode in with
> the peak of industrial production."[2]

The proliferation of bootlegging taverns (Kansas being a dry state) and other suspect establishments in the town caused consternation for local law enforcement and public health officials. The new establishments and the "Victory Girls" they attracted were regarded as a serious threat to the students and good citizens of Lawrence, evidenced by the rising incidence of sexually transmitted infections.[1] While the sorority sisters were unlikely to venture into the more notorious establishments, they were aware of the heady atmosphere in the community.

Military service remained a very real prospect for male premed students throughout the decades covered by the interviews. The Selective Service Act and the "Doctor Draft" sought to ensure an adequate supply of health professionals for the military

DOI: 10.1201/9781003539568-6

throughout WWII and the Korean and Vietnam Wars.[3] Our interviewees spoke of the many ways in which military service impacted personal and career decisions for themselves and their male classmates, boyfriends, and husbands. In the years following WWII, interviewees described competing with the influx of male applicants funded by the GI Bill for places in premed courses, medical school, or internships. Later, women were accused of highjacking medical school or college places that would have allowed a young man to claim draft deferment. More than one interviewee was told, *My friend got sent to Vietnam because you took his place.*

Throughout their college years, our interviewees picked their ways across campuses that must have resembled construction sites. Colleges and universities expanded rapidly to accommodate the postwar influx of students and the federal and other infusions of funds to support education and research. They were aware of the Cold War's impact in stimulating the education of scientists, but also of the chilling effect of anti-Communist fervor.[4] *I didn't like being pressured or forced to do things like the loyalty oaths during the McCarthy era.* On the Lawrence campus, the threatening atmosphere of McCarthyism led to the shutdown of a left-leaning student newspaper after 25 years of publication.[5] Later, students were inspired by Kennedy's Call to Service and Johnson's War on Poverty. One of our interviewees joined the Peace Corps, one spent her summers working in impoverished Appalachian communities, and another took the Foreign Service exam as a backup plan if she was not admitted to medical school, *because I felt called to do something useful.*

The city of Lawrence and the KU campus are usually depicted as bastions of liberal ideas in a very conservative region. The campus was a regular stop for politicians, radicals, and public figures when crossing coast to coast. In 1968, Robert F. Kennedy opened his presidential campaign at KU, where over 20,000 enthusiastic students and others jammed Allen Fieldhouse.[6] In contrast, after a more muted welcome in 1970, the counterculture Yippie leader Abbie Hoffman stated, "This place is a drag; I'm going to Dallas."[7]

Kansas has strong abolitionist credentials from its foundation as a free state and the sacrifices of "bleeding Kansas" during the Civil War. Lawrence was almost destroyed, and 150 men massacred by Quantrill's Confederate guerrillas in 1863, because of the city's reputation as a bastion of anti-slavery movements. Despite this history, Lawrence was still largely segregated when our first interviewees attended KU in the early 1940s.[8] The medical school had been forced by the state governor to allow African American students to complete their clinical education in 1938, and the first Black student graduated in 1941, just as our oldest participant was being refused admission to premed studies.[9] The Medical Center continued to have segregated wards and facilities until the mid-1950s. On the Lawrence campus, Black students were still relegated to the back of the classroom by some professors in the 1940s.[10] In 1943, student government groups voted to allow Black students to attend university dances, but the soda fountain at the Student Union refused them service. A women's residence was refused permission for a Christmas dance in 1946 because it was interracial.[11] Integration of residence halls began following WWII, but progress was slow. As one KU alumna explained: "All my roommates were Negro; all the rest of the dorm was White. I don't recall that being a problem. It was just the way it was in 1954."[11] By 1965, discrimination led to protests that culminated in a march and occupation of the Chancellor's Office. Over 100 students were arrested.[11] Unrest continued in Lawrence, influenced by regional and national events, especially the 1968 Kansas City riots that caused six deaths and millions of dollars of damage.[12] A community center in Lawrence, Afro House, financed in part by KU and intended to nurture Black culture, was suspected of supporting Black Panther and other radical groups.[13] The 1970 police shooting of a young man associated with Afro House precipitated "five days of often-bloody clashes between local police and student antiwar and civil rights protestors, which resulted in two deaths, countless injuries and a campus that resembled a battle zone."[14,15]

Not all the violence was related to Civil Rights. The campus and the "Hippie Haven" neighborhood in Lawrence were centers for militants and activists of all types. By one account,

> "approximately 600 radicals lived in town, of which no more than 200 were highly motivated. Of these, perhaps only a few dozen were actually dangerous. In addition, there were probably 1,000 individuals – students, faculty and townspeople – who were available when the need for a show of force arose."[15]

Protests, disruptions, and violence, including arson, escalated during the long hot spring and summer of 1970, described by an interviewee as a *tumultuous time, lots of upheaval, Vietnam War, and social unrest. Lots of tension on campus.* A "week of rage" in April mainly directed at the Vietnam War culminated in the firebombing of the Student Union, with over $1 million in damage.[16] An interviewee recalled, *My husband worked at the bookstore. He and his friends rushed to the fire to try to rescue as much as possible – it was terrible.* By May, rising local and national tensions, especially the Kent State campus shootings, led to the suspension of the semester. Graduation ceremonies were canceled.[16,17] Ironically, a makeup graduation celebration on the 50th anniversary was also canceled, this time due to the COVID-19 pandemic. As one interviewee complained, *I never got to graduate properly, even the second time!* The class of 1970 was finally honored at the 2022 graduation ceremony.

Antiwar and civil rights protests and disruptions continued in the autumn term of 1970, but things were somewhat calmer. The last serious violence was a firebombing of the Computations Center in December 1970.[17] Advocates for other causes began to be heard. One interviewee recalls, *There was lots of interest in feminism on campus.* In February 1972, 30 feminist activists known as the February Sisters staged a sit-in as a "means of obtaining the resources to meet the pressing needs of women."[18] The occupation lasted for 13 hours, ending after KU administration agreed to consider their six demands, which included improved affirmative action and employment practices, provision of childcare facilities, establishment of a women's studies program, and improved health services for female students.[18]

Most interviewees recalled focusing on their studies to secure the grades required for admission to medical school, rather than participating in political action. They described navigating disruptions and often feeling afraid – as well as the stress of constantly having to respond to the concerns of worried parents. At that time, many Kansas families steered potential students away from KU because of its radical reputation. Even in more conservative colleges, the national spirit of protest and revolt could not be avoided or quashed. One interviewee, who attended Kansas State University, reported, *I enjoyed it but in junior year got really restless. I was involved in anti-Vietnam movement and transferred with a friend to LSU. Changed majors, then realized I needed to return to K-State to graduate.* She added that the attraction was with how *LSU was more of a party school!* Others embraced the excitement of the times. A Kansas girl who attended college in New York recalled, *New York in late 1960s was exciting. I heard James Baldwin, Malcom X, and others. During the student protests of 1968, students protesting on behalf of Harlem residents occupied the Columbia University building, but we kept it clean (as opposed to other student groups who trashed occupied buildings) and were supported by community. I was not one of the occupiers but was a runner, bringing food and supplies to those involved in the sit-in. Good thing my mother didn't know! I was a TA and well-known to staff and faculty. I missed an important final exam because of the sit-in, but lab techs stood up for me and persuaded the professors to let me take the exam so I could get into medical school.*

Colleges Attended

> "Kansas students are also provincial, particularly with respect to their educational backgrounds. They have had little experience or knowledge of the world of higher education beyond their immediate geographic region."[19]

The largest group of interviewees (17/37, 46%) attended KU in Lawrence. Ten (27%) graduated from other Kansas institutions, namely, Kansas State and Wichita State Universities or smaller public or private colleges. The remaining interviewees attended a diverse group of institutions across the United States, from Radcliffe College in Massachusetts to Pomona College near the Californian coast, and from Hamline University in Minnesota to Tulane University in New Orleans. Two attended all-female colleges. Some graduated from prestigious and expensive institutions, including William and Mary, Duke, Barnard, and Washington University (St. Louis); conversely, three attended community colleges to acquire as many credits as possible at the lowest available cost.

Making the Leap to College

Transitioning to college was exciting, but challenging. Several interviewees recalled the shock of adjusting to the college environment. This was most marked for those from small communities who entered the large KU–Lawrence campus and for those who were the first members of their families to attend college. The challenges went beyond the large numbers of fellow students or complexities of college schedules; for many young women from conventional homes and small communities, KU–Lawrence was an alien environment. During the period covered by the majority of our informants, KU–Lawrence transitioned in the perception of many Kansans from the shining intellectual city on the hill (Mount Oread) to "Berkeley on the River Kaw," a haven for hippies, troublemakers, and revolutionaries, who indulged in drugs, orgies, and other unspecified vices.[1] Several of our participants recalled family pressure in the late 1960s and early 1970s to attend the more conservative Kansas State University or remain at home and attend Wichita State University, rather than risk exposure to the evil influences rampant on the Lawrence campus.

KU–Lawrence was a big adjustment from a high school class of 8 to 5,000 in the 1941 freshman class.

Major culture shock. Wow, it was the first time I had lived in a town – I grew up on a farm! Lawrence in late 1960s was vibrant, lots of political action. Vietnam was dragging on, and KU had a major weed scene!

At least one interviewee felt overwhelmed and almost immediately decided to abandon her attempt at higher education. *After my first week at KU, I went home to the farm and told my parents I wasn't going back to school. The conversation went like this. Mother: "What do you plan to do?" Me: "I'll get a job." Mother: "What kind of job, wrapping butter at the creamery? That's about all you are qualified to do! And where will you live? You're not going to live here!" Dad: "You need to give this more thought. Deep down, you know what you should do. You decide what that is, and I will support your decision." I went back Sunday afternoon. The first semester was hard. Going from a small town and small school to a large university and not knowing anyone was difficult. Things improved as I made good friends. That weekend conversation with my parents was pivotal. If they had not exercised tough love, I may have followed a very different path.* The countless learners and faculty mentored by this woman during her long and distinguished academic career owe a great deal to her parents' *tough love* that weekend.

Living arrangements were crucial in making friends and adjusting to college life. Those who did not live in dorms or sororities found the transition to college particularly difficult.

I was aware of other girls in premed but didn't know any in college. Felt at a disadvantage as not in a sorority.

Sororities were generally described as facilitating friendship with like-minded young women and providing supportive environments for academic success. Our oldest participant, who entered KU in 1941, was a notable exception.

I lived in sorority. My friends thought I was crazy to do medicine. Everyone thought I was crazy and said, "Don't do it!"

Roommates and close friends were especially important for those who described themselves as shy, introverted, or overwhelmed by college.

I focused on studies in college. Not many friends, except a roommate who had similar priorities.

I was a very focused student, nose to the grindstone. I hung out with like-minded people and got honors.

Friends and others were okay with a girl doing medicine. Large classes, I felt overwhelmed.

More extroverted types relished the intellectual stimulation of new circles of friends and embraced the academic and political turmoil of the times.

College in New York City was a wonderful social experience. It was FUN. We spent hours drinking tea and talking – thought we were the great philosophers. I was smart in high school but in college realized there were a lot of other smart people around and I was just average.

Sororities could provide practical assistance and mentors as well as encouragement to aim for medical school. Throughout the period covered by our interviews, college accommodations for male and female students were strictly separated, and female residents were subject to curfew and various regulations, presumably to protect the good moral reputations of the young ladies.[1]

There were a few female premed students – about eight and we became friends, supported one another.

Good support from my sorority. One sorority sister ahead was going into medicine, plus two contemporaries, so I wasn't the only one.

I was in a sorority. The women's movement was just beginning, so I was not discouraged by peers to aim for a career. Lots of interest in feminism on campus. Several friends/sorority sisters were pre-law.

Several participants mentioned that the fraternities and organizations for their male classmates provided more resources, mentors, and insider information for aspiring medical students and were not above a little cheating to gain an advantage.

The guys in the fraternities studied together and had access to exam books and notes from previous students. Male classmates in fraternities also used write-ups from previous students to skip on physics experiments.

Several women recounted using boyfriends, sometime future husbands, to access information and resources about medical school requirements.

The male students seemed to have more contacts and be better organized about planning careers. My boyfriend in a fraternity seemed to know which classes to take for medicine, how to find the premed advisers, make contacts, etc.

I found out about requirements for medical school from my boyfriend (later husband), who went to medical school a year ahead.

I was greatly helped by an older male friend who was premed: He laid out the path.

The pipeline of information from the medical school to the fraternities in Lawrence was well-known and even recognized by the chair of the medical school admissions committee. "Committee members had favorite questions for applicants. . . . These questions were probably in the files of every fraternity house in Lawrence."[20]

The scholarship halls on the Lawrence campus were fondly remembered by several interviewees. These four halls each accommodated about 40–50 female students. They provided low-cost accommodation for women with good academic records but required residents to contribute to running the institution by undertaking various domestic responsibilities.[21] Fittingly for our interviewees, the first scholarship hall for women was endowed by a woman who had been forced to curtail her education because of financial problems in her father's medical practice. She held on to her convictions of the importance of education for women after she became wealthy. "My sympathy has always been with the girls who must travel up-hill and my dream to aid self-supporting girls to get an education."[22] Our interviewees who lived in a scholarship hall described their financial problems and the need to *live as frugally as possible*. Several recounted making their own clothes. Others worked in various part-time jobs to finance college, and one recounted with pride, *I finished in 3.5 years to save money*. For many of this group, scholarship hall was the only means to obtain a college education. Beyond this basic support, the hall's uniquely female and academic environment had a profound impact on residents. Interviewees spoke of the peer support, academic encouragement, and practical advice from fellow residents and associated personnel – as well as having a lot of fun. The culture of the hall encouraged focus on academic priorities and helped residents balance maintaining the necessary grades with enjoying the college experience amid the many distractions of campus life. Above all, the hall normalized aspirations for a young woman to enter medicine or another profession. Several interviewees credited living in scholarship hall with building their confidence to attempt application to medical school.

If you had the grades and the financial need, scholarship hall provided inexpensive board, and everyone had to help run the house, cooking, etc. I like to cook. Lived around a lot of female nerds and creative souls (in theatre, arts etc.) – had a lot of fun. WOW!

One of the house sponsors was a pediatrician who had three children and was encouraging about medicine. When I was struggling over chemistry, she said, "Don't worry, you don't need chemistry to do medicine."

Scholarship hall was absolutely the best training – we did all our own cooking, cleaning. Lived frugally. Made my own clothes.

Being in a scholarship hall in Lawrence, I saw many women intending to go into medicine and other professions. It provided confidence. I saw it was possible. Scholarship hall opened my eyes.

Similarly, the two interviewees who attended all-female colleges believed that environment had facilitated studying and fostered confidence in young women to enter the professions without many of the distractions of a co-ed campus.

Courses, Classes, and Grades

Our interviewees entered college with great enthusiasm for learning and strong motivation to serve others. They had been outstanding students in high school, especially in science, and had absorbed solid values from their families and communities. Each participant spoke of a strong work ethic and sense of responsibility for the privilege of a college education. Most carried the aspirations of their families for each daughter to achieve her full potential – even if family financial support was lacking and enthusiasm for her becoming a physician was sometimes tenuous.

About half of the group entered college intending to apply for medical school or with a strong interest in a medical career. Among the others, about half had considered medicine but had been discouraged, or interest had waned. These individuals frequently cited insecurity in their abilities or lack of encouragement, reporting that medicine was perceived as *a stretch or an elite thing.* Few of this group had clear career goals beyond *something in science, probably research or teaching.* Two planned to become medical technicians; a few were considering careers in literature, music, or other non-science-based occupations. The broad range of initial interests is reflected in the diverse subjects studied and the many reports of changing college majors. About one-third (13/37) reported changing majors during college, and six graduated with minors or extensive credits in languages, music, literature, or other non-scientific subjects. For the earliest participants, studying non-science subjects may not have been completely motivated by a love of learning. Until the mid-1960s, the admissions requirements for the University of Kansas School of Medicine (KUSM) clearly sought the Renaissance Man.

> "Broad and diversified collegiate education is required. Medicine is concerned with people rather than with disease . . . the humanistic as well as the scientific.
>
> College Course Requirements: Chemistry 13 hours (5 inorganic, 3 quantitative analysis, 5 organic), biology 6 hours (must include zoology lab), physics 6 hours. In addition, facility with one's native tongue as well as with a foreign one is the mark of an educated man. Requirements: 10 hours English, 8 hours language (modern, Latin or Greek). College courses must NOT duplicate medical courses such as anatomy."[23]

In the early 1940s, our oldest participant described studying English, German, and algebra in addition to (unofficial) premed courses, despite the prevailing wisdom that *women were supposed to do home economics and things they could use.* Even with a heavy schedule, she excelled academically and was an honor student and a member of Phi Beta Kappa. She commented on *taking PE for credit to lighten the load.*

Another early graduate recalled having a *heavy load. Gave up band as I couldn't manage the time for away events with coursework.*

Nevertheless, even as premed courses and medical school admission criteria became more focused on the sciences in the 1970s, several interviewees spoke of undertaking liberal arts college courses purely out of interest or for the joy of learning.

I did well in all of the premed courses but also liked arts and humanities – I liked everything, took everything!

I majored in English literature and writing – found my soulmates. Also did courses in psychology, anthropology, and medicine prerequisites.

Interviewees frequently credited non-science courses with helping sustain their spirits during the grueling premed coursework. In addition, several commented on how much courses in the arts, literature, and languages had contributed to their lives.

Several graduates from the 1970s reported that KUSM had unusually strict admission requirements in mathematics and science. The requirements for calculus and several branches of chemistry posed challenges and caused consternation for several interviewees – some still shuddered at the memory.

KU had more requirements for physics and calculus than other schools.

Only time I was ever somewhat discouraged was calculus.

Really liked physiology but found chemistry difficult.

Friends really helped to get through organic chemistry and physics.

Sometimes, completing premed coursework required a complete change of trajectory. Two completed masters degrees, and several were enrolled in graduate programs when they decided to switch to medicine. Faculty were sometimes instrumental in this career decision; others regarded medicine as an inferior discipline.

In my senior year of pharmacy, a professor suggested research or medicine. I hadn't really thought about it. He thought I had more ability than doing retail. I had won a big award, had done research as a job working in a lab for graduate students, and I didn't like it, so I circled back to consider medicine.

As a senior, I was still unsure where I was headed, seemed destined to do a PhD in chemistry but didn't really want to work in a lab. A male classmate said, "Why not do medicine?" I thought about it and took an additional year to get the required courses. The faculty considered medicine "dirty science" – compared to PhD, "pure science."

Seven interviewees graduated from college and worked before returning to complete the requirements for medical school. Several described heroic efforts to complete premed courses while working full-time, supporting their husbands' careers, and managing a family. In addition to working as a teacher and raising children, one lady had a full-time job as a pastor's wife. *I taught high school biology and chemistry and drove 20 miles each way to take refresher courses at KU–Lawrence, including organic chemistry and biology.* Perhaps the most determined interviewee completed premed requisites, despite significant health problems, while her surgeon husband was assigned to the Panama Canal Zone. *I took all the prerequisites for medical school at Canal Zone Community College – the reason they offered them was, they had a big med tech program. I was very ill with hepatitis B in Panama and spent two weeks in the hospital. Had to catch up with all my classes, labs, and take the tests.*

Whether taking a direct or circuitous path, applicants had to successfully complete all the required premed courses, plus any additional credit hours required for the college degree. Widespread rumors circulated among students that certain non-premed courses were regarded either favorably or, conversely, with suspicion by the Admission Committee. Oral histories of faculty members in the 1950s and 1960s indicate some truth in these rumors, but they hindered and confused rather than helped applicants.[20] Would a non-science course be perceived as indicating broad intellectual interest or a lack of focus on science and medicine? Even more stressful confusion surrounded non-academic activities, hobbies, interests, and all the other items included in a curriculum vitae – would time spent developing non-academic credentials be worthwhile? Time was the undergraduate's most precious commodity. Any time diverted from studying could detract from grades, and excellent grades were essential for success in admission to medical school. For our conscientious participants, any shortcomings in grades could erode confidence and even sabotage aspirations to become a physician.

I felt compelled to get all A's!

I did very well in my major – straight A's – but I had to appeal my last course grade to raise it from a B++ to an A−. Not sure what the difference was, but it seemed crucial at that time.

Took difficult science courses – inorganic chemistry, calculus – and didn't excel. Had doubts about medical school and ability to do the work needed.

Especially among the earlier graduates, the group expressed a strong theme that medicine was an unusual ambition for a young woman. *I was a bit of a maverick.* Many believed they had to try harder and perform better than their male classmates to have a chance of admission to medical school – a perception that was probably correct.

I was still unsure about getting into medicine as a woman and was frequently the only one or one of very few women in premed classes.

Measuring themselves against their male classmates, however, frequently resulted in "light bulb moments" when female students realized they were just as good, if not better, than the men.

As college progressed, I realized I could compete with the guys and got more comfortable with doing medicine.

One of my male classmates was accepted to med school, so I thought I might apply as well. Had thought about it briefly back in high school but never seriously considered it as an option for a girl.

Didn't do science in first year – it was not a good direction for a woman. But the place was loaded with premeds, so I thought, "Why not?" Took science courses starting in second year and worked in a microbiology lab on work-study.

Women who excelled academically could be threatening to male classmates, especially as potential competitors for places in medical school. One interviewee described an attempt to sabotage her performance. She was desperately short of money and almost more concerned about having to ask her parents to fund replacing the missing equipment as about damage to her grades.

I was working on a four-hour chemistry experiment and stepped out for something. When I returned, some of the equipment was missing. This was a huge deal, as you had to pay for anything you broke or lost, and I was worrying how to tell my parents. Then the guy at the next bench returned the equipment he had hidden. We were both applying for medical school, and he admitted wanting to sabotage my grade!

Teachers, Advisers, and Mentors

Our 37 interviewees encountered multiple faculty members during their college years. They had vague and generally neutral recollections of interactions with most college faculty members, but two contrasting faculty attitudes stood out. As expected, we heard accounts of negative attitudes and behaviors toward female students, especially those aspiring to study medicine. Conversely, we heard many more stories of supportive, helpful, and even inspirational faculty members and others who were positive influences on the journey toward medical school. In both positive and negative groups, almost all the faculty members were men, reflecting the overwhelmingly male professoriate of that time. Most, but not all, were in the sciences, but few were directly related to medicine.

Negative interactions varied from being ignored to frank harassment. Echoing the theme of the "waste" of education on girls, an early graduate commented, *The professors kind of ignored us. They thought we were going to flunk out.* Another early graduate got the clear message that her presence was inappropriate in a premed class. *I was the only woman in the required comparative anatomy course. The lecturer took rollcall every session, calling out "Mister" when it was my turn. He also addressed me as "Mister" if I had to speak in class – my classmates still call me that at reunions!*

Other faculty members were more subtle in their disapproval of women aiming for medicine. *Excellent teachers in science, but rather discouraging about medicine.*

Official sources of advice and practical assistance for aspiring female medical students were woefully lacking. Our oldest participant recalled the idea of medicine being dismissed in the 1940s but gleefully described how she worked around the system.

I applied for premed but was told women can't do premed, so I asked them what classes premed had to do . . . [pause] and then I did them!

The discouragement encountered by later graduates was less absolute, but even in the 1970s, our interviewees encountered ingrained attitudes about appropriate roles for women.

When I inquired about getting into the honors program, I was told by one kindly older gentleman professor, "No reason for you to do honors – just find a husband and get married."

Similarly, when consulted about improving academic competitiveness, an adviser suggested changing from premed to a less-demanding schedule, rather than strategizing how to improve grades. *My grades were not great. Somewhere between second and third year, I spoke to the adviser for medical school, and he was discouraging because of my grades. I decided to do it anyway. If you don't try, you don't know. I was determined.*

Sexist attitudes were described as *normal. It was the '60s.* The most egregious report concerned a senior administrator. *I needed a letter from the assistant dean to get into medical school and was told I could get it if I met him at a bar. I went because I needed that letter. It never sounded like a date – more like a proposition. It is just the way it was.*

Conversely, many more interviewees, especially in the later classes, spoke appreciatively of faculty members who had been particularly helpful.

Faculty really encouraged us.

Good professors all along, some really inspiring.

Fantastic inorganic chemistry teacher (male) did letter of recommendation.

Very encouraging German professor (a refugee from WWII) who believed women can do anything.

Sometimes a faculty member was influential at a critical time during college.

I married in my junior year, and medicine didn't seem possible. Influential professors (male), especially in chemistry, really encouraged me to do medicine and not drop the idea.

Encouraging faculty. Took lots of home economics, but my adviser told me to do the sciences.

While *good, supportive teachers, both male and female*, were reported from all types of colleges, outstanding female professors were more commonly mentioned by participants who had attended smaller institutions and community colleges. *At community college, I had really good female teachers, especially in calculus – a brilliant and devoted teacher. Also, the science teacher was very good. He had done research for the government before becoming a teacher. Inspiring for my career.*

Only one participant, who attended a small liberal arts college out of state, recalled *several female professors*. Even among the alumnae who attended college in the early 1970s, a more typical comment was, *I encountered no female mentors or role models*.

Aspiring female physicians could occasionally find role models during college coursework. *There was a young woman postdoc who had a young family and always seemed very happy. She loved her work and was good at it. Perhaps I saw her as a model for "you can do all of this."*

Even more rarely, a faculty member facilitated mentorship for a female premed student.

One of my professors introduced me to a pediatrician in Lawrence who invited me to her home to talk about a career in medicine. She was helpful and encouraged me to apply for med school.

Private Lives

None of our interviewees were married upon entering college, but a few were in committed relationships, and one was a nun. Ten married before graduation from college, including the (by then) former nun, and several were engaged. Most husbands were also students, some in premed or already in medical school. One interviewee married a professor. Only one interviewee described pregnancy during college, and this was in the last year of her undergraduate studies. *I waddled into MCATs nine months pregnant. Everyone thought that was pretty funny.* They were less amused when her water broke during zoology lab. *I continued with classes and was dissecting a cat when I went into labor.* She subsequently divorced and proudly announced, *I was the first unmarried mother knowingly admitted to KU Med!*

As for most college students, our interviewees faced the challenges of navigating relationships and the social attractions of university life. This must have been especially challenging in the charged atmosphere of the 1960s and 1970s.[1] Much has been written and said about the "sexual revolution" of the period, although some commentators conclude that sexual behaviors did not change greatly from those documented by Kinsey, Masters, and Johnson and others in the previous decade. They attribute the reputation of the 1960s and 1970s for flamboyant sexuality partly to greater openness to public discussions of the topic, and partly to sexual behavior being co-opted by other revolutionary movements.[1,24,25] For many ordinary Americans, sexual liberation became enmeshed in the counterculture of hippies, protesters, women's liberation, and a legion of destabilizing forces with the common purpose of destroying accepted values and societal norms. What began in 1945 with Reich's book *The Sexual Revolution* as a call for healthy relationships and freedom from sexual repression became "hijacked, and eventually derailed by a combination of greed, lust, and immaturity to become code for hedonistic, irresponsible, and destructive sexuality."[25]

Amid all the noise and confusion about sexual revolution and moral backlash, our interviewees had little to say about dating and relationships on campus. We did not directly address the topic, but some information was volunteered in response to open questions about college experiences. Most conveyed that they were focused on their studies and prioritized getting the grades expected for medical school admission over social activities. *One boyfriend complained I was too busy studying to be available for dates.* She and other interviewees commented that *there were lots of other girls around – plenty looking for Mrs. Degrees, especially with a nice premed, future doctor husband!* Disappointing experiences with the college dating scene provided one participant with a strong incentive to live an independent life: *My experiences with dating in college were dismal. It seemed I might never marry or have children. I wanted an interesting, well-paid profession that would make it possible to travel and pursue interests outside my career.* A few interviewees described themselves as *quiet, shy,* or even *a bit of a nerd* as undergraduates, but others were more flamboyant. *I liked guys, and guys liked me.*

Summary and Reflections

College was a crucial transitional experience for our interviewees. They expressed strong themes of growing maturity and confidence in several aspects of their lives, including their aspirations to become physicians. For some, college affirmed intentions to enter medicine, others described college as nurturing nascent aspirations and helping them overcome their *impostor syndrome*, and still others credited college experiences with originating the idea that medicine was a possible career choice. For a few of the last group, the realization that they could *reach for medicine* came as a shock, and they needed the reassurance and support of friends, instructors, and family to proceed. This is in keeping with the literature on the impostor syndrome and studies in the 1960s indicating that women appeared to need more validation of academic achievements and potential than men.[26–29] "Though better grade-getters, women honor students felt less adequate in their field than the men honor students."[29]

We were surprised by the few references to problems with participating in science and premed courses, as this is a common theme in much of the contemporary literature and was prominent in our earlier discussion with senior female physicians.[28–32] Those participants who described such problems were among our older participants, suggesting that attitudes toward women in science-based classes changed during the 1960s. While it is tempting to attribute this to the post-Sputnik emphasis on education in science, the multiple societal changes of that time, including the rise of feminism, suggest more complex reasons for the change. While most of our interviewees were able to participate in science courses, few felt actively mentored or encouraged, especially regarding medicine as a career. Our participants rarely recounted helpful formal advising for medicine – validating the scathing criticism of the anti-medical state of college counseling for women at that time.[28–30] "College vocational counsellors are the single most potent force steering women away from medicine. They exaggerate the difficulties, inspire false fears of professional handicaps . . . and indicate that the odds are not worth fighting."[28] Possibly more significant than the poor quality of official advising, our interviewees regretted the support of the quasi-formal networks, resources, and sponsorship that typically *laid out the pathway* and provided information, encouragement, and support for their male classmates. As in other areas of their professional lives, our interviewees typically tackled challenges alone, finding individual solutions to successive problems and neither expected organizational accommodations nor resented the lack of institutional support. As demonstrated by their stories, they even took mischievous delight in working around a regulation (*I found out what the premed courses were and did them anyway!*) or accessing information and resources through male friends.

In keeping with their backgrounds and high aspirations, our participants expressed strong themes of focusing on their studies. They *took heavy loads* and *difficult courses*. As described in the motivation chapter, the range of requirements for medical school meant that at least one subject was problematic for most interviewees. Several shuddered or smiled ruefully when describing their struggles to attain a good grade in a challenging class that *did not come easily*. Prioritizing studies may explain, at least in part, the relatively few comments about social life and dating. Some comments appeared to validate the literature reports that high-achieving female students, especially those in the sciences, are perceived as threatening to male colleagues, thus complicating personal relationships.[28] We also wondered if the self-derogatory comments about being unattractive were in part projections of the long-standing myth that women aspiring to study medicine must be asexual or at least unfeminine and unattractive.[28,29] Our interviewees were no shrinking violets, but perhaps the intense demands of coursework plus their determination to achieve MD rather than Mrs. Degrees inhibited more exuberant social activities. Possibly, they felt it prudent not to discuss youthful indiscretions of 50 years previously during the interviews.

The need to present pristine academic and personal credentials to medical school admissions committees almost certainly influenced their attitudes toward participation in the various movements that roiled campuses and communities during the 1960s and the 1970s. The history of that period remains controversial, but even the most careful retrospective analysis cannot do justice to the prevailing confusion and distress, especially for young people. Idealistic participation in an apparently virtuous activity, such as desegregation, could be interpreted as "dangerous, communistic treason."[4] In addition, many movements evolved during the 1960s and the 1970s from altruistic motivations to become more polarized, extreme, and even violent. This left many initial supporters stigmatized as either sympathetic to dangerous radicals or as dupes who might be emotionally unreliable as professional colleagues. Any record of participation in a controversial movement, no matter how sincere or virtuous one's intent, was a potentially dangerous factor in the competitive selection process for medical school. Most aspiring medical students felt safer keeping their heads down and focusing on their studies.

Despite all the academic, personal, and other challenges of this particularly difficult time, the strongest theme expressed by our interviewees about their college years was *FUN*. This was described in various ways in response to an open question: *What was college like? Tell me about your time in college.* Multiple comments across all years and all institutions attested to relishing the college experience – challenging work, good friendships, and plenty of fun.

They did not convey the obsessive focus on grades and exclusion of all activities that could not contribute to medical school admission described in the literature.[28,32–34] The only reference to the paranoia and cutthroat competition that were reported to be characteristic of premed students was the attempted sabotage of a chemistry experiment by a male classmate. We heard little evidence of the reportedly universal "premed syndrome," that is, excessive concern with grades, extreme competitiveness, and lack of sociability.[34]

We recognize that potential biases could have influenced participants to provide more positive recollections than their college experiences merited. Our participants were successful in college and may have suppressed, forgotten, or been unwilling to share unpleasant, negative, or embarrassing memories. Nevertheless, they freely shared negatives in other areas of the interviews, and the body language of the interactive interviews was consistent with positive recollections of challenging but happy times. They emerged from college showing little of the "crippling effects of undergraduate education on women" described in a 1968 publication.[28] Conversely, our participants

TABLE 6.1

Examples of Responses to Open Question about College

	Year of MD Graduation
I really enjoyed college.	1967
College was a wonderful experience.	1970
LOVED college.	1971
Great science program and wonderful social experience. It was FUN.	1972
College was a lot of fun, especially the upper-level courses. I wanted to keep studying for years!	1973
I had a lot of fun – WOW!	1974
I liked everything, took everything!	1974
I loved it.	1975

Note: Institutions represented in quotes: Duke, Ottawa, Tulane, KU, Wichita State University, Barnard College, Kansas State University, College of William and Mary.

conveyed that, by the end of college, they were apprehensive but cautiously optimistic that they were prepared for the next hurdle on the path to becoming a physician – admission to medical school.

REFERENCES

1. Bailey B. Sex in the heartland. Cambridge (MA): Harvard University Press;1999.
2. University of Kansas School of Medicine Class of 1948 Yearbook.
3. Anon. Analysis of doctor-draft regulations. J Am Med Assoc. 1953 Nov 28;153(13):1201–2.
4. Schrecker EW. 1986. No ivory tower: McCarthyism and the universities. New York (NY): Oxford University Press.
5. Anon. KU history: plenty hot, but not scorching. Available from: https://union.ku.edu/plenty-hot-not-scorching
6. Anon. KU history: charisma amidst the chaos. Available from: https://union.ku.edu/robert-f-kennedy-coming-visit
7. Anon. KU history: Hoffman's huff. Available from: https://union.ku.edu/college-degree-useless
8. Monhollon RL. Taking the plunge: race, rights, and the politics of desegregation in Lawrence, Kansas. Kan Hist. 1960:138–159.
9. Anon. Rejecting rejection. Available from: https://union.ku.edu/discrimination
10. Anon. KU history: gather together. Available from: https://union.ku.edu/gather-together
11. Kenneth Spencer Research Library Blog. 'We're all going to jail, to jail': the university and civil rights in 1965. Available from: https://blogs.lib.ku.edu/spencer/were-all-going-to-jail-to-jail-the-university-and-civil-rights-in-1965/
12. Wall D. 1968 Kansas City race riots: then & now. Available from: https://www.kshb.com/longform/1968-kansas-city-race-riots-then-now
13. White R. Police killing of black KU student in 1970 reflects today's racial climate. University Daily Kansan. 2016 Jul 24.
14. Metz C. 1970: racial unrest sparked deadly violence. Lawrence Journal-World. 2010 Apr 21. Available from: https://www2.ljworld.com/news/2010/apr/21/1970-racial-unrest-sparked-deadly-violence
15. Harvey D. KU history. Available from: https://union.ku.edu/rick-tiger-dowdell
16. Towns WC. KU history fire and smoke. Available from: https://union.ku.edu/union-firebombing
17. Introduction. 1970: the year that rocked KU. KU Libraries Exhibits. Available from: https://exhibits.lib.ku.edu/exhibits/show/the-year-that-rocked-ku/introduction
18. Harvey D. KU history sisters act. Available from: https://union.ku.edu/womens-rights
19. Becker HS, Greer B, Hughes EC, Strauss AL. Boys in white. Chicago (IL): University of Chicago Press;1961.
20. Friesen SR, Hudson RP. The Kansas School of Medicine eyewitness reflections on its formative years. Kansas City: University of Kansas School of Medicine;1996.
21. Scholarship halls. KU student housing. Available from: https://housing.ku.edu/scholarship-halls
22. McCool JH. For the girls who must travel uphill. Available from: https://union.ku.edu/girls-who-must-travel-hill
23. Bulletin of the University of Kansas. KU School of Medicine catalogue. Information for applicants 1958 (same information multiple years). Accessed via Archives of the Glendenning Library.

24. Hills R. What every generation gets wrong about sex: sexual revolution then and now: hook-ups from 1964 to today. Time. 2014 Dec 2.
25. Anapol D. What ever happened to the sexual revolution? Psychology Today. 2012 Aug 15.
26. Bravata DM, Watts SA, Keefer AL, Madhusudhan DK, Taylor KT, Clark DM, et al. Prevalence, predictors, and treatment of impostor syndrome: a systematic review. J Gen Intern Med. 2020;35(4):1252–75.
27. Weir WD. Honors and the liberal arts college. In: Cohen JW, editor. The superior student. New York (NY): McGraw-Hill;1966.
28. Lopate C. Women in medicine. Baltimore (MD): Johns Hopkins Press;1968.
29. Walsh MR. Doctors wanted: no women need apply: sexual barriers in the medical profession 1835–1975. New Haven and London: Yale University Press;1977.
30. Morantz RM, Pomerleau CS, Fenichel CH. In her own words. Westport (CT): Greenwood Press;1982.
31. Walling A, Nilsen K, Templeton KJ. The only woman in the room: oral histories of senior women physicians in a Midwestern City. Womens Health Rep (New Rochelle). 2020 Aug 24;1(1):279–86.
32. Bowers JZ. Special problems of women medical students. J Med Educ. 1968 May; 43(5):532–7.
33. Wolf SG. I can't afford a 'B'. N Engl J Med. 1978 Oct 26;299(17):949–50.
34. Conrad P. The myth of cut-throats among premedical students: on the role of stereotypes in justifying failure and success. J Health Soc Behav. 1986;27:150–60.

7

Getting in the Door: Admissions

"The interview is a serious affair. . . . They comport themselves on this solemn occasion not as boys but as men. The teachers of medicine who interview them look at them seriously and anxiously. They ask themselves and one another, 'Will this bright boy really make a medical man?'"[1]

Applying to medical school has always been a daunting task, presenting significant emotional, academic, and practical challenges. Emotionally, applicants must muster the self-confidence to believe they have the ability to enter "the finest of professions."[1] Freshmen medical students at the University of Kansas School of Medicine (KUSM) in the 1950s described medicine's awesome reputation, sufficient to discourage the faint-hearted potential applicant. "Medical school is a kind of little plateau; it's the very tops in most people's minds. . . . We've got so much at stake here it really isn't funny."[1] For women, applying to medical school in the 1950s, '60s, and '70s required overcoming years of negative feedback about women in medicine, often compounded by internal doubts or the impostor syndrome. Those who had the courage to apply knew they risked failure in an unpredictable high-stakes process with many elements over which they had no control. At most US medical schools, a quota for female matriculants of 5–10% was stated or assumed.[2,3] The system was certainly hostile toward women. In evidence to a congressional subcommittee in 1970, nearly 80% of deans of Northeastern medical schools stated they "accepted men in preference to women unless the women applicants were demonstrably superior."[3] The antipathy towards women entering medical school is vividly illustrated by other statements. For example:

"Hell, yes, we have a quota; yes, it's a small one. We do keep women out when we can. We don't want them here – and they don't want them anywhere else, either, whether or not they'll admit it."

(Medical School Dean 1961)

"Yes, indeed we take women, and we do not want the one woman we take to be lonesome, so we take two per class."[3]

(Senior Administrator 1968)

It is hardly surprising that, during the 1960s, fewer than 10% of women who entered college as premeds finally applied to medical school. Our interviewees were among a determined group of survivors who proceeded to the next set of challenges in the journey toward becoming physicians.[4]

DOI: 10.1201/9781003539568-7

Preparing the Application

For most of the period covered by our interviewees, the acceptance rate for qualified female applicants was less than 50%.[4,5] Then as now, applicants must achieve excellent grades in both the required subjects and a range of other courses selected to impress the admissions committees of the targeted schools. As medical schools differ in culture and priorities, insider information about the preferred credentials was highly valuable but, as our ladies discovered, best accessed through fraternities and support networks for male premeds.[4] Insider information was especially critical in addressing the hidden curriculum of hobbies, interests, and volunteer, and leadership activities expected of applicants. The long-standing belief that KUSM favored those aiming to become rural family physicians was well established. "A standing joke that students, almost to a man, announce on their applications that they are interested in becoming general practitioners in a small town in western Kansas."[1]

The 1971 Yearbook cynically reveals other beliefs about what to emphasize in applications and how students perceived the values held by the institution, or at least the admissions committee:

> "Hints on how to fill out your application. State I am NOT interested in money. I want to be a GP and practice medicine in a small town in Western Kansas. Proficient in several languages, have multiple physician relatives (especially faculty and state legislators). Received awards from Young Republicans, Youth for Christ, KU, and research organizations. Not applying elsewhere. Ambition to learn from Dr. X."

Our interviewees strove to create an application that conveyed an acceptable personality, social responsibility, commitment to worthy causes, and other appropriate attributes, as well as outstanding academic ability and the physical and emotional stamina required for medicine. The desired impression had to be consistently reinforced throughout the application, especially in the applicant's personal statement and letters of recommendation.

Then as now, letters of recommendation were required from professors, physicians, and similar individuals who could attest to the applicant's suitability for medical education – and hopefully add insights that help distinguish this individual from the large pool of qualified applicants. Our interviewees spoke of struggling to identify suitable referees and to persuade them to write appropriate letters. Advisers were rarely helpful, and interviewees repeatedly described feeling at a disadvantage compared to their male classmates, who usually had plentiful mentors or helpful upperclassmen. As mentioned in the previous chapter, some women obtained information about good referees through boyfriends. One recalled being sexually propositioned by an assistant dean in order to secure a required letter. With little or no ability to influence the content, they worried that letters could be unhelpfully bland or that reviewers could read inappropriate nuances into any item or turn of phrase. In particular, they were concerned that letters could stress their feminine qualities rather than the "masculine" attributes associated with success in the competitive field of medicine. Conversely, they dreaded being portrayed as too masculine, aggressive, or demanding. Hopefully, they obtained letters that better presented a young woman's potential as a physician than some 1974 examples:

> "An attractive, mature, personable young lady who is a pleasure to have around and has no 'hang ups' sometimes associated with female physicians.
>
> A very pleasant and friendly individual who is delightfully feminine at all times.
>
> Intelligent, mature, pleasant and dependable – she is also an excellent cook."[4]

The admissions process is still fraught with uncertainty but hopefully has improved to increase transparency, clarify criteria, and improve equity for applicants from minority groups.[5,6] As members of a potentially troublesome minority, each of our participants struggled with many unanswerable questions. Should she stress academic record and risk being seen as too *nerdy*, lacking the stamina, social skills, and practical abilities necessary for medicine? Would experience in volunteer activities be seen as advantageous or indicate lack of dedication to studies? How could a lower grade best be presented to do least damage to an application? How could she express being totally dedicated and committed to helping others without appearing naïve? Would evidence of initiative and leadership be interpreted as valuable or as indicating an uppity young woman and potential troublemaker? In the period of protests and campus disruptions, applicants faced very real dilemmas. Would being active in the Civil Rights or peace movements be advantageous or grounds for an instant rejection? What did one say if they asked if she was a feminist? How many women would they take? Above all, what did the admissions committee *really* want?

Anticipating the priorities of admissions committees was (and remains) a preoccupation of potential applicants. Information and recommendations from advisers, faculty, classmates, and others are often ambiguous or even conflicting.[7] Among students, rumors and myths run rampant about the secrets of success and fatal flaws that could condemn any application. The guidelines produced by medical schools often leave potential applicants wondering about the expectations and the institutional vision of an ideal applicant.[7] A young woman in the 1970s who perhaps already struggled with the confidence to apply to medical school must have wondered how to satisfy the high expectations in multiple areas and what to prioritize in her application.

The confusion and contradictory advice are not surprising, given the long history of debate over preparation for medical school. The emphasis on hard science following the 1910 Flexner Report was followed by calls for a more humanistic approach as early as the 1930s.[8] In the period when many of our interviewees were navigating the admissions process, the debate about the most desirable credentials in applicants was particularly heated and was shifting toward greater emphasis on the *soft* or qualitative personal attributes of applicants.[7,9,10]

Unfortunately, consensus on which personal attributes should be prioritized in select-ing potential physicians is challenging. Attempts to define desired attributes of appli-cants ended up with limited consensus on a list of ten categories.[12,13] The items, such as "character and integrity, personality and attitude, work habits and motivation to study, and personal effectiveness," are challenging to define and impossible to validly and consistently measure.[10–15] Nevertheless, during the 1960s and the 1970s, there was great interest in incorporating personality inventories, psychological screenings, and other qualitative assessments of applicants.[10–15] This enthusiasm waned in the 1980s, partly because of inconsistent performance by the assessments, but mainly because faculty were reluctant to surrender personal intuition and judgment in the critical task of selecting medical students.[10,12,13]

With so many controversies and difficulties in agreeing on the attributes of a good physician, let alone how to assess them in applicants to the profession, confusion and stress over the application process are easy to understand. Our interviewees pri-oritized achieving the excellent grades and scores on the national Medical College Admission Test (MCAT) that are essential in any application. Working out how to excel in the other components of medical school application was much more compli-cated. Each applicant strove to make all components of the application convey ideal-ism and dedication to medicine while convincing readers that she had the necessary abilities and stamina to manage the demands of medical education and a career as a physician. Striking the right balance between high aspiration and pragmatic reliability was especially challenging for women. They were blatantly held to a higher standard for admission.

> "We subject women candidates, and possibly with some justification, to a more searching scrutiny in the admissions process than male candidates. We are willing to gamble that we can foster motivation in a male, but we insist that the women have a proven motivation."[2]

Our participants sought out every available resource to demonstrate their qualifica-tions and strengthen their applications.

I got letters of recommendation from the governor and my congressman.

I knew they were taking 10% women, and I was determined to be one of the 10%!

The majority of our interviewees needed every advantage they could muster as record numbers of men applied to medical school during the late 1960s and the early 1970s. The postwar boom in applications fueled by the GI Bill had peaked in 1949, then ebbed somewhat during the 1950s. A strong resurgence began in the early 1960s. Application numbers increased by 33% between 1961/1962 and 1964/1965.[5] The 1949 record was matched in 1964, but numbers continued to escalate each year and peaked at 43,624 in 1974.[16] Applications then declined to a nadir of 26,721 in 1988, causing some consternation about the lack of quality applicants and the increasing proportion of women in the applicant pool.[16–18] This pattern has been attributed to Vietnam draft deferments for students in the health professions.[19] The majority of our interviewees applied for medical school between 1966 and 1971, the period of most intense competition for places. For male applicants, the stakes were high – failure to be admitted to a postgraduate program in a health profession risked being drafted into military service at the height of the Vietnam War.[16,19] In the opinion of at least one of our participants, avoiding the draft was more important to her male competitors than any aspiration to becoming a physician.

Vietnam was very active. There was a lot of competition for admission to medical school since it was a way for men to avoid or delay military service, extra pressure, to get into medical school as a way out of the military. Some of them didn't really want to be physicians.

Those applicants who successfully passed the triage of grades and written application materials waited anxiously to be called for the final step of the process, the personal interview. The process for selection of interviewees from the pool of qualified applicants was unclear and the source of multiple rumors. As mentioned previously, at most state-supported medical schools, residents of the state are a significant advantage.[20] Our participants who applied in 1971 and 1972 also hoped for some advantage based on the rumors about medical schools being forced to admit more women due to Title IX and federal regulations.

My husband was a third-year medical student at KU, so I was able to talk with medical students and prepare. They thought KU was going to accept more women, and this gave me greater confidence for acceptance.

I found out that KU had a big federal grant to train more doctors and had expanded criteria to admit more women and people who wanted to change careers.

The Admissions Interview Format

Then as now, the personal interview was the most critical component of the application process.[21] Despite copious evidence of the poor reliability and validity of interviews in selecting applicants, faculty members at almost all US medical schools have always insisted on the right to make personal assessments of potential medical students.[6,9,10,17] At KUSM, some of the challenges and political pressures were evident in the 1950 Murphy Plan that shaped the development of KUSM for decades.

> "The Medical School still continues to have serious problems in the matter of admissions. These problems all stem from the fact that many more applicants wish to enter the Medical School than can be handled with available or even projected facilities. In such a highly competitive situation, feelings become strained and the Admissions Committee of the School finds itself often under severe personal as well as organized pressures. Such circumstances demand that extreme objectivity be maintained in choosing the class. Three criteria are applied in the selections 1) academic record, 2) score of the medical college admissions test, and 3) reaction of an interview committee of the faculty

to the applicant. . . . We will continue to resist political, medical, or other pressure. . . . Our first and major obligation is to the state of Kansas and we, therefore, select 90% of our class from among bone fide Kansas residents."[22]

The term "reaction" suggests the onus was on the applicant to convince the committee of his or her credentials. In practice, the committee had the initiative and controlled the interviews. The dean from 1952 to 1960 had great confidence in the system, possibly because he had so much power over decisions.

"We had, I believe, the best admissions procedures of any medical school. The admissions procedure was compressed into a few weekends. Three faculty members met with three applicants for 30–45 minutes and then the applicants met briefly with my assistant dean and with me. Late in the evening and into the early morning we went as a group to sort out the results of the interviews."[22]

The dean could even insert a late applicant. In an anecdote that powerfully explains the paranoia about grades among applicants, he recounted active sponsorship of a male applicant.

"He had been told by his premed adviser that there was no use in applying because he had one B on an otherwise straight A record. He took it upon himself to seek an interview with me (he had not applied) and I saw to it that he filled out his application and was screened by the Admissions Committee."[22]

Members of the admissions committee were confident that they selected the most appropriate individuals. The committee chair during most of the 1950s expressed faith in the committee's decisions but revealed the priorities for academic performance, inherent biases, and the ability of senior administrators to override the entire system for a favored applicant.

"I doubt that conscious or unconscious prejudice had much influence. Of course, some committee members expressed a preference for 'straight arrows.' Whatever prejudices existed surrendered to grade point averages. So did biases in favor of candidates, except in regard to a very few known as 'gold armband' applicants because of administrative intervention."[22]

Despite his assertions of lack of prejudice, the committee chair had no hesitation in using very revealing language about applicants. He described an applicant from a poor background as "unacceptable, a typical dirty-cut American boy."[22] He also documented comments about women and Jews that now seem unbelievable.[22] Such comments may have passed muster in the 1950s, but this individual showed no insight, regret, or concern in describing these attitudes and practices 40 years later, knowing they would be published in a collection of oral histories about the medical school.[22]

"Women applicants were welcomed, especially if they were relatively plain or a little masculine in appearance. But when someone like the Calendar Queen came through, some members were uneasy."[22]

In fairness, his views were shared by leaders of other medical schools at that time. The dean of another school is quoted as saying, "When a very feminine-looking gal comes in, I might wonder if she's fit for medicine."[4]

The admissions interviews were conducted over the Christmas break, often disrupting family plans and requiring applicants to get to Kansas City at a time when travel could be hazardous due to bad weather. *I flew back from Panama to downtown KC airport at Christmas and arrived in a snowstorm for the interview. I was shaken up, nervous, and really tired.*

Until the mid-1990s, KUSM utilized a bizarre three-on-three interview system for admissions committee interviews. A panel of three faculty members interviewed three candidates simultaneously. This format was highly unusual. Over 70% of US medical schools used a one-on-one process. Almost all the remaining schools used either a group format (one interviewer with a group of applicants) or its reverse, the panel interview, in which one applicant faced questions from a small group of interviewers.[21] When our participants were attempting to gain admission, the interview with the committee members (all male) was followed by a personal meeting with the dean or his deputy. We found no evidence that KUSM used structed interviews or made other attempts to standardize questions in order to improve the validity of interviews during the period covered by our participants. Questions appear to have been determined purely by the interests or whims of the faculty interviewers.

> "We interviewed as a group of three faculty members questioning three applicants. Faculty members had favorite questions. What is the difference between a profession and a trade? Who is your favorite fictional physician? Why? What is your favorite comic strip? Why? (My personal favorite question) These questions were probably in the files of every fraternity house in Lawrence."[22]

(Admissions Committee Chair 1953–1959)

In the 1950s, the dean removed the question "Where do you want to practice medicine?" from the application form and rather naively assumed "by its elimination saved hundreds of applicants from responding fictitiously, 'In a small town in western Kansas.'"[22] The question continued to be asked in admissions interviews for decades. The belief that pledging aspirations to become a rural GP is essential for acceptance has remained entrenched in generations of KUSM applicants.[1]

The Admissions Interview Experience

Why should we give YOU a man's place?

About one-third of our participants applied only to KUSM. For many of these women, the interview was especially stressful as they could not afford to go to any other medical school – KUSM offered their only hope of becoming a physician. Others indicated that finances played a major role in their applications.

Knew I had to pay my own way, so I only applied to KU.

Only applied to KU, mainly for financial reasons.

Applied to KU and several other places that sounded good but expensive, so I was really hoping for KU.

Family support and familiarity with the area were important in decisions about medical schools. The group conveyed a strong theme of calculating how to optimize resources and support while minimizing distractions and stressors, especially about finances. They were very focused on being able to prioritize their studies and felt great pressure to succeed.

Applied to KUSM because concerned about finances and my modest MCAT scores, but mainly because I was a Kansas girl, and this is where I belonged.

Applied to KU as Mother wanted me to come home. Plus, I was very anxious about making it in medical school.

Applied to KUSM because of strong family ties to Kansas. Low tuition (about $1,000 per year) and could live with relatives.

Many ladies described weeks of stressful anticipation and entered the interview with *trepidation.*

I remember that day vividly. It was miserable. I was very insecure.

I don't remember much except being very nervous.

Some even joked that they had repressed the painful memories of the ordeal.

I don't recall the interview maybe I have blacked it out!

One participant interviewed despite upheavals in her personal life. *A lot going on in my life at that time. Just had a baby and got divorced. It was very emotional, and I was just taking one day at a time.*

Without the pipeline of information and network of support enjoyed by many of their male premed classmates, rumors only increased stress levels for female applicants. *I had heard about women being asked terrible questions.* This was most marked for applicants in the 1950s and the 1960s. Many of those applying in the early 1970s had heard speculation about Title IX and new federal funding regulations *forcing KU to take more women and Blacks because they had a big grant.* Nevertheless, they remained anxious and distrustful about how female applicants might fare in the interview process. They did not expect equitable treatment with their male classmates. During an interview at another medical school, one participant was told, *Everyone knows women need to apply to more schools than men. Six would have been okay if you were a man. It's harder for a woman.* Another participant recalled a competitor trying to increase her stress by undermining her confidence – apparently without success.

While waiting for my medical school interview, one of the men sitting next to me was really cocky, rude. Putting me down, saying, "You don't have a chance," etc. – really obnoxious. Never saw him again, so he didn't get in, AND he told me he only applied to KU!

Nerves could overtake applicants in very different ways. One woman recalled being too overwhelmed to give a good account of herself. *I was very insecure, bashful. Not anyone's fault but my own. I didn't like the idea of sitting in front of someone. I had a tendency to lose my voice. I have no idea what I said and was sure they were not impressed.* Conversely, one of her future colleagues became excited and garrulous. As she had taken a red-eye flight from the East Coast the previous evening then driven over 200 miles from Wichita to Kansas City in bad winter weather, she was understandably full of adrenaline. *My interview was after a late-night flight from NY to Wichita then the drive to KC, so very tired and nervous. I dropped my purse, and everything spilled out just as I got into the room. The dean said, "Okay, you're nervous. Just talk." I talked about dreams of going into medicine to help children, to start at the beginning to change society. Not sure who else was there or what else they talked about – anyway, they bought it!*

Our participants recalled being asked a wide variety of questions during their admissions interviews, some of which seemed to have little relevance to becoming a physician. *They asked this weird question about navigating around New York City – maybe it was something to do with problem-solving.*

The strongest focus of questioning concerned their commitment to medicine, in particular, their ability to practice despite current or future family responsibilities. As late as 1990, national studies confirmed that female applicants were frequently asked about plans for marriage and children, whereas males were predominantly asked about plans for specialization.[23] As discussed in an earlier chapter, throughout the decades during which our participants applied for medical school, it was widely believed that women were twice as likely to drop out of medical school, many would leave medicine when they married, and the those who remained in practice would be at least one-third less productive than their male colleagues.[3] Recruiting women appeared irresponsible to medical school deans in times of worsening physician shortages and a projected crisis in medical "manpower."

"How can you justify more of them? The girls are just looking for something to do until they get married. We have to train two or three to get one who will practice medicine."[3,4]

Our participants interviewed from 1944 to 1972. Throughout this period, they recalled the preoccupation with the *waste of resources* in training a female physician. Questions probing different aspects of this issue dominated the interviews. (See Table 7.1 for additional examples.)

TABLE 7.1

Additional Quotations Regarding Admissions Interviews

There was a theme of wanting to admit people who would give many years to medicine. They weren't hostile – just ignorant.
Why should I take up a man's place in med school when he was going to work harder afterward?
So discouraging – the message was not to get married or have children.
Major background concern seemed to be that women wouldn't practice full-time. Questions about having children and managing career and family.
They asked several questions that are probably illegal now. Asked plenty about plans to marry, have children, and what would happen. Asked if I would quit training or practice if I got married, or got pregnant, or had a baby. Talked about taking a man's place in medicine – all that stuff.

The general theme of my interview questions was around "Why should we spend money on you if you're only going to go off and get married? Will it be worth it for the state to invest in your education?" In the interview and throughout my training and career, I perceived that any question of being part-time or not matching male colleagues in time/effort was fatal to success.

The usual questions: Why should YOU go to medical school? Are you REALLY going to practice? The implication was about taking up a man's slot.

The gist was the stereotypical female taking up a valuable spot then . . . flitting off, getting married, and having kids and not practicing. Kind of ironic, as there were 13 girls in the class and we all graduated and went on to practice, but five of the guys dropped out!

Sometimes the questions were very personal and probed specific scenarios. Applicants parried awkward questions to the best of their abilities.

The dean asked, "Do you think you will ever want to be married?" I replied that I very much wanted to be married, but it would take a very special kind of person to be married to a woman physician. They laughed – I found out later he was married to a woman physician!

First question was, "What would you do if your husband was in the military and stationed overseas?" I was dumbfounded. I was a bit of a pacifist (anti-Vietnam), so why would I marry a guy in the military? And second, why would I marry a guy who was not supportive of me and my career? I also remember questions about why medical school instead of research.

They asked a lot of questions, including: "What would you do if you married a man who didn't want you to practice medicine?" I said I hoped I would know him better than that before I married him. They laughed. After the group interview, I met with the dean's representative. He asked very pointed personal questions. I felt intimidated.

Several interviewees recalled being given the scenario of conflict between the needs of a sick child at home and of patients in the hospital.

I was asked about family/work duty conflict, but the men were not. What would you do if you had a sick child at home and were called in for a sick patient?

The few married women were asked about their husband's opinions of women entering medicine, his willingness to support her decision, plans for future pregnancies, and arrangements for childcare and domestic duties.

They asked questions about my husband being able to support me during medical school and who would look after my child while I was a student. I wore a baggy dress so they wouldn't realize I was pregnant again!

Within the general theme of value in using state funding to educate female physicians, some participants recalled specific questions about intent to practice in Kansas.

They asked one question about marrying someone who did not want to live in Kansas.

They were very interested in what you planned to do. There was an exodus from Kansas at that time. They were very interested in family medicine and plans to stay in the state.

Predictably, other questions concerned non-medical interests, and some probed familiarity with literature and current affairs. Nervous interviewees sometimes answered immediately and honestly, but then worried about the impression they had conveyed.

I was asked about my favorite TV show and answered without thinking, Mr. Rogers, *as I watched that with my kids. The psychiatrist on the panel thought that was great.*

They asked about the most recent book I had read – honestly, it was War and Peace. *I don't know if they believed me!*

Was asked a lot about literature and reading, including weird questions like, "Do you think there really was a Walden Pond?"

I was asked several questions about mentors or role models. There was a specific question about how Margaret Chase Smith became a senator. I knew more about it than they did – I think they were surprised by my answer.

At least a third of our participants recalled being questioned about their clothing. Some remembered this as a general question to male as well as female applicants; others were sure it was only asked of the women. None of those who recalled this line of questioning believed that their appearance was inappropriate. *It was serious – no miniskirts or anything like that – Sunday clothes.* Most had *dressed up* for the interview, and one made a dress for the occasion.

I made my own clothes. The dress I wore for the interview was the last one I made – after that, I was too busy.

One question came out of left field: "Why did you wear that dress?" There was nothing unusual about the dress, and I'm sure they would never ask a guy about what he was wearing.

I interviewed five days post-partum. They asked us all (the guys too), "Why are you wearing what you are wearing?" I told them it was the only thing that fit!

They asked, "Why did you wear that outfit?" I have no idea why or what I said.

Overall, our participants had surprisingly positive impressions of their interviewers: *They were very nice.* Several recalled attempts to lighten the atmosphere or humorous interactions between interviewers. The panel members seemed to appreciate applicants who stood up for themselves but were quick to detect and shut down overconfidence. A participant described one of the male applicants in her group being a *bluffer* – talking too much and being opinionated, trying to impress. In a discussion about a contemporary political writer, he was caught out by one of the professors and brusquely told, *You know nothing about this!* After that, she felt more relaxed and freer to speak.

The interviewers were three male professors who all seemed old.

One of the interviewers was a psychiatrist – and he had a cigar!

The interview was provoking but surprisingly supportive. I was scared I was being pretentious being a female and did not do as well as I hoped. They were supportive and kind – seemed to appreciate my concerns.

I was scared of the interview, but it wasn't too bad. Don't remember many of the specific questions, but they were very interested in what you planned to do. I thought they were all respectful, and getting in was an awesome decision about my future.

Don't remember a lot but got the impression one of them seemed to be asking trick questions. He made a snarky remark when I said I wanted to help people, but I put it back to him and the other two laughed.

The usual questions: "Why should YOU go to medical school? Are you REALLY going to practice?" The implication was about taking up a man's slot. One of the interviewers said, "Don't let him throw you with that question. He's married to a doctor, and they have six children!"

Most believed the interviewing panel took their responsibilities seriously, but one of our participants was not impressed.

I was surprised how superficial the questions were. They asked very little, and the questions had no depth. My impression was that the interviewers did not take it seriously and had already decided who was in.

Most left the interview relieved but uncertain.

I was so glad to make it out without embarrassing myself.

I have no idea what I said and was sure they were not impressed.

Group interview (three interviewers and three interviewees) was unnerving. Never sure what they were looking for. Came out with no idea how well you had done.

One fortunate applicant was given very positive immediate feedback in her personal interview with the dean following the group session.

The dean asked, "What would you do if you were accepted to KU today?" (I also applied to Tulane.) I said I would accept. It would be great to know over Christmas with my family that I was accepted. He said, "Committee really liked you. They wanted to pin you down today."

The others had to wait to learn that the interview had been successful, and that they had a few months to prepare to enter KUSM the following summer.

Felt very privileged to be accepted.

Let me in for some crazy reason!

I thought getting in was an awesome decision about my future.

REFERENCES

1. Becker HS, Greer B, Hughes EC, Strauss AL. Boys in white. Chicago (IL): University of Chicago Press;1961.
2. Bowers JZ. Special problems of women medical students. J Med Educ. 1968;34:532–7.
3. Walsh MR. Doctors wanted: no women need apply: sexual barriers in the medical profession 1835–1975. New Haven and London: Yale University Press;1977.
4. Lopate C. Women in medicine. Baltimore (MD): Johns Hopkins Press;1968.
5. Johnson DG. The study of applicants, 1964–65. J Med Educ. 1965 Nov;40(11):1017–30.
6. Kreiter CD, Axelson RD. A perspective on medical school admission research and practice over the last 25 years. Teach Learn Med. 2013;25(Suppl 1):S50–6.
7. Gross JP, Mommaerts CD, Earl D, De Vries RG. Perspective: after a century of criticizing premedical education, are we missing the point? Acad Med. 2008 May;83(5):516–20.
8. Reinke EE. Liberal values in premedical education. J Assoc Am Med Coll. 1937;12:151–6.
9. McGaghie WC. Perspectives on medical school admission. Acad Med. 1990 Mar; 65(3):136–9.
10. Benbassat J, Baumal R. Uncertainties in the selection of applicants for medical school. Adv Health Sci Educ Theory Pract. 2007 Nov;12(4):509–21.
11. Weingartner RH. Selecting for medical school. J Med Educ. 1980 Nov;55(11):922–7.

12. McGaghie WC. Qualitative variables in medical school admission. Acad Med. 1990 Mar;65(3):145–9.

13. Albanese MA, Snow MH, Skochelak SE, Huggett KN, Farrell PM. Assessing personal qualities in medical school admissions. Acad Med. 2003 Mar;78(3):313–21.

14. Gough HG. Nonintellectual factors in the selection and evaluation of medical students. J Med Educ. 1967 Jul;42(7):642–50.

15. D'Costa A, Schafer A. Results of a survey of non-cognitive tests used in medical schools. Washington (DC): Association of American Medical Colleges;1972.

16. Hall FR, Mikesell C, Cranston P, Julian E, Elam C. Longitudinal trends in the applicant pool for U.S. medical schools, 1974–1999. Acad Med. 2001;76:829–34.

17. Cuca JM, Sakakeeney LA, Johnson DG. Medical school admissions process: a review of the literature 1955–76. AAMC;1976.

18. Jonas HS, Etzel SI. Undergraduate medical education. JAMA. 1988 Aug 26; 260(8):1063–71.

19. Singer A. The effect of the Vietnam War on numbers of medical school applicants. Acad Med. 1989 Oct;64(10):567–73.

20. Nowacek G, Sachs L. Demographic variables in medical school admission. Acad Med. 1990;65:140–4.

21. Edwards JC, Johnson EK, Molidor JB. The interview in the admission process. Acad Med. 1990 Mar;65(3):167–77.

22. Friesen SR, Hudson RP. The Kansas School of Medicine eyewitness reflections on its formative years. Kansas City: University of Kansas School of Medicine;1996.

23. Marquart JA, Franco KN, Carroll BT. The influence of applicants' gender on medical school interviews. Acad Med. 1990;65(6):410–1.

8

Medical School 1944–1975: Construction, Curriculum, and Controversy

Medical education in the United States changed dramatically in the three decades covered by our interviews (1944–1975). The University of Kansas School of Medicine (KUSM) and other medical schools expanded physical facilities, repeatedly changed curricula and teaching methods, and struggled with multiple social, political, economic, and other pressures from both internal and external forces.

When our first participant graduated in 1948, the dean's preface to the class yearbook described an institution that had struggled to survive but had cautious hope for the future.

> "The School is just emerging from the educational and service stage of its development, when it struggled to obtain the bare physical facilities to provide space and equipment for a laboratory for the education of doctors and nurses. Now it is entering into a period when it will also actively contribute to medical science."[1]

He significantly underestimated the dramatic changes of the following decades.

The renaissance of KUSM was led by the first two postwar deans, Franklin Murphy (1948–1951) and W. Clarke Wescoe (1952–1960). Incredibly, they were 32 and 30 years of age, respectively, on appointment as dean – the term "boy dean" was not always used in admiration![2] The ambitious Murphy Plan in 1950 tied the development of the school to the needs of the state and determined KUSM development for decades.[2] The plan aimed to make KUSM a major state resource and source of pride for all Kansans. It directly impacted our interviewees, especially in the changes it initiated in class size, admissions, and curriculum.

Construction: Building and Growing

"Construction seemed constant. . . . it produced one new building each year."[2]

The boy deans led an ambitious building program. "From early 1950s to mid-1960s facilities doubled in size."[2] To finance the expansion, they secured multiple grants through the Hill–Burton Act, a federal program to accelerate hospital construction; successfully lobbied for increased state funding; and secured major philanthropic donations. In the 1940s, the budget was under $750,000; by 1960, it approached $10 million. In addition to managing the complex political and economic issues of

DOI: 10.1201/9781003539568-8

expanding the medical school, the deans were personally involved in construction issues. The challenges of removing, renovating, or expanding the existing buildings were exacerbated as the original plans had been lost, leading to several nasty surprises and innovative urgent adjustments by architects and structural engineers. On at least one occasion, the foundations of a major building were almost undermined by the new construction! As Dean Wescoe recalled: "There was not a day during my deanship when a major construction project was not in progress. Perforce, I became a sort of amateur architect and an assistant clerk of works."[2]

Dean Wescoe even ran into unique political problems due to creative funding by a thrifty (or devious) predecessor.

> "It was decided that the outpatient facility needed to be expanded and it was decided to build fourth and fifth floors on to this building. There was a slight problem because Topeka (State government) did not have any record of there being a first, second and third floor. Were they to build on air? It was said that Dean Wahl had the first three floors built from funds he had saved at the Medical Center and had never requested funds from Topeka. As far as Topeka was concerned, there were no three lower floors although they had been in use for 15 years. I am sure the "pols" had never heard of a director who saved state money."[2]

Unfortunately, the outcome was legislation requiring the Medical Center to return any surplus funds to the state, resulting in enduring resentment and mistrust. Rumors still circulate that multiple buildings on the Lawrence campus were paid for by Medical Center earnings and that "the State highway department received a good share of these funds."[2]

By 1955, the *Kansas City Times* commented:

> "The medical center is fast becoming one of the top tourist attractions in the state. The medical center continues to grow. The 15-acre site now has 17 buildings. . . . A small city itself with more than 4,000 persons, counting 1,500 employees, 600 students, and 1,600 staff members plus patients going in and out daily."[3]

Campus construction was complemented by expansion of other local hospitals that participated in clinical training, especially a new Kansas City Veterans Administration Hospital, completed in 1952. The Murphy Plan's emphasis on serving the state and requirements for student experience in rural areas stimulated statewide hospital construction, even in small communities, with the hope of attracting physicians. The "standing joke that students, almost to a man, announce on their applications that they are interested in becoming general practitioners in a small town in western Kansas"[4] gained a cynical comment from 1964 graduates: "My vision of Paradise is a Hill–Burton hospital all my own."[5]

A second long-range plan for facilities development was submitted to the Board of Regents in 1960. "During the period of mid 1960s to 1980s, the size of KUMC facilities doubled again!"[2] The centerpiece of the second expansion was a new teaching hospital, approved in 1971 and completed in 1979. "The largest building construction project ever undertaken by the State of Kansas and probably by anyone within the State. It was also the first hospital revenue bond financed project by the State."[2] This huge project required the acquisition of large tracts of land adjacent to the campus, the closure of two streets, and the demolition of over 100 properties, including "the infamous One Block West Beer Tavern and Dance Hall, a significant hazard and nuisance to the neighborhood."[2] The senior administrator describing the project did not comment on any loss to the social life of the students with the demolition of the tavern. More importantly, he ignored the impact on students of the removal of a large swath of affordable housing within walking distance of the Medical School. The neighborhood was run-down, and our oldest participant recalled, *It could be dangerous walking around the old hospital – women could be approached.*

Our interviewees described navigating the disruption and mess of construction throughout their time at KUSM from the 1950s to the 1970s. In addition to winter mud and summer dust, the demolition and construction generated alarming noise and vibration that interfered with learning and patient care. "Sometimes the entire building shook as another dynamite charge went off."[2] The new buildings were greatly needed. Quonset huts were still serving as temporary facilities in the early 1960s, and the only accommodation available for the new Department of Family Medicine in 1971 was a dilapidated nearby motel.[2] The available campus buildings were crowded, badly organized, and in poor condition. The environment was certainly not conducive to learning. Anatomy teaching and laboratory sessions had to contend with laundry carts being incessantly pushed up and down the halls. At one stage, the chairman of Anatomy "padlocked the laundry door during the day while experiments were in progress. This led to administrative repercussions at many levels."[2] For many years, air-conditioning was only available in the surgical operating rooms. In 1953, at the peak of a summer polio epidemic, Kansas City recorded 17 days with temperatures over 110 degrees Fahrenheit. Conditions must have been very uncomfortable for patients as well as learners. In the on-campus Bell Memorial Hospital, not all rooms had basic facilities. In 1952, the hospital charged $8.50 per day in a multibed (four to six) in a room, $9 if the room had a sink, and $10 for a single room with toilet and shower.[2]

The new Student Union Building was completed in 1953, and the library in 1958. A participant recalled the party atmosphere when student and faculty volunteers formed a human chain to move all the books from hand to hand from the old library to the new location. Almost all campus buildings were connected by a system of tunnels. A female intern described seldom being outdoors all winter. "We rarely left the Medical Center; lived in the nurses' dorm, had meal tickets for the cafeteria, and social events were in Battenfeld auditorium, so we just used the tunnels mole-like and seldom came above ground."[6] Even with all the new construction of the 1950s and the 1960s, a 1972 matriculant was *surprised how shabby the buildings were.*

Curriculum, Curricula

"Medical education is not just a program for building knowledge and skills in its recipients. . . . it is also an experience which creates attitudes and expectations."[7]

Medical schools have a long tradition of making continual incremental changes in their educational programs with periodic major reforms that cause great controversy and upheaval. For most of the period covered by our interviews, the curriculum was similar to that of other contemporary US medical schools, with the first two years focused on basic sciences (such as anatomy, biochemistry, physiology) and the senior years taken up with clinical studies. The third year consisted of required rotations through the major clinical specialties (e.g., internal medicine, surgery, pediatrics, psychiatry). The final year allowed students more latitude for elective experiences in areas of personal interest. The KUSM senior students also had a few required courses, especially the rural preceptorship. The school was very proud of this innovative rural experience introduced around 1948. It was intended to provide both a maturation (real-life) experience for the student and powerful evidence of the institutional commitment to preparing physicians for the rural areas of the state.

"Each one of our students, following completion of the junior year, will spend eleven weeks participating in the practice of medicine with a man in general practice in a community in Kansas of 2,500 people or less. The preceptors were hand-picked by a faculty committee from a panel submitted by the Kansas Medical Society. This program is a signal step forward in medical education, providing as it does for a student eleven weeks of medical reality without in any way reducing the time spent in Medical School."[2]

Administrators lauded the program, especially to legislators, and boasted that it had been copied by other US schools. The students writing the 1958 Yearbook found it less inspiring: "A change of climate and rest cure on preceptorships in the Great American Desert."[8]

Despite multiple curricular changes, the rural preceptorship endures but has been modified over time. Currently, the requirement is four weeks of primary care in a small community, and about one-third of preceptors are women.

In describing their medical education, our interviewees focused on three major curricular changes – the move of first-year classes from the Lawrence campus to Kansas City in 1962, the development of the regional campus in Wichita in the early 1970s, and the experimental three-year curriculum of the early 1970s. Their student perspectives provide interesting contrasts with faculty recollections of these events published in oral histories and curricular documents from the medical school archives.[2]

Campus Consolidation (1962)

Prior to 1962, all medical students spent the first two years on the Lawrence campus and were predominantly taught by non-physicians. The tightly scheduled classes and overwhelming material to be mastered isolated them from other Lawrence students, and distance limited contact with upperclassmen and medical school faculty in Kansas City. "Boys in White" (a sociological study of KUSM students in the late 1950s) describes a brutal learning environment.[4] Male medical students clustered in three fraternities that provided some validation and support, but "independents" (unaffiliated men, often married) and the few female students were on their own. The 1948 Yearbook (the class of our first interviewee) reflects the difficult atmosphere of the mid-1940s despite its jocular and rather immature tone.

> "The men lived in the hostelries of Nu Sigma Nu, Phi Beta Pi, or Phi Chi. The women in a second-story walk up on Oread Avenue. We became inured to the hardships of bearing continuously the odor of 1% phenol and the contempt of certain co-eds who 'could hardly wait for the MEN to get home.' We overcame early grade-anxiety, repressed dissection-room nightmares, learned to sleep despite crammed-brain insomnia, and moved somewhat more confidently into sophomore year. In 1946 the class migrated to the city between one and two dozen lighter than its fighting weight, said unfortunates having been pulled down by the Lawrence jackals of rote."[1]

During the years in Lawrence, students constantly complained about the poor facilities and intense academic pressure. "Boys in White" documents the students' mounting frustration and poorly repressed resentment toward the faculty, culminating in a short walkout from an anatomy lab session.[4] The 1958 Yearbook describes their experiences:

> "Our first year was 1954 in Lawrence, Hayworth Hall. After an intensive orientation, we were subjected to massive inoculations of biochemistry, physiology, anatomy and related subjects. Constant pressure – only 60% passed the first biochem quiz. 5 students "got the axe." The lecture hall was very uncomfortable. It had a large fan – alternating hypothermia at back and stifling discomfort at front."[8]

The teaching facility, known as the anatomy shack, was a rebuilt WWI barracks that burned down in the 1940s. The replacement was far from ideal. A 1960 alumna recalled, *First year in Lawrence was overwhelming. Things were very different. Nowadays, anatomy begins with ceremony to honor those who donated bodies, and it is all very respectful. NOT in our day – they just took us to the basement and pulled cadavers out of a vat. It was not respectful. Surreal, traumatic.*

Students who survived the rigors and discomforts of the first two years in Lawrence transferred to the Kansas City campus, where they were joined by students from two-year schools in Missouri and the Dakotas for the clinical years. Completion of new facilities on the Kansas City campus finally enabled the basic science departments to move from Lawrence in 1962. This closed a long chapter of bitter political wrangling and criticism of the Medical School. Over 50 years earlier, Flexner had deplored the "severed halves, for all practical purposes the university conducts two half schools."[2]

The Wichita Campus (1973)

Uniting all four classes of students on the Kansas City campus addressed only one of the long-standing feuds about the location of the Medical School. At the beginning of the 20th century, several cities (each with powerful legislative support) had vied to become the site of this state-supported institution. Pressure to participate in medical education intensified after the closure of proprietary medical colleges in Wichita and Topeka.

> "The final legislative decision in 1899 to put the first two basic science years in Lawrence and the clinical years in Kansas City created warring factions that continued to plague the medical school administration. In the minds of some Wichita physicians, the dream of a local medical school never disappeared."[2]

The process and motivations for establishing the Wichita campus remain subject to partisan interpretation. Whether intentions were devious or virtuous, by the 1960s, providing medical education in Wichita appeared to offer mutual benefit to that community and the Medical School. Prior to the completion of the new hospital, the Kansas City campus was limited in the number of patients available for teaching and had antiquated facilities. The Wichita hospitals and clinics provided care to copious numbers of patients in modern facilities. Education in Wichita also appeared more likely to encourage graduates to settle in the central and western parts of the state – always a concern of state legislators in funding the Medical School. The Wichita hospitals had long-standing independent internships that were largely staffed by KUSM graduates, and most local physicians were KUSM alumni. Nevertheless, members of both the Kansas City faculty and the Wichita medical community resisted attempts to establish programs for medical students. Some of this resistance concerned the quality of medical education, but political and financial considerations were certainly prominent. The entire debate reflected decades of rivalry and distrust between the two largest cities in the state. The final agreement for a Wichita branch of KUSM approved by the Board of Regents in 1971 hinged on the support of the three principal Wichita hospitals plus the Veterans Administration but required the intervention of the mayor of Wichita, the governor of the state, and multiple other politicians and stakeholders. Rumor holds that recalcitrant faculty leaders were promised new facilities on the Kansas City campus to secure their support of the Wichita campus. Whatever pressures, inducements, or promises were involved, following "five turbulent gestational years and a barrel of meetings," the first group of 14 students transferred to Wichita for selected clinical experiences in 1973.[2]

While officials cited the altruistic educational and community benefits of establishing clinical training in Wichita, the initial students often had more practical motivations. Most had family or intended to settle in the area. Even the Wichita campus dean recognized they were "eager for study, but also affordable housing, jobs for spouses, and free hospital food."[2]

I did many electives in Wichita as I wanted to return to the area.

In Wichita, I had inexpensive apartment and free food at the hospitals. Graduated with only about $3,000 debt!

Wichita offered many advantages, but being in a small, highly visible group of students also had some drawbacks.

Small group, brand-new program, we were treated like special people – not run-of-the-mill. We were treated very well – we got free food in the hospitals! Didn't get all the grunt work (compared to KC students). I did not enjoy the OB experience, but we got to deliver babies under resident supervision. It was very hands-on, exciting. Wichita didn't have the "have to wear skirts" rule. No female residents, and no on-call accommodation for women. I slept in the nuns' infirmary. We were a little more isolated, not able to form close friendships.

The Wichita medical community was overwhelmingly male and had a reputation for being conservative. The attitude of many older physicians toward female students was described as *blatant male chauvinism, frank discrimination.* One interviewee recalled a senior Wichita physician stating, *It's not normal for women to be doctors,* and being advised not to consider applying for an internship as they *don't accept women* and *women have no business being doctors.* Initially, in Wichita, *female students were not allowed to do surgery.* Another Wichita student described being required to drive the 250 miles to the Kansas City campus to present cases – and her treatment by the Kansas City chairman.

I had a very good experience taking obstetrics at St. Francis Hospital in Wichita, where I was able to deliver babies myself and had direct contact with a resident in obstetrics and a KU faculty member. I had to present a case back at KU to the chief of obstetrics and was humiliated in front of my classmates for wearing street clothes, which he forbade among students and residents. He said, "At least she won't grow a beard." For the next trip back to KU to present another patient, I sewed myself a white business suit so I would look presentable traveling with the resident and faculty member. Women were treated SO differently from the guys.

The Wichita campus was only one of a range of ambitious projects developed during the late 1960s and early 1970s to address the anticipated critical shortage of physicians. In addition to expanding facilities in Kansas City and opening campuses in Wichita and Topeka, plans were developed to double class size to 200 students per year and accelerate training through a new three-year curriculum. The plans met with limited success. Facilities on the Kansas City campus have continued to expand, with the centerpiece of the new hospital opened in 1979 and multiple new facilities and renovations since. The Wichita campus has grown to a full four-year campus with over 200 students, but Topeka has not developed as a major teaching site. The combined class size eventually reached 200 per year. The three-year medical student program was "given a quick trial and burial,"[2] but not before it had a major impact and caused great consternation for about half of our interviewees.

The Great Curricular Experiment (1971–1975)

Around 1968, a group of faculty members began planning a new three-year curriculum to "appropriately train a rather large number of health science personnel to meet the sharply increasing demands for health care."[2] The rationale for the new curriculum, and many of its proposals, could be appropriately repeated today. After considering several revolutionary proposals and counterproposals, the faculty approved a model in which basic sciences, such as anatomy, physiology, biochemistry, and microbiology, would all be taught in 18 months, followed by two years of clinical experiences.[8,9] The intended emphasis was on integrating material across disciplines and correlating scientific information with clinical conditions. Then as now, entrenched practices and deeply held convictions about priorities in medical education are difficult to reconcile, and consensus in a large medical faculty is almost impossible to reach. Changing educational programs requires overcoming multiple political, practical, economic, and other challenges. The degree of discord and uncertainty about the accelerated curriculum can be seen in the official 1971–1972 catalog of the school of medicine, when even the earlier start date had not been approved by the faculty by the time of publication of information for matriculants. "The class entering in 1971 will probably begin medical school in late August. However, it is possible that classes may start in mid-July."[10] Prospective students must have wondered what was going on!

Despite ambitious intentions, the "new" curriculum introduced in 1971 did not consist of innovative multidisciplinary courses integrating basic and clinical sciences but was very similar to the previous four-year program, with everything compressed into 3.5 years. Few changes were made in the basic sciences programs to reduce content for the shorter time available or to link material across courses. The compressed clinical experience focused on required courses and provided few opportunities to explore different medical specialties or take electives in areas of special interest. Our interviewees who were involved vividly recalled the overload, frustration, and stress they experienced as *guinea pigs in an educational experiment.*

I was in the experimental three-year curriculum. Preclinical was intense. Eighteen months of the sciences without a break. No chance for electives to help decide career.

Part of experimental three-year curriculum pushing things together really tight. We had no time off. We didn't have enough elective time to explore medicine. It was not a good idea. It was supposed to increase the number of doctors for western Kansas. Everything was crushed together. We didn't have time to do research or externships, so we applied for internships before we had enough experience to know what was available.

Curriculum just crammed everything into three years. Solid, no breaks, no vacation, brutal. Everyone took it very seriously. There was a rumor our classes had more divorces than any other class. Nine months of solid pathology.

Curriculum was intense. One and a half years basic sciences and, four days later, started one and a half years of clinics with no breaks.

Our interviewees described student disappointment and frustration with teaching methods as well as the excessive content and pace of the new curriculum. The intensive passive lectures and multiple examinations seemed regressive after the more liberal experiences of their senior years in college. During the first 18 months, students spent hours in lectures every day and felt treated like children.

Early on was discouraged by the course structure, being alphabetical, having to sit there. It felt like grade school. "Rinky-dink."

Intense. Lots of classes and studying. We sat alphabetically in class. Questions were not encouraged.

I didn't like the teaching method. They just threw out the information at you, with no indication of what was really important or how to prioritize it. It was impossible, too much.

So many tests, and everyone was very competitive. Exams every alternate Saturday morning for 16 weeks, so weeks of no sleep on Friday nights. There was one infamous pathology professor who said "nobody passes" his test. It was multiple choice, and I think only about 10% passed. How could that go on year after year? It was wrong, stupid.

I expected medical school to be hard as college courses had been, but medical school was not just difficult coursework – it was a hostile environment.

Some of our interviewees recounted that a few faculty members seemed determined to prove the new curriculum would not be successful by failing as many students as possible.

Some faculty were angry and frustrated with administration over this new curriculum to have us graduate in three and a half years. The infectious disease instructor wanted to make the point that it was a stupid idea, so he wanted to flunk a lot of the class to prove it couldn't be done. We were sweating bullets.

Med school was hard. The hardest was pathology. The professor was a fiery, hot-tempered Italian who prided himself on making it as difficult as possible. Two of our class flunked and had to repeat the course. I had six weeks of tutoring but got through.

Some leading faculty members were particularly scathing about attempts to introduce innovative teaching methods to replace the heavy schedule of traditional lectures.

> "The witchcraft craze of New England could be equaled in intensity only
> by the mania which struck academicians, creating and aura of unrest in our
> educational institution. Our faculty was suddenly hit by a string of nomadic
> educators. . . . Terms were hurled at us in a manner suggesting that none of us
> had ever given serious thought as to how one could best deliver information
> to students or stimulate them to learn for themselves."[2]

Our interviewees recalled a few bright spots in the new curriculum when they could envision becoming physicians.

First two years were mostly in the classroom and felt like college. However, I greatly enjoyed the few courses where there was patient contact, like home health and physical examination.

Several mentioned a new course, sex in medicine, although it had some unintended effects.

We had sexuality and medicine for a whole week. They showed all these pornographic films in the big auditorium. They were not really pornography, just very graphic, but were actually considered professional films for the purpose of teaching the subject. (This was about 1971.) My partner came in late, when the lights in the auditorium were off, and was so engrossed watching the movie he sat unintentionally on my lap! They said the reason for having the class was that people would come on to us in medicine and we had to learn to separate their inappropriate sexual advances from their legitimate medical issues. There were sessions on different aspects of sex in medicine – sex for pregnant women, sex for quadriplegic patients, masturbation, etc. Some of it was interesting, useful.

The intense coursework and increased failure rates resulted in many students *getting out of sync* and being unable to graduate within the 3.5-year time frame. Those who did graduate early often had difficulty securing an internship or residency position, as these traditionally always start in July. One interviewee made full use of her "gap" period.

I couldn't start residency till the following July, so wanted to travel and get more experience in another country. England was the easiest. Was at Queen's Square National Hospital for Nervous Diseases (neurology) and worked briefly with Dr. Roger Bannister, the famous runner. Was also on a rotation at Hammersmith (Royal Postgraduate Hospital) for cardiology. Had a wonderful experience with Dr. John Goodwin, a world's expert in cardiomyopathy. Both world-class institutions. Culture was SO different. Attendings worked up patients in a huge amphitheater and gave dissertations on findings. Scholarly, amazing physical exams. Had first CT in the world. Incredible experiences. Very civilized experience. Morning and afternoon rounds with break for coffee/tea and cakes/biscuits (cookies) with the team. Registrars seemed old – stayed on through their 40s, hoping for a senior position. Very experienced. Famous faculty. Traveled around UK and the European continent before starting internship.

The accelerated curriculum was abandoned shortly after the period covered by our interviews, and the curriculum returned to the classical four-year format. Despite multiple curricular innovations and reforms in subsequent decades, the first two years of medical education at KUSM still focus on mastering the basic sciences, while the third and fourth years concern clinical experiences. Nevertheless, the aspirations of the accelerated curriculum are evident in the current educational program. The basic sciences are taught as integrated courses, with extensive clinical correlations that draw on multiple basic sciences to enable students to understand the scientific basis for normal function and the development of disease. Throughout the curriculum, the much-despised teaching methods of the "nomadic educators" are normal practice, and KUSM has an active group of medical educators who contribute to research and innovation in medical education. Perhaps the accelerated curriculum was ahead of its time; perhaps it failed because of inadequate preparation and hasty implementation in the face of entrenched opposition. No studies have examined how well the shortened curriculum prepared KUSM students for internship and future practice; our interviewees certainly had long and successful careers. Nevertheless, several shuddered or sighed in describing the legacy of resentment, sadness, and regret from the great curricular experiment.

Controversies: *The Times They Are A-Changin* (Bob Dylan 1964)

In addition to the internal turmoil of construction and curricular change, our interviewees recounted how KUSM was impacted by the many external upheavals of the period, including the Civil Rights movement, the feminist revival, and student protests over the Vietnam War and other issues.

When our first interviewees were medical students in the 1940s and 1950s, most facilities in Kansas, including hospitals and clinics, were segregated. Only a few years earlier, the dean had argued against the admission of Black students on the grounds that White patients would object to the presence of "colored staff and students."[11] The first Black student graduated in 1941 only at the insistence of the state governor.[11] In the early 1950s, Black patients were still restricted to a single rather run-down building that had "Negro Ward" carved into the stone lintel above the entrance. A faculty member who taught our first interviewee recalled:

> "Racial segregation was very prominent. All Black obstetrical and gynecological patients were kept on the second floor of the Negro Ward. There was a baby boom, so we had to keep many of the Black patients on litters in the hallway. White obstetrical and gynecological patients were kept in a separate area of the hospital. Although there was a small number in those days, Black house staff and students were not permitted to take care of White patients."[2]

Despite official policies, faculty members in the off-site psychiatric facilities began desegregating patient care around 1950. "Without asking anyone's permission, and fully expecting complaints, I admitted our first Black. No one said a word."[2] In the main hospital, desegregation followed a more complicated path. The dean recalled discussing desegregation with a delegation from the NAACP of Kansas City in 1952 and using the polio epidemic of the following summer to house all patients who needed ventilators (iron lungs) in a single ward, regardless of race.

> "The only room large enough was in the Negro Building. For the first time patients of both races were housed in the same room. After the emergency was passed, the building continued as an integrated facility; there was no public clamor and no sign of public protest."[2]

The only objections came from the same NAACP leaders who had advocated deseg-regation. "We have come because you are taking our hospital from us. After some dis-cussion about having it both ways, agreement was reached and so ended segregation at KUMC."[2] Memories about the date and process of desegregation differ, as another faculty member recalls receiving a directive several years later from the same dean to "desegregate this place!" Arriving as the Chair of Obstetrics and Gynecology in 1959, he found one building designated for Black patients:

> "If beds were unoccupied in the white areas, yet no opening in black beds, the black patient was put in the hall. Segregation was ended by sheer will-power. I slept in the hospital and personally put patients in the beds that were open. The walls of the Black Delivery Room were of vitrolite – easily broken and hence this room was closed: labor and delivery were put together."[2]

This chairman also withdrew students from community hospitals that had separate facilities for White and non-White patients, causing "a great deal of consternation among the obstetricians in Kansas City."[2] While patient facilities were slowly deseg-regated in a piecemeal fashion, the Medical School remained an overwhelmingly White institution. The 1958 Yearbook shows only two Black men (and four women, all White) in a class of 104. All the faculty, interns, and residents pictured are White.[8] Yearbooks throughout the 1960s show only one or two Black members of the faculty or house staff. A Black pediatrician was the director of a pediatric community clinic during the 1968 race riots in Kansas City,

> "There was burning and looting in the area of the clinic over a period of two days and one night. The staff departed, rightly fearing for their physical safety; but Dr. B volunteered and remained as the sole guardian of the clinic, frequently standing in the open doorway of the clinic building. The clinic was not attacked or molested in any way, thanks to Dr. B."[2]

Several White faculty members actively supported the Civil Rights movement – one had taken part in the Selma march. A Black interviewee recalled the dean in the early 1970s being very supportive of minority students. *Dr. Waxman really worked with the Black organizations. He came to us and allowed us to voice our concerns and hopes for additional help. He intervened for me a couple of times.*

During the 1960s, faculty members initiated programs to attract and support learners from minority groups. These programs were bolstered by grants under the National Health Professionals Educational Assistance Act of 1963. This legislation, along with multiple other policy and funding opportunities and programs, was cited by our appli-cants as facilitating entry to medical school for women (as members of a minority group) as well as non-White individuals. Nevertheless, in 1974, the organization rep-resenting Black students made a formal complaint of

> "Willful and unlawful acts of discrimination toward black medical students at the University of Kanas Medical Center in an attempt to systematically eliminate them from medical school and depriving them of an opportunity of achieving a medical education, through individual acts, conspiratorial efforts

and inciting the Kansas University Medical Faculty to discriminate against black students."[12]

The core issue was the high failure rate among minority students, many of whom had been admitted with lower MCAT scores through the minority programs. The situation deteriorated into rancorous accusations of racism and academic discrimination principally directed at one outspoken professor. After two trials, he won a libel action against four minority students in 1975, but this was reversed by the Kansas Supreme Court in 1981.[12] The legacy of bitterness and mistrust, especially toward one department, complicated efforts to enhance the recruitment and professional success of Black students for decades.

To Protest or Not to Protest?

Whatever their personal beliefs and passions, medical students faced significant constraints in expressing opinions on political or social issues during the 1960s and the 1970s. Despite the revolutionary sentiments of that time, when Bob Dylan's song lyrics could proclaim *"the times they are a-changin'. . . . Your sons and your daughters are beyond your command,"* medical students were very much under the command of rigid and often unsympathetic authorities. Yearbooks convey a mixture of distrust, disrespect, and even disdain toward authority and institutions. These attitudes were pervasive among students nationwide at that time and often erupted into protests and violence. The administration is typically portrayed in yearbooks as remote, mysterious, powerful, and uncaring – or even cynical and vindictive – toward students. "Nobody really knows who runs this hole."[13] The national fervor of student protests peaked at the time when KUSM students were struggling with the new curriculum and had almost no free time for personal activities, including volunteering to support cherished causes. In addition to their demanding studies, medical student life was tightly regulated by formal and informal standards of professional behavior. Dress codes were strictly enforced. Special attention was given to hair. At a time when long and/or untidy hair was regarded as a sign of a hippie, beatnik, drug user, protester, or some other form of troublemaker, all students were required to be neat and tidy. Any student with unruly locks or a male with beard or facial hair could be excluded from clinics and was likely to receive verbal abuse or worse from faculty members in classrooms, clinics, or other venues. A faculty member complained, "The widespread period of student unrest in the 1960s was also felt of our campus. Clothes became sloppy, and language disrespectful. Perhaps it was part of a belligerent attitude of all youth against the rest of society."[2]

A critical element of student frustration was their total dependence on faculty members for grades, letters of recommendation, and offers of internship positions. At that time, assessment of students was predominantly subjective, and clinical grades were almost entirely based on the faculty member's perceptions of the individual student. The impression a student made on a few powerful faculty members could influence his or her entire career. Female students especially struggled with the paradox of standing out from the crowd versus risking being seen as too pushy or being embarrassingly *put in one's place*. Nobody wanted to risk being labeled as a troublemaker or a *radical*.

Frustrations over the new curriculum and other issues reached a peak in the winter of 1968–1969. Local tensions were aggravated by national reports of FBI and other government agencies keeping files on student leaders who were suspected of being potentially dangerous to national security. The national atmosphere of fear, anger, and paranoia resulting from protests and the response by authorities, polarized relationships, making it difficult to negotiate even straightforward issues, such as notifying students of their grades.

During the Winter of our Discontent as it was described in our yearbook, there was a major incident. It was sort of a sit-in rather than an occupation. We asked to have a meeting to discuss several issues, most importantly a request that we heard about from UC Berkeley to see our "dossiers." We had never been told our MCAT scores, so we had applied to medical school blindly and simply asked to see our scores. We were getting ready for the first part of the National Boards and were curious about how we had done on our most recent standardized test. We also wanted to know if there was incriminating evidence on any of us "rabble-rousers." I was active in the Student American Medical Association so I would have been considered one of the radicals.

Among the range of student concerns was being addressed disrespectfully by faculty and staff, including the operators of the almost-continual overhead paging system. The agreed resolution seems to have overlooked the possibility of any female medical students – and provided one of the few moments of light relief in a tense situation.

One issue concerned how students were to be addressed. After a survey, decided they could be called "medical student" or "Mister." I remember being paged overhead as Mr. Martha S! I spoke up to say I preferred "student doctor" rather than "Mister," and to gales of laughter the issue was settled. I was the only female attending the meeting. Women were treated SO differently from the guys.

Not all faculty members had a low opinion of students. The acting dean in 1970 described an innovative approach to improving relationships.

"Two of the student radicals showed up in my office about five o'clock, and they said, 'Dean, tomorrow we're going to burn down the Student Union.' I said, 'Let me tell you something. If you're going to burn anything down, you start at the Northeast corner of the campus and you burn every single building. Because if I come in here tomorrow and hear that you've only burned the Student Union, you're going to be in serious trouble.' They laughed and then with a kind of devilish look in their eyes, they said, 'How about going up to Jimmy's Jigger and having a beer?' This was kind of a dare, you see, to get the Dean up there. I said, 'OK.' So we went up and we walked in, and the girls were dancing on the bar, and everybody saw the Dean. I had a beer with a bunch of the students. They said, 'Have a second.' They were daring me, they wanted to see how far they could go. I said, 'All right.' I got about halfway through that second beer and all of a sudden, I got this premonition of impending doom. So, I said, 'I'm sorry, I've got something I've got to do back at the office' and I left. I got about halfway down the street, and I heard these sirens. The police raided Jimmy's Jigger. Well, I could just see the headlines the next morning: 'KU DEAN ARRESTED IN RAID IN JIMMY'S,' and how that would go down with the Regents. You know, it would have been a disaster."[14]

The dean went on to illustrate the significant role played by the proprietor of Jimmy's Jigger in providing students with sympathetic support as well as alcohol. "Of course, Jimmy had a terrific role to play with the students. He was the father counselor. I always thought they should have awarded Jimmy an honorary degree or something."[14]

The Vietnam War directly impacted many students personally, but there were few protests at KUSM, and students were inhibited from participating in overt antiwar activities. *I was actively antiwar in college and then joined the Peace Corps. I remained committed to the cause in med school, but I don't remember much antiwar activity of the med students.*

I believe the sit-in was in April 1970 because of the bombing of Cambodia during the Vietnam War. I think there may have been something about it being at the same time as an exam in pathology. I remember sitting in the classroom when we were told that if we went to the sit-in, it would affect our grade. I tuned all of that out, because I didn't want to go to the sit-in, because I didn't think that was the best way to protest. I certainly didn't want to affect my grade in pathology. I was having difficulty in that class, anyway.

My sophomore year was 1969–1970. There were riots on the Lawrence campus. There was talk about our med school class boycotting class in protest. I don't remember whether there may have been one or two classmates who did boycott. I wasn't in favor of the Vietnam War, but I wasn't going to jeopardize my medical career. I figured I could express my antiwar views in other ways.

The antiwar protests on the Lawrence campus continued to have repercussions for the medical students after the catastrophic events of 1970 described in the previous chapter. The 1972 graduation *was postponed because of unrest on the Lawrence campus. They wanted to have a week after school was out to clear the campus and search for bombs.* One of our interviewees had only three weeks' notice to change wedding plans!

The working environment within the Medical Center was not always harmonious. Dissatisfaction with pay and working conditions was widespread during the 1960s and occasionally resulted in industrial action, mostly disrupting housekeeping and food services. The most serious strike occurred in the summer of 1967. The Medical Center was picketed; normal functions, including food services, housekeeping, and facilities maintenance, were severely impacted; and hospital admissions were curtailed. Students were deprived of services and expected to *pitch in* to help keep the hospital running during the four-day stoppage.

On a lighter note, the atmosphere in the Medical Center cleared somewhat in 1964, when the dean of the Medical School convinced the Board of Regents to ban the sale of cigarettes in all state colleges and universities, resulting in the memorable newspaper headline: "Regents ban sale of fags on campus."[2] The dean enjoyed cigars, so pipes and cigars were excluded from the ban. The hospital gift shop protested vigorously as cigarette sales generated its greatest profit. Smoking remained prevalent at the Medical Center for decades. After its dedication in 1947, students and others regularly met up at the Glendenning Memorial Fountain in the central courtyard to smoke, socialize, and seek respite from all the challenges of studying medicine in turbulent times.

REFERENCES

1. University of Kansas School of Medicine Yearbook Class of 1948.
2. Friesen SR, Hudson RP. The Kansas School of Medicine eyewitness reflections on its formative years. Kansas City: University of Kansas School of Medicine;1996.
3. Major RH. An account of the University of Kansas School of Medicine. University of Kansas School of Medicine;1968.
4. Becker HS, Greer B, Hughes EC, Strauss AL. Boys in white. Chicago (IL): University of Chicago Press;1961.
5. University of Kansas School of Medicine Yearbook Class of 1964.
6. Holmes G. On safari. Lima (OH): Fairway Press;1998.
7. Flexner A. Medical education in the United States and Canada. Carnegie Foundation for the Advancement of Teaching. Bulletin No. 4;1910.
8. University of Kansas School of Medicine Yearbook Class of 1958.
9. Report to Curriculum Committee 1969 (Archives).
10. University of Kansas 1971–72 Catalog School of Medicine (Archives).
11. Anon. Rejecting rejection KU history. Available from: https://union.ku.edu/discrimination
12. Scarpelli v. Jones :: 1981 :: Kansas Supreme Court Decisions :: Kansas Case Law :: Kansas Law :: US Law :: Justia. Available from: https://law.justia.com/cases/kansas/supreme-court/1981/52-482-1.html
13. University of Kansas School of Medicine Yearbook Class of 1972.
14. Transcript of interview of Dr. Charles Brackett by Deborah Hinkle for oral history project. 1991 Jun 21. Accessed through KUSM Archives.

9

Medical School: Practical Issues

Being accepted into medical school was the culmination of years of hard work and overcoming multiple challenges. Several interviewees remembered surprise at finally achieving the goal of becoming a medical student. For some, admission had become their singular purpose. They were so focused on getting into medical school that they could not think beyond admission and had formed only vague concepts about themselves as medical students or even physicians in some distant future. As the implications sank in, some interviewees recalled feelings of panic and waves of self-doubt. After striving so hard for this goal, would they be able to fulfill their ambitions? Would they *really* become physicians? Would they flunk out?

Our interviewees felt great pressure to justify their acceptance into medicine. The literature of the 1960s and the 1970s insisted that female students were twice as likely to drop out of medical school as their male classmates.[1-5] The belief that women lacked the stamina or determination to succeed in medicine was prevalent throughout the decades covered by the interviews.[1-5] All our interviewees were determined to prove themselves academically and clinically in the robust environment of the clinics and hospitals. Some of those matriculating in the 1970s reported perceiving even greater pressure than earlier cohorts due to allegations that they had only been admitted due to legal, political, and financial pressures on the institution to increase diversity.[2,4,6] Many women in this group also felt burdened by accusations of taking the place of men, who could have deferred being drafted and sent to Vietnam. Interviewees from all three decades commented that although the impostor syndrome had not been described at that time, it was highly prevalent in young women preparing to enter medical school.[7]

They let me in for some crazy reason!

I was a bit surprised to be admitted! I got a shock when I went to medical school.

It was like that joke about the dog who chases cars and doesn't know what to do when it catches one. I thought, "Wow, NOW I gotta GO!"

Acceptance into medical school had serious practical implications. The potential medical student faced finishing up her college requirements, moving to Kansas City, finding suitable accommodation, and identifying a way to pay for medical education. As they came to terms with the realization that they would really be medical students within a few months, resolving these issues became urgent. Most received notification of acceptance in January or February. A few were wait-listed and recalled the anxiety of waiting for news and the frustration of being unable to make plans or commitments.

DOI: 10.1201/9781003539568-9

Members of the first class of the new curriculum in 1971 also recalled multiple rumors and great uncertainty about what to expect, including the actual start date! When it was announced that classes would start at the beginning of July, matriculants had to scramble to finish college and be ready to start medical school without the traditional summer break.

Some women were well-prepared in financial and other practical matters; others had deferred or avoided making plans for a variety of reasons. The explanations offered by our interviewees clustered in two overlapping areas. Some recalled being so over-loaded with finishing college, completing all the necessary paperwork, and managing personal issues that they had little energy or time to plan further into the future. A few were getting engaged or married during this period, and one was distracted by delivering her first baby and simultaneously divorcing her husband! Others had avoided planning as they had never been confident of being accepted into medical school. Some of these women joked that they had superstitiously avoided planning in case overconfidence *hexed* their applications. *It always seemed like a long shot. I didn't want to tempt fate. I thought I would work out the details if I ever got in, make it work somehow.*

Paying the Bills

Finance was the most pressing concern. Almost all interviewees commented on the low cost of the University of Kansas School of Medicine (KUSM), especially for in-state residents, and contrasted their experience with the large debts incurred by current students. As in college, the group expressed a strong theme of living frugally and being very careful with money. Nevertheless, paying all the necessary educational and living expenses was a significant challenge for most of our interviewees. *Financed a nickel here and a dime there. Scholarships, beg, borrow, steal.*

Financial challenges left indelible impressions – most interviewees had no hesitation in describing how they paid for their medical education, and some recalled exact sums and other financial details even after 50 years or more. They primarily relied on funds they had generated themselves through saving, part-time work, and scholarships. Several had saved throughout high school and college, often working multiple jobs to finance their own medical education. Some continued working during medical school. The group conveyed a strong theme of self-sufficiency.

I paid for med school mainly from savings. Always working and saving since grade school, high school, babysitting, etc. I worked summers throughout college. This was the beginning of the women's movement. When I was in high school, my mother encouraged me to apply for a job for the summer in the office of Dr. Jane Berry, a pioneer in women's studies. Worked with faculty on multiple projects, research, grants – often meeting end-of-year deadlines. Wonderful experience. In college, I always worked. I was a very good typist. Typed theses, dissertations, etc. They had to be very carefully done – lots of exact requirements. Also worked after classes in the psychology department with office work for the Chair. Also had small scholarship from KU and loans (I paid them all off) plus help from parents.

I financed medical school by working as a med tech part-time and during summers. Mostly paid my own way.

Took on various jobs and loans to finance my education.

Just over half of the group used some form of loan, but very few reported loans as their principal source of funding. The women who used loans usually came from families who could not provide any financial support. *I financed with loans. My parents were not in a position to pay. Not as expensive as it is now, and I made arrangements to pay off loans over ten years once qualified.*

Financed with loans. Cost was not that onerous – paid back quickly once I was in practice.

Most of the women who took out loans used them to supplement other sources of funding. The majority of loans were for relatively small sums and were promptly repaid after graduation, often through service commitments that forgave student debt.

Financed with savings, loans, grants – graduated with small debt that I paid off within three years.

Financed through loans, summer job as nurse's aide. Money was always tight.

Financed by one grant, two loans (repaid by National Health Service Corps Commitment), plus Father's part-time work.

Financed from savings and a loan. Always vey frugal and saved, expecting to go to graduate school. Always worked in summers and lived at home during college. Med school was cheap, and I lived as cheaply as I could. I owed $4,650 at 3% interest when I graduated. It was forgiven while I was working for the Indian Health Service.

Medical school was cheap! I think it was $1,000 a year for three years. Had small scholarships and survivor benefit from Father (deceased) through Air National Guard. Borrowed $3,000. Graduated with about $3,000 debt!

Financed from savings (always worked summer jobs and during college) and loans. Much cheaper then. I think about $3,000–4,000 total loans for med school.

About one-third of participants mentioned scholarships in financing their medical education. Several were merit-based awards from sororities or local organizations supporting the education of women; others were related to programs incentivizing physicians to practice in rural communities. One woman benefited from an award to her husband.

I was only able to stay in school to start my junior year in June because the Medical Society of Sedgwick County had started a medical student loan program for Sedgwick County students with no strings attached to encourage grads to come back to Sedgwick County. Each month I was sent enough money for expenses. It was a lifesaver.

I used savings and some scholarship money awarded because of honors in college. My husband had a scholarship from a Kansas community, so I had room and board covered and only had to worry about tuition.

One interviewee relied on a national program to support minority students in medicine. *I financed medical school through a Robert Wood Johnson scholarship for minorities (women were a minority group then) that paid tuition – I think it was $500 per year. I would never have been able to do it without that scholarship.*

Some interviewees described examples of the widespread financial discrimination against female medical students at that time.[8]

I had a close friend who was depending on a local scholarship from her home county, but she was refused the scholarship as the widow of the donor would not allow it to be given to a girl. She dropped out.

Other recollections illustrate the very different attitudes to male and female students seeking financial assistance through the Medical School. *I was very careful with money. I had a small fellowship from a sorority. I heard my male classmates talking about getting student loans easily and spending them on cars, vacations, mountain climbing equipment, and all kinds of fancy unnecessary things, but when I asked for a student loan, I was not warmly received. The administrator told me to ask my mother for the money. My mother lent me $300. I paid it back from my first paycheck as an anesthesiologist. I am not sure if I was refused a loan because I was a woman or if men just know how to ask. Women tend to accept being turned down and get on with it.*

Even a female student in desperate financial need was treated unsympathetically by those responsible for student financial aid. *My father had died, and I ran out of money sophomore year. Was going to drop out, get a job, earn some money, and try to come back. Sold my textbooks – I was broke. I went to the student financial aid office to request a loan and was told that they did not loan money to female medical students, only single males (i.e., guys without wives to support them). Got a scholarship from the county medical society and a job for three months at a hospital and saved money.*

Most families provided some financial support, but the degree varied enormously. A few paid all expenses as the family was strongly invested in education. *Father paid for medical school. He felt it was his duty to "play it forward" to his children as his parents had paid for his education.*

Many participants were moved by the efforts families made to contribute to medical school expense and were still appreciative of their sacrifices. One described her father taking an additional part-time job in order to make medical school a reality for his daughter. Conversely, a few families were unable to provide any significant support. Only one participant felt her parents had been able but reluctant to support her financially. *Med school in those days was pretty cheap. Financed mostly with scholarships and a few loans. Parents didn't help much – their priority was on my brother's education.*

The majority of families tried to provide some type of financial assistance. This generally took the form of gifts or loans, sometimes supplemented with the use of a vehicle or accommodation with family members during term or vacation. The most unusual family support was the use of farmland. One interviewee revealed that her distinguished academic career was founded on a long hot summer cultivating corn.

KUSM was only possible because it gave two good scholarships, plus I got a low-interest loan from a local women's organization. I still needed family support, but things were tight. The summer before med school, Father had a contract to grow corn for a popcorn factory. He had a few extra acres that were difficult to work, so he said I could keep the proceeds from whatever I could grow. I spent the summer raising corn on my assigned acres. Popcorn paid some of my medical school – at least in the beginning!

Most commonly, parents directly paid some or all of the tuition, and some families also contributed to other educational and living expenses. Even with parental support, the women felt the need to contribute to meeting their own living and educational expenses.

Tuition was $500 a year! I think with books, accommodation, and everything, the entire four years cost me less than $10,000! My father supported me, and I worked a small job for extra money.

My parents did not believe in loans for college. They paid my tuition for medical school as well. It was $400 per semester, and only a three-year program, so very inexpensive! For the rest of my financial needs, I worked nights as an EKG technician. Did 16-hour shifts for $1.60/hour – that was a mistake. I should have taken out loans or something but had a strong family belief in paying your way and not accumulating debt. I could have used that time better studying or sleeping.

Women who were married as medical students felt financially advantaged. Even if their husbands were also students, expenses could be shared.

I married at end of first year. His folks paid our housing, and I used his books, so I really only had to cover tuition!

Financed mainly with savings, maybe a little help from my husband's and my parents. It wasn't expensive.

Father paid tuition until I married in final year. Then I used loans as my husband was in pharmacy school.

Financed from my husband's magnificent salary! I think it was $14,000 or $15,000 a year as a surgery resident. Tuition was $1,042 per year. We lived very frugally.

The most financially secure interviewee was married to a young lawyer. *Financed by my husband's salary as a county prosecutor. We bought a house and had an Irish nanny live-in. Tuition was about $150 per semester.*

Even more than in college, almost all participants recalled being short of money and living as frugally as possible. *I was always very short of money. I ended with the same shoes I started with.*

Lived like a pauper!

Food was frequently mentioned. Students could purchase meals in the hospital cafeteria, but most female students prepared their own food to save money. One of the more enterprising interviewees struck a deal with some male classmates. *The boys next door liked to hunt. I offered to cook whatever they killed in return for a share. My father hunted, so I was used to preparing venison and game and all that kind of thing – it worked out pretty well.* Prior to its recent gentrification, the neighborhood had few eating establishments, especially for young women on limited budgets. Nevertheless, dates might take one further afield and provide better food in a nicer ambience. *Sounds terrible, but I never turned down a dinner date!*

Rented a house a block from the med school with two classmates. No car – we walked or used buses for transport. We all had jobs. I did babysitting. One roommate worked at Safeway and brought home food that was being thrown away. We spent $5 a week on groceries and cooked all our meals at home. Came home for lunch – couldn't afford the cafeteria. I loved to cook. I lived very frugally.

I think I lived on $5 a week – ate a lot of canned corn! Paid my own way from savings built up since college. I had zero left when I started internship.

Those on tight budgets were often distressed by unanticipated fees or expenses.

Financed by parents plus savings. School insisted we buy microscopes that we didn't use, maybe only in one class. I borrowed, shared with a pathology resident. They also said you have to buy all these books – but you really didn't need to. The teachers provided most of what you needed. The books were mostly for reference, and they were VERY expensive. My parents could fork out, but it was a lot of money. Some classmates struggled with loans and other ways to finance these additional expenses.

Those who transferred to the Wichita campus for years 3 and 4 were delighted to discover the lower rents and free meals in the hospitals. *In Wichita, I had an inexpensive apartment and free food at the hospitals!*

Living Arrangements

Accommodation was a significant budget item, and choice was limited in the area around the Medical Center. Students could be kept late on the wards and called in at night for emergencies. Conversely, several rotations required very early starts to cover ward duties. As few students had access to a vehicle, everyone needed to live within walking (or running) distance of the Medical Center. Medical, nursing, and other students competed with staff and others to find affordable housing that was close to the Medical Center and hopefully clean, in decent repair, and habitable throughout hot Kansas summers and frigid winters. Arriving from safe college and home environments, some women were surprised and shocked by having to consider personal risk in finding accommodation. For the first time in their lives, they had to worry about safety in walking to and from the Medical Center, especially at night, and if their possessions would remain secure when they were not at home.

The areas to the north and east of the Medical Center were pretty sketchy and not very safe. Everyone tried to live south.

I was concerned about safety when we had to come and go at night – a guy might not have been so concerned.

The environment was not friendly. It could be dangerous walking around the old hospital, especially at night. Women could be approached when walking.

The community in which the Medical Center is located was based initially on heavy industry, including ironworks and a coal mine. Many of the houses were built for lower-income workers and had not been well maintained as the area deteriorated. In the decades covered by our interviews, the area provided limited housing options for single women with constrained budgets. The neighborhood had few purpose-built apartments, but several houses had been subdivided into smaller rental units that were keenly sought after by students and Medical Center workers. Some of the available accommodation was less than desirable.

Had an apartment with my best friend, who was in nursing school. After she graduated, I had a small house that had been condemned but was cleaned up by the landlord. My parents gave me old furniture for the house.

Rented a small house with two classmates one block from the Medical Center. There was no air-conditioning. It was very miserable. The lowest point was during third year, 106 degrees in August.

Our interviewees described using a variety of housing options during their times as medical students. Most recounted moving several times in quest of cheaper and/or better accommodations or to gain privacy and uninterrupted time for studying by living alone. *Shared an apartment close to school with a student who was a few years ahead then always moving to find a cheaper place.*

Several initially lived in the nurses' dormitory. Although convenient, this was an older building with limited amenities and had the drawbacks of restrictions on male visitors and a 10:00 p.m. curfew – the housemother recorded any latecomers. Everyone who recalled living there moved out after a semester or two.

First year lived in nurses' dorm, then shared an apartment close to the Medical School.

Lived in the old nurses' dorm, and it cost about $31 a month.

First semester lived in nurses' dorm, then got a studio apartment and lived on my own.

In 1970, additional on-campus accommodations became available when women were permitted to occupy one of the three floors of the Student Center Dormitory.

> "Until this year, the dormitory was a residence for male medical students. With the new arrangement men and women share a sun deck and recreation room. An added convenience for the girls is the comfort of air conditioning, a luxury unavailable in the Women's Residence. (For this reason, the cost of living in the Student Center is $10 a month more than in the Women's Residence.)"[9]

Lived in nurses' dorm with nurse roommate. Then in a co-ed dorm in the Student Center, where I had room to myself. Convenient, right on campus, close to library, etc. Safe to walk to library, etc. I was very focused. In senior year, I sublet apartment across from the school from a friend who wanted to move in with his fiancée.

Several interviewees described sharing accommodation with classmates for at least part of their time in medical school. One recalled being helped by the institution to find accommodation and roommates before matriculation.

I thought the medical school was very helpful. I received a letter asking if I would like to share an apartment with three other women. We had a nice apartment nearly right across the street, so I didn't have to worry about finding a place, etc. I didn't know what to expect.

More commonly, female students made their own arrangements to share with friends or classmates.

Roomed with two girls from class.

Lived alone for two years, then with a friend from Lawrence who was also a medical student.

Initially lived in apartment close to Medical School with cousin (a more senior student), then shared an apartment on State Line with a roommate.

Rented from a third-year student, then shared a house with two female classmates.

Shared different apartments with a college friend who was a schoolteacher.

While several interviewees described seeking to live alone in order to study without inter-
ruptions, especially in their senior years, one group of classmates lived in a very sociable
apartment across the street from the med school. *We were the party house. We even had
a party when everyone had to come dressed as a disease. Another group offered more
tranquil relaxation. I was close friends with one girl and a gang of guys. We had a house
with a garden to grow vegetables, so we would hang out there to get away.*

Transport

Transportation was not a major expense but at times provided challenges. During
most of their training, medical students who lived close to the Medical Center did
not need a vehicle. Students spent many hours per day (and night) in the classrooms,
clinical facilities, and libraries of the Medical Center. They ate most of their meals
in the hospital cafeteria and socialized in events held on campus or the homes of fellow students. The principal student "watering hole," Jimmy's Jigger, was and remains
directly across the street from the Medical Center. This establishment is such a fixture
of the KUSM student experience that it had its own section in every class yearbook,
garnering as much coverage (and more pictures) than several academic departments.
The 1971 Yearbook referred to Jimmy as the "Dean for Student Activities." Although
their lives were focused on a small area around the Medical Center, students had to
travel for rotations at affiliated sites as well as for family and personal reasons. Only
two mentioned having cars. Both were mothers of young children. One commuted
every day from home in a nearby town. The other was a single mother, who recalled
her vehicle as a necessary but expensive liability. *The four years were very difficult.
Babysitting problems, vehicle kept breaking down. Took one day at a time.*

When necessary, the majority of students relied on lifts from the few who owned
vehicles or used public transport. Classmates were not necessarily very helpful, and
public transport could be inconvenient and uncomfortable.

No car. We walked or used buses for transport.

The guys didn't share information or offer transportation – we just walked.

*My lowest point was during a pathology rotation at Menorah Hospital. Wonderful
rotation, but I had to take two buses and change buses in a bad neighborhood. Waiting at the bus stop for my second bus in 106 degrees in August, I asked myself, "What
am I doing here?"*

Safety when traveling may have been less of a concern for some women in the late
1960s than it is now.

I would hitchhike home to visit my parents.

Comparisons and Reflections

The experiences of our participants provide interesting similarities and contrasts with the literature concerning female medical students in the three decades covered by our interviews (1945–1975).[1–8,10,11]

The heavy reliance on family and personal financial resources correlates with a federal report in 1965 on how medical students financed their education. Compared to the national picture, however, our participants reported lower use of loans.[11] This may reflect a tendency for female medical students to be less willing than their male classmates to take on student debt. Writers in the 1960s attributed this to women being reluctant to graduate with "a negative dowery because it hinders her chance of finding a good marriage partner and/or cause an interminable delay in planning a family until all debts are paid."[5] We have no evidence that our participants were influenced by either of these considerations in electing to avoid using loans to finance their medical education. Our impression was that they and their families were reluctant to incur debt due to a strong ethos of self-sufficiency. It is tempting, but possibly fanciful, to associate this mistrust of loans with family experiences of foreclosure and hardship in the Great Depression and Dust Bowl only one generation previously.

The most striking contrast between our interviewees and the literature is in the prevalence and severity of financial difficulties. Whereas only half of the 1950–1970 female graduates of an East Coast institution reported financial concerns,[10] almost all our participants were seriously concerned about money throughout their medical education, and some almost dropped out because of financial difficulties. They told stories of making their own clothes, scrounging food, finding the cheapest possible accommodation, and *stretching every dollar.* Even speaking in 2020 as prosperous retirees, they vividly recalled their impecunious student days. Several sighed and *wondered how [they] did it.* In contrast, national data for the period show that most medical students came from families with higher incomes, and articles expressed real concern of "a possible increase in the systematic skewing toward children of upper-income families."[12] Further, experts confidently stated in 1968 that "various studies indicate that the women come from even more financially secure backgrounds than the men."[5] This does not appear to be the case for our interviewees. We have no data on the financial status of their male classmates, but the "Boys in White" study of male Kansas medical students in 1958 suggests they were supported by relatively prosperous families.[13] In addition, class yearbooks from the period covered by the interviews make few references to financial difficulties.

Could the male students have worried less about money than did their female classmates? They probably had greater access to resources and were more sympathetically treated by financial aid offices. The anecdotes from our participants about unhelpful offices of student financial aid and denial of scholarships based on gender resonate with reports from a 1969 national survey of "secretive and discriminatory" practices in financial assistance to medical students.[8] In particular, this scathing national report concluded that women were assumed to be supported by their parents, whereas men were considered independent; women couldn't claim husbands as dependents, but men could claim wives; and single men got a $200 allowance for dating, whereas claims for childcare were treated as if an indulgent luxury.[8] The report also noted greater availability nationally of school-supported accommodation for male students.[8] This was the case at KUSM. The male classmates of our interviewees also enjoyed significant support from the three fraternities associated with the Medical School.

Finally, in our institution and nationwide, "the male student is more likely to be financed by his wife than the woman by her husband."[11] The medical students' wives were a recognized component of KUSM medical education. They had a flourishing organization that sponsored activities and mutual support. Every class yearbook contained a section devoted to the "medical dames," with multiple references to their hard work in supporting their husbands to meet the many challenges of medical education. The chivalrous writers of the 1971 Yearbook referred to the wives as "the broads who made it possible." Financial support by wives was assumed and endorsed by students and the institution. We were puzzled by multiple references to PHT certificates being awarded at the senior picnic or even at graduation and dismayed to be informed that the abbreviation indicated "Put Husband (or Hubby) Through!" The practice was so pervasive that the term did not need explanation in the contemporary yearbooks. We hope most medical student marriages were based on more than financial support and had higher aspirations than expressed in the 1958 Yearbook.

> *Becoming a doctor will cost you a lot*
> *Some may have the money, and others may not*
> *If your bankbook is empty, here's what you can do*
> *Just find you a wife who will work your way through*

REFERENCES

1. Johnson DG, Hutchins EB. Doctor or dropout? A study of medical student attrition. J Med Educ. 1966;41:1099–269.
2. Braslow JB, Heins M. Women in medical education: a decade of change. NEJM. 1981;304:1129–35.
3. Bowers JZ. Special problems of women medical students. J Med Educ. 1968;43:532–7.
4. Walsh MR. Doctors wanted: no women need apply: sexual barriers in the medical profession 1835–1975. New Haven and London: Yale University Press;1977.
5. Lopate C. Women in medicine. Baltimore (MD): Johns Hopkins Press;1968.
6. Spieler C, editor. Women in medicine. 1976 Report of a Macy Conference. New York (NY): Josiah Macy Jr. Foundation;1977.
7. Clance PR, Imes SA. The imposter phenomenon in high achieving women: dynamics and therapeutic intervention. Psychol Psychother Theory Res Pract. 1978;15(3):241.
8. Campbell MA. Why would a girl go into medicine? Old Westbury (NY): Feminist Press.
9. University of Kansas Medical Center Bulletin. 1970 Oct;22(1).
10. Williams PA. Women in medicine: some themes and variations J Med Educ. 1971;46:584–91.

11. Altenderfer ME, West MD. How medical students finance their education. US Department of Health, Education, and Welfare. Public Health Service Publication No. 1336;1965 Jun.
12. Jolly P. Diversity of US medical students by parental income. Association of American Medical Colleges. Analysis in Brief;2008 Jan;8(1).
13. Becker HS, Greer B, Hughes EC, Strauss AL. Boys in white. Chicago (IL): University of Chicago Press;1961.

10

Medical School: Into the Man's World

"A US medical school is a 'male world' . . . an inhospitable world for a woman. . . . Foreign women physicians who have studied in our medical schools have commented on how hostile the environment is for a woman student."[1]

(Bowers 1967)

First Impressions

I started in 1970 – scary. I was terrified but wanted to do well.

Our interviewees vividly recalled their first days at the Medical Center (KUMC). They described a gamut of emotions. Excitement and eager anticipation alternated with anxiety, fear of failure, and concerns about loneliness and social isolation. Everyone was determined to succeed but worried about the academic and other challenges ahead. They had all heard about the brutal pace and volume of learning in medical school. Although they had done well in college, they worried how they would fare in a class of competitive high achievers. Those who did not have particularly strong backgrounds in science were especially concerned.

Entered in 1971. My major impression was of being scared.

Most of the class had been science majors. One friend had a masters in microbiology, another a masters in comparative anatomy from Cornell University. Most of the students were Phi Beta Kappa. I felt slightly behind in science initially but worked hard and did well.

Really struggled and worked hard to get in. In college, you are used to being in the top 10%, but things were different in medical school – everybody had been at the top of their class.

In addition to academic concerns, our interviewees recalled being anxious about personal and social issues. They were curious about their classmates and hoped they would find friends and fit in with other students. Those who were shy quickly realized that medical school required a robust attitude.

I was excited, scared, and nerdy, always had my nose in a book. I was so timid and shy but found out being shy doesn't work in medical school!

DOI: 10.1201/9781003539568-10

I vividly recall the class lining up on the steps of the Murphy Building on the first day. Medical school was very exciting, loved it – a heady business, but big adjustment. First time I had left home. I needed to concentrate on studies and grow up at the same time. I was a homebody. It was a lot to contend with. I was very shy, insecure, and didn't know anybody in medicine. No doctors in the family, and limited contact with physicians growing up.

Despite years of preparation and anticipation, several remembered feeling *scared and overwhelmed* in their first days at the Medical Center. This was particularly the case for women who had attended small colleges, especially if they also came from small towns or rural areas.

After senior classes of 15–20 in college, the class size was daunting.

I was incredibly naïve. I felt like I came from a little town and a little college and would be right in the middle of the class – and I was.

Incoming medical students who had attended the University of Kansas (KU) in Lawrence knew several classmates and others on the Kansas City campus. Students who were not KU graduates felt at a disadvantage.

Many of my classmates knew one another from KU undergraduate or other colleges. I only knew a few of the men who had gone to Rockhurst High School.

It felt hostile, hot, uncomfortable, not welcoming, especially for non-KU grads. KU grads all knew one another.

Women in the Male Environment

"Medicine is man's work. . . . [T]he medical profession itself remains overwhelmingly male. In this book we shall talk mainly of boys becoming medical men."[2]

The interviewees recalled being acutely aware of plunging into a male environment. Although they expected few women among their classmates, the reality took many by surprise.

It was scary, exciting. First class was in this huge auditorium. Only 11 girls and 144 men. I had never been in such an overwhelmingly male environment.

All our interviewees entered large classes with few women. *Thirteen women in class – the classic 10%.* During the decades covered by our interviews, the University of Kansas School of Medicine (KUSM) consistently fell well below the nation in the percentage of women graduates – in some years reaching only half of the national average.

In Table 10.1, the number of KUSM female graduates ranged from a low of 2 (2.0%) in 1964 to 30 (20%) in 1975. In keeping with the national trend, the number of women

TABLE 10.1

KUSM and US Female Graduates by Year of Interviewee Graduation

	KUSM Number Female Graduates	KUSM % Female Graduates	US % Female Graduates
1948	5	9.0	7.1
1958	4	3.8	5.1
1960	5	5.1	5.7
1964	2	2.0	6.1
1965	4	4.0	7.3
1967	7	6.9	7.5
1968	4	4.0	8.0
1970	7	5.9	8.4
1971	7	5.8	9.2
1972	9	7.2	9.0
1973	9	7.6	9.1
1974[1]	28	11.7	11.1
1975	30	20.0	13.4

Note: Two classes graduated in 1974 due to overlap of three- and four-year curricula.

Sources: Braslow JB, Heins M. Women in medical education: a decade of change. *N Eng J Med.* 1981 May 7;304(19)1129–35; Dube WF. Women students in US medical schools: past and present trends. *J Med Educ.* 1973 Feb;48(2):186–9.

graduating from KUSM began to increase slowly in the late 1960s and jumped dramatically around 1974.

I entered in 1968. Eight women in the class. It was a banner year for KU to have eight women. Previously they had, like, two. They thought I was the first Black woman, but my family looked at all the old class pictures and picked out several Black women.

As discussed in Chapter 2, the increasing diversity in admissions owed much to external pressures, including the women's rights movement, but was strongly driven by legal actions against US medical schools over the admission of women, equal rights legislation such as Title IX, and non-discrimination criteria introduced by federal and other funding agencies.[3–6] The federal requirements directly impacted many of our interviewees as KUSM applied for several large federal grants in the early 1970s and scrambled to meet the new antidiscrimination criteria.[7] At the same time, the school came under increasing pressure from the state legislature to expand the class size and prepare more graduates for primary care, especially in rural areas.[8]

The combination of increasing local and national pressure resulted in the admission of many more students from minority groups, especially women, and several older students pursuing second careers in medicine. The classes of 1974 and 1975 were larger and very different from those of previous years. Our interviewees from those years were aware of being part of a *revolutionary group*. The introduction of the experimental three-year curriculum resulted in two graduating classes in 1974. The class 1974A completed the traditional four-year curriculum; their colleagues in 1974B were in the first class to graduate from the three-year program. Several interviewees from the 1974 and 1975 classes commented that their admission owed more to political and financial pressures than to institutional enthusiasm to increase the number of women in medicine, but at that time, they were only vaguely aware of the actual federal mandates and other external influences on the Medical School.

I arrived 1971. About 15 women in a class of 150. Huge increase for KU – previous class had, like, three women. Medicare had been introduced the previous year, and one of the federal requirements was at least 10% women.

I was in the three-year curriculum. Experimental class – very different from previous classes in more women, minorities, older students. Previous class had about seven women. Lots of characters in our class.

Thrilled to get in. We were the first big class of women – 22 of us. The previous class had about 6, and before that only a few.

I was admitted July 1972 to the three-year curriculum. Most unusual class – about 40/160 women (25%) and more Blacks and older students. The majority were still the traditional White males. My husband in the class of 1971 warned me there would be very few women and that I would be the only married woman, but I met another married woman on the very first day, and we became close friends.

Surprised by the large class, the number of women and coloreds. I think we had about 30 women. I had never seen or heard of a minority doctor.

Unusual class: 33/200 were women, better representation than previously, several Black classmates, and two classmates over 40 years of age.

The male environment was not simply a matter of numbers. The Medical School mirrored the medical profession in being an unambiguously masculine institution throughout the period covered by the interviews. This is well illustrated by the "Boys in White" study of medical student culture (based mainly on the KUSM class of 1958) that justifies exclusion of any considerations of female students by their small numbers and outlier status.[2] Even our interviewees from the class of 1975 with 20% women entered a world in which all physicians and medical students were assumed to be male. This was made clear from the first day of orientation. *During the welcoming address and all the talks, the speakers referred to men and their wives, etc., like there were no women in the room. On the first day, all students were required to give blood and urine for lab tests. The only urine collecting glasses were for guys – not designed for women to use.* After the fairly liberal attitudes of colleges in the late 1960s and the early 1970s, many felt they had entered a more restrictive and old-fashioned environment. Initially, some wondered if the institution had just not realized that female students might have different needs from their male classmates. Most female students quickly concluded that the medical school was at best an uncaring, and at worse a hostile, environment.

After KU, medical school was much more regressive in attitudes toward women.

Paradoxically, the institution promoted itself as "modern and progressive" based on increasing numbers of female students. An article in the December 1971 official newsletter boasted about KUSM admitting the largest ever number of women and compared the institution favorably to other US schools in "lack of male bias."[9] The article has a condescending tone, including the assumption that most of the female students would become pediatricians, and conveys a general bemused tolerance, illustrated by the subtitle "Skirts and Long Hair More Prevalent Than Ever."[9] In contrast to the jolly picture of happy and grateful co-eds conveyed by the article, the perception of most of our interviewees was that the Medical School *believed it had done enough by condescending to admit them. Nobody had thought through any of the implications of having more women or made any preparations for female students. The attitude was that [women] should be grateful to be there and behave [themselves], not make trouble – definitely not be asking for any special treatment or basic accommodations.*

From current perspectives, it is difficult to grasp the realities faced by female medical students in the decades covered by our interviews. They formed a small, highly visible minority that was incongruent with institutional expectations, norms, and values and thus likely to upset the status quo (deliberately or not). Women in US medical schools were distrusted and suspected of being troublemakers or overly demanding of special treatment. They were vulnerable to being marginalized, victimized, or suppressed, especially when the numbers were small.[10,11]

> "Women who enter the domain of medicine, which has been male defined, are likely to find that their presence is jarring and upsetting to others. First, women are unexpected and therefore feared as unpredictable. Second, their personal 'female' characteristics and qualities (which may be stereotypically imputed or actually theirs) are incongruent with those expected and valued for a physician."[10]

Prior to the 1970s, the few women in medicine could be stereotyped and expected to remain in acceptable roles and behave in ways that did not disturb the smooth functioning of the institution. "A stereotype of the woman doctor as 'hen medic' developed; hen medics were not necessarily mannish, but they were clearly unfeminine, that is unattractive and unmarried. These women doctors were seen as dependable because they were free from competing priorities."[10] The 1970s saw the admission of large numbers of young women who resisted being stereotyped and could pose a threat to long-established practices and assumptions. Against the turbulent background of that time, any student requests for change were likely to be perceived as instigated by radicals and troublemakers (including disruptive feminists); hence, any calls from women for accommodations or complaints about mistreatment were likely to meet with suspicion and/or resistance from institutions unwilling to show any signs of weakness. As cited earlier, all students from minority groups were expected to be deeply grateful for admission and not presume to ask for any further concessions from the institution or colleagues. Our interviewees were certainly not troublemakers, but they struggled to succeed in an environment designed for and governed by men. As in the majority of US medical schools of that time, masculine beliefs, attitudes, and perspectives determined and maintained the institutional culture of KUSM.[7,10] They permeated all aspects of the lives of students, from politics and policies to practical details of daily operations. Conflicts and intransigence over accommodations for women could arise over any issue, even personal matters, such as clothing.

Practical Issues: What Should I Wear? Where Can I Change? Where Do I Hang My Purse?

> "The student is symbolized by the uniform he dons at the beginning of the third year: the white shirt, trousers, and jacket he will wear through the remainder of his undergraduate and postgraduate medical training."[2]

Medical students were expected to always dress appropriately and required to wear a uniform in clinical situations. For third- and fourth-year students, the uniform was worn at almost all times, including at night calls. The required short white jacket and trousers were adapted for female students by the substitution of a straight white skirt (not too short) and hose. Uniforms for male students could be purchased in the student bookstore, but women had to find their own.

KU system was designed for males. It wasn't easy for them either, but women didn't fit in all sorts of ways. For example, uniforms (skirt and jacket) were required. Men could buy uniforms from the bookstore; women had to make them ourselves or get a seamstress to make them.

During the 1970s, when fashion reflected the revolutionary mood of young people, the Medical School tightly controlled the clothing worn by students. Even the 1975 graduates reported women were forbidden to wear pants or trousers. Perhaps because not wearing a bra was associated with radical feminism, the regulations for women included stipulations about underwear!

We were not allowed to wear pants. Had to wear dresses or skirts and always pantyhose, in case of "perineal fallout." I don't know what they were expecting!

They instructed us on our underwear – we had to wear bras!

Skirts were often impractical, as students were kept busy with ward tasks and were physically active. Examining and manipulating patients, performing tests and treatments, resuscitating patients, delivering babies, and multiple other activities required greater freedom of movement than could be easily and modestly achieved in a knee-length straight skirt. The attention to women wearing short skirts at all times was perceived by our interviewees as impractical, inappropriate, and *creepy* on the part of lewd-minded male faculty members and others.

Women always had to wear skirts. The rules were especially enforced on OB-GYN rotations. Ridiculous, as you were always clambering over things or bending down, and unless you wore ridiculously long skirts, it was embarrassing.

I was examining a patient in one of the big open wards at the VA hospital. When I straightened up, every eye was trained on my behind – they had all enjoyed a good view when I was bending over the patient.

One professor of OB was VERY insistent on dresses, NOT pants. He liked to look at the women's legs.

For surgery, we had to wear surgical dresses. On one occasion, I couldn't find a small surgical dress, so I put on a large one. The professor stopped the surgery, called me out for being "dressed inappropriately," and sent me out to find a smaller dress. This same professor insisted female students wore dresses or skirts.

One redoubtable mother came up with a solution and browbeat the dean into accepting it. *Women were not allowed to wear pants, had to be skirts. My mother went to Dean Waxman. Complained about her daughter having to climb on beds or resuscitate people with other able people being able to look up her skirt! She told him this is how it is going to be – she will wear culottes, and so will the other women. He said, "Okay, but they still can't wear pants." She made culottes for all seven women in the class.*

The regulation to wear pantyhose was never relaxed, even when the temperature was over 100 degrees, and much of the Medical Center lacked air-conditioning. Wearing hose was particularly uncomfortable and impractical on orthopedic rotations, when students were frequently assigned the messy tasks of applying or removing plaster casts. *On orthopedics, I was told I had to wear pantyhose. Putting on plaster casts, my hose and legs and everything got covered in wet plaster. Cutting casts off meant they got permeated with dust. I asked a resident to get me a pair of scrub pants to wear under my dress, but the nurse in charge told me I couldn't wear pants. I had to go back to the head of ortho for permission to wear pants.*

Some women in a 1974 class used clothing to protest negative attitudes to women, especially the showing of *Playboy* and pornographic images during lectures. They were quickly reprimanded. *In the first year, there was a lot of* Playboy *stuff going on. A classmate drew a picture of a uterus and ovaries as a stag's head with antlers and the caption "Death before Dishonor." My friend and I embroidered a copy of the picture on our lab coats (never worn in public, only seen in the KUSM labs). Well, this GREATLY offended the professors – we were notified it was inappropriate!*

Other women used clothing to express individuality – but only when safe to make minor protests against the system. *Regulations were less strict at the VA – I sometimes wore a hat with big sunflowers just to make the old vets smile. They could be in hospital for weeks.*

Clothing issues for female medical students were most problematic in the Departments of Surgery and Obstetrics and Gynecology. These departments were the strictest about enforcing the uniform code for routine clinical work and had stringent rules about attire in the operating rooms. Male students had access to a plentiful supply of surgical scrubs and use of the physicians' changing facilities and lounges. Female students were required to wear surgical scrub dresses – never pants – and nursing supervisors could be obstructive in providing dresses and allowing use of the nurses' changing areas. Women in the first groups of students to transfer to Wichita encountered great hostility from the senior surgical nurse supervisor at one of the hospitals. One student was told to buy her own surgical scrubs. She complained to the hospital administrator, citing illegal discrimination and hinting about legal action. The supervisor then issued her with two surgical dresses *so tight they fit all my curves, but I wore them anyway. Never looked so sexy.* Early female students at another Wichita hospital described changing in a public restroom after being barred from both the physicians' and nurses' changing areas. The intervention of a senior surgeon was necessary to allow female students to use the nurses' changing facilities. Even then, students were not welcomed and encountered difficulties in securing surgical dresses, hair coverings, and other necessary equipment.[12]

Despite modest and grudging accommodations, the overall surgical environments on both campuses changed very little over three decades. The comments of a 1975 graduate were identical to those of a member of the 1948 class.

There were no accommodations for women. We changed in nurses' locker rooms and had to wear surgical dresses.

In addition to the unfriendly environment, using the nurses' facilities put the female students at a significant disadvantage. The physicians' locker rooms provided more than space for changing and storing clothes; they incorporated areas for relaxation, discussion of cases, networking, and informal consultations among physicians. The space provided a valuable acculturation experience for future physicians and unparalleled opportunities for learning and mentorship. It also offered plentiful free food!

Women changed in the nurses' locker room. The guys used the doctors' locker room – it had treats and coffee, etc.

Where Can I Sleep?

During the third and fourth years, students were regularly required to remain in the hospitals overnight for admissions or to respond to inpatient needs. The students and interns needed places to sleep between calls. The most typical arrangement was a small room (often a converted patient room) adjacent to the patient care areas, operating rooms, or delivery suites. Accommodation was basic, consisting of two or four bunk beds, a desk and chair, and a telephone. Most rooms had an adjacent small bathroom with a shower.

In the 1940s and 1950s, our earliest interviewees reported being required to sleep in the nurses' dorm and recalled being locked out when trying to return from the wards in the early hours of the morning. *The housemother was NOT pleased to be woken up, especially if this happened several times during an obstetric case, when I had to check frequently on a woman in labor all night.* Individuals came up with their own arrangements. *On OB, one female classmate slept on a gurney in the hall as the dorm was too far when patients needed frequent checks.* Over time, the regulation was increasingly ignored, and the women shared accommodation with their male class-mates and interns. *When on call, female students were supposed to sleep in nurses' dorm – a long way from the wards – but they mostly slept in bunks in the call room, where the male students slept. Awkward, but never any problems.* All participants from the 1960s onward recounted sharing overnight accommodation with male col-leagues. Some commented that they mostly slept in surgical scrubs to save time and avoid issues over changing in mixed company. They recalled few problems, apart from some embarrassment or teasing, and saw the sharing as part of the expectations of proving they had the right attitude to be medical students. Some perceived that *the guys were more embarrassed than we were.* Apparently, some of the male students' wives were not pleased with the arrangements.

On OB-GYN rotation, four of us shared a call room, three guys and me sleeping on bunks. It was a bit uncomfortable at first, but we got over it. These three fellows and I celebrated the end of the rotation by going out for a beer. My classmate's wife was upset that he came home late. She even remembered this at our tenth-year reunion.

On call, slept in the same room as the guys and changed in the bathroom.

None of our participants recalled any attempts to enforce regulations concerning sleeping arrangements or to mandate separation of male and female students. Con-versely, when approached about providing accommodation for female students and residents, one senior administrator is reported to have commented on the perceived promiscuity of young people in the 1970s, saying, *They all sleep together, anyway, outside of the hospital.*

It Was Just the Way It Was

Sexism was rampant.

Sexism and casual misogyny were pervasive in US society during the decades cov-ered by our interviews. As traditionally male enclaves, medical schools may have been more overtly sexist than other environments, but they were by no means unique. Interviewees who had careers prior to medical school reported that the atmosphere was better for women in medicine than in other professions or in business. *I was a secretary after college. The only way you were going to work your way up was on your back.*

I think things were better for women than in other fields, like business.

Pervasive gender-based discrimination and sexism were vividly documented in a 1973 survey of 41 US medical schools as "an unremitting recital of Bad Things."[11]

Attitudes and behaviors that are now considered unacceptable or even repulsive were then accepted as normal and often tacitly encouraged by faculty and others. Even the female students did not regard the sexism as abnormal for that time. *There was a lot of sexually inappropriate behavior that I really only recognize retrospectively.* The class yearbooks convey an immature "frat house" image with frequent sexist or lewd comments and illustrations, especially of nurses in provocative poses. The 1969 Yearbook even had a *Playboy* theme with a highly sexualized cartoon of a scantily clad female student on the cover.[13]

When I see some of the things in our yearbook now . . . they were inappropriate, but I was involved in putting together the yearbook and wasn't paying attention or they didn't seem inappropriate at that time. Our interviewees conveyed the general understanding that women who voluntarily entered a traditionally male domain were regarded as *fair game* and *knew what they were getting into.* Indeed, the ability to handle gender-based harassment and worse was regarded by both the male and female students as part of training, an essential way for women to prove they had the right attitude and stamina to become physicians. Sexist comments and behaviors were regarded as distasteful and annoying but were expected as part of the training process. *Throughout training, we tolerated a lot of comments. During lectures, negative comments about women were very prominent, especially in sexualized areas. As a female in our time, we thought, "I'm only being prudish, or it's just the way it is." We put up with it.*

Gender-based hazing began on the first day of freshman orientation when an announcement was made that *male students were offered $15 for sperm donation – plus lewd comments about what the girls could do to earn $15.* In lectures and teaching sessions, all students were referred to in masculine terms and expected to participate in the robustly masculine culture. *I thought the approach was like the Marines – to break you down then build you back up in the expected image. It was derogatory, verbally abusive. A female approach was not valued. Playboy* images and pornographic material were common in slides and presentations as well as in posters and other materials, such as invitations to events. *Very first lecture, they showed slides of* Playboy *pictures, you know, topless. Nothing to do with the topic or context – maybe just to help the guys feel more relaxed? Also, the nurses invited all the new med students to a dance. The posted invitations from the nursing student body depicted the nurses using* Playboy *pictures as images of the nursing students. After all this* Playboy *stuff, we put up pictures of men from* Playgirl *in the student locker room. This caused great consternation among some of our male colleagues! We had to take them down.*

Comparisons and Reflections

Our participants vividly recalled their first impressions of medical school and their attempts to adjust to the unique environment they had worked so hard to enter. Although they knew classes would be large and male-dominated, the reality came as a shock, especially for those who had enjoyed small, student-centered classes with good representation of women during their final years at college. The institutional size, masculine culture, and uncompromising regimentation were daunting. The incoming female students knew they would be members of a minority that was not necessarily welcomed, could be resented, and was vulnerable to unfair treatment. They recognized that their colleagues, faculty, staff, and administrators held mixed and probably negative views on women in medicine. Studies such as those showing women were *twice as likely to drop out* were universally accepted, meaning, that even the most supportive faculty members believed that women were likely to fail or just give up.[14] Contemporary studies also concluded that women physicians would contribute significantly less to society; hence, the female medical students represented a waste of resources and denial of education to a man at a time of escalating physician shortage and mounting pressure on schools to train more doctors.[4,5,14] The female students of the 1960s and the 1970s were haunted by the "low value/poor productivity" issue throughout their careers, from premed counseling to retirement, but it probably was most openly expressed and had the greatest impact as they strove to establish themselves among their medical school classmates. Nevertheless, our interviewees conveyed a theme of being prepared for challenges and difficulties with comments like, *I knew what I was getting into*, or, *I was determined to show I could succeed.* They epitomized the priority characteristic for female students described in a 1976 review: "Until recently, toughness of character has been the first prerequisite."[15]

Writings about women medical students show an interesting contrast between the earlier post-WWII years, when women were a very small percentage of each class, and the period after the mid- to late 1960s, when the percentage of female students began to increase. The earlier group epitomized a non-threatening minority that served to make the institution look and feel unbiased and modern. As a medical school dean commented in 1967, "it would not look good to have so few women."[5] The trade-off for such tokenism was that the minority should be suitably grateful, behave appropriately, not cause any problems, and conform to the expected stereotypes. The stereotype conveyed to the earlier female medical students is strongly reminiscent of the "dilettante lady physician" of the 1890s who was decorative, amusing, and posed no real professional threat to her male colleagues.[4] The 1966 Macy Conference on Women in Medicine referred to evidence that "many women openly admit that they enjoy their minority status. It accounts for the certain niceties extended to each girl and gives her a sense of being special . . . particularly when they felt they had maintained a clearly feminine role."[5]

Conversely, as they required better qualifications to succeed in the admissions process, the female students frequently outperformed their male classmates academically. This conflicted with expectations and acceptable behavior. Overt and more subtle strategies to contain women's performance and control their behavior are well documented at all levels of medical schools at that time. It is also clear that some women adjusted their own behavior in order to conform to the expected feminine identity.[5,11] A speaker at the 1966 conference reported her experience:

> "It isn't right for a woman to have her hand up first with the right answer. It is probably a sorry state of affairs to say that sometimes I kept my mouth shut. . . . I am not sure this is right. It may reflect the social standards that are imposed on us and accepted while we are in med school."[5]

Survival strategies to avoid attracting attention or invite backlash in their professional or personal lives could have the tragic consequence of sabotaging academic performance. The 1966 conference includes an anecdote from a male student:

> "One of the girls, an exceptional student, had been engaged to another medical student who stood much lower academically than she. Apparently, the two had difficulties over this discrepancy, or at least the girl feared trouble, because on the last pathology exam she had tried to fail herself – succeeding only in getting a low grade – in order to block her chances of getting honors. 'That's what I can't stand about women medical students! They're always lousing themselves up, holding back their intelligence so that no one will think they're competing'."[5]

The women medical students of the later 1960s and early 1970s enjoyed larger numbers but still faced the stark reality of being identified as members of a minority group carrying multiple negative stereotypes and disadvantages. Indeed, their larger numbers could have increased antagonism, as some research suggests that when a minority reaches a critical mass of 15% of a population, it influences the majority culture, potentially triggering backlash and strategies to contain and control the minority.[6] The female students of the late 1960s and the early 1970s carried the additional burden of proving themselves in an institution where many believed that political and other external pressures had forced the admission of inappropriate students from minority groups. This was a national issue. A woman matriculating into a Californian medical school in 1973 observed:

> "I was surprised and delighted to learn that women had captured 40 of the 146 spots in the class. . . . Our class also had ten percent minorities. The older, darker, female students were lumped together under the heading 'nontraditional' students. We represented the aftershock of three political earthquakes: the civil rights movement, the feminist movement and the Vietnam War. Even those among us who had not marched or protested and yearned to shed the 'nontraditional' label knew that our presence in that class was related to factors beyond our individual endeavors. We shared a new collective consciousness."[6]

Our interviewees clearly expressed that they took any advantage that was offered in order to get into medical school and regarded the low expectations, negativity, and impostor accusations as stimuli to excel – *to show them!* They may have selectively remembered youthful bravado and suppressed, minimized, forgotten, or chosen not to discuss self-doubt, mistreatment, and distress. Most had learned in college to navigate, rather than directly confront, challenges. In medical school, they continued to utilize strategies of adaptation rather than confrontation, as shown in their descriptions of managing dress codes, on-call arrangements, sexist behaviors, and other aspects of an institution that had somewhat grudgingly admitted more women but made no efforts to accommodate their needs. Like our interviewees, we have no way of knowing if this striking neglect of female students on the part of the institution was deliberate or just lack of insight. Did those who controlled medical schools want to make life as difficult as possible for female students? Did they just not realize that women might differ from male students in some respects? Did they believe that being allowed to become medical students was such a privilege for women that they would not dare complain and would solve any issue that arose by themselves?

Most interviewees presented their stories about dress codes, on-call sleeping arrangements, and sexist behaviors as humorous anecdotes that illustrated the ridiculous things that happened in *the bad old days*. Only when asked for more information or to reflect on the incidents did they express sadness, anger, and some resentment. In retrospect, several attributed the institutional focus on dress codes to the need to demonstrate control over students by exerting authority over all aspects of their lives. This was particularly important during the decades of student protests, when any relaxation of regulations regarding student behavior could be interpreted as institutional weakness. For female students, challenging dress codes or sexist behaviors could be viewed as indicating "radical feminism" – a label that even distinguished female physicians found handicapping.[16] As a result, female students were forced to wear an impractical uniform and tolerate gender-based abuse for decades.

Our interviewees made no mention of group action or collaboration with other women to address problems or confront inappropriate language or behavior. Apart from the incidents of the *Playgirl* posters and when two friends cooperated to embroider a uterine-inspired symbol on their lab coats, the women addressed issues as individuals, and each took responsibility for solving her own problems. Our interviewees indicated several reasons for the lack of organized action by the female medical students. Most commented that they did not have the time or energy to organize like-minded classmates, analyze issues, strategize about solutions, and attempt to negotiate with an unsympathetic but powerful administration – and doubted if such negotiations would be tolerated, let alone be successful. They stressed that a woman had to be resourceful, independent, and self-sufficient to prove herself in medicine, and solving her own problems was one way to demonstrate these qualities – and prove she would not be a drag on her colleagues by expecting special treatment or having too many needs. This resonates with a 1967 survey of female medical students who were unsympathetic to special accommodations for women, citing "the stringent process of natural selection is necessary to ensure that those girls who reach medical school are prepared to give what the training demands."[5] Similarly, the KUSM women were very aware that any request for special accommodations bolstered suspicions about their commitment to medicine and willingness to make sacrifices for the profession. *The whole atmosphere was "married to medicine." You're not a good doctor if medicine doesn't always come first.* In addition, the women faced multiple different issues or had unique circumstances that limited the utility of sharing solutions and resources. They felt there was no single issue of such importance as to inspire a critical mass of students to risk taking action as an organized group.

In the 1960s and the 1970s, medical schools were intolerant of student activism of any type, and there was little sympathy for student "rights." For students and others without power, the risks of speaking out or having the reputation of a troublemaker were high. An outspoken woman was likely to be stigmatized as a "radical feminist," with real negative consequences, such as being dismissed or prejudicing letters of recommendation for internship or residency positions. In addition, individuals could not be certain of support from fellow students, as all were calculating the potential damage to their academic survival and professional prospects from any negativity in their records. Both the KUSM women and national surveys in the 1960s and the 1970s show that female medical students distrusted their female colleagues to support moves to address sexism and improve the environment. The national surveys indicate significant discord and antagonism among the female students between those who took a feminist and reforming approach and their colleagues who were more accommodating to the status quo.[5,11] A 1973 book minimizes the many positive responses to a survey about women's experience in medicine to convey a bleak picture of rampant mistreatment and discrimination as "an unremitting recital of Bad Things."[11] The same author dismissed women who chose to attempt to assimilate rather than change the culture as "proselytes" in a 1974 article.[17] All medical students, especially women, were very aware of the risks associated with causing trouble or being perceived as *too pushy*. In this environment, it is understandable that women generally tried to solve issues on their own or *kept my blinders on and ignored things, kept marching forward*. They needed all their ingenuity, adaptability, resilience, intelligence, and humor to navigate the large cast of characters and multiple experiences of medical school.

REFERENCES

1. Bowers JZ. Special problems of women medical students. J Med Educ. 1968;43:532–7.
2. Becker HS, Greer B, Hughes EC, Strauss AL. Boys in white. Chicago (IL): University of Chicago Press;1961.
3. Braslow JB, Heins M. Women in medical education: a decade of change. NEJM. 1981;304(19):1129–34.
4. Walsh MR. Doctors wanted: no women need apply: sexual barriers in the medical profession 1835–1975. New Haven and London: Yale University Press;1977.
5. Lopate C. Women in medicine. Baltimore (MD): Johns Hopkins Press;1968.
6. Martin T. When the personal was political: five women doctors look back. Lincoln (NE): iUniverse;2008.
7. Friesen SR, Hudson RP. The Kansas School of Medicine eyewitness reflections on its formative years. Kansas City: University of Kansas School of Medicine;1996.
8. Medical Faculty Proposes Plan to Alleviate Doctor Shortage. University of Kansas Medical Center and School of Medicine Bulletin. 1969 Dec;21(2):1–2.
9. Skirts and Long Hair More Prevalent Than Ever: Women in Med School Increasing Each Year. University of Kansas Medical Center and School of Medicine Bulletin. 1971 Dec.
10. Bourne PG, Wikler NJ. Commitment and the cultural mandate: women in medicine. Soc Probl. 1978;25(4):430–40.
11. Campbell MA. Why would a girl go into medicine? Old Westbury (NY): Feminist Press;1973.
12. Walling A, Nilsen K, Templeton KJ. The only woman in the room: oral histories of senior women physicians in a Midwestern City. Womens Health Rep (New Rochelle). 2020 Aug 24;1(1):279–86.
13. University of Kansas School of Medicine. Yearbook Class of 1969 Play Document.
14. Johnson DG, Hutchins EB. Doctor or dropout. J Med Educ. 1966;41:1107–274.

15. Spieler C, editor. Women in medicine. 1976 Report of a Macy Conference. New York (NY): Josiah Macy Jr. Foundation;1977.
16. Morantz RM, Pomerleau CS, Fenichel CH. In her own words: oral histories of women physicians. Westport (CT): Greenwood Press;1982.
17. Howell MC. Sounding board: what medical schools teach about women. NEJM. 1974;291(6):304–7.

11

The Basic Science Years: Classes, Consternation, and Cadavers

"In becoming medical students, the boys enter upon one of the longest rites of passage in our part of the world . . . that series of instructions, ceremonies, and ordeals by which those already in special status initiate neophytes into their charmed circle, by which men turn boys into fellow men, fit to be their own companions and successors."[1]

Although the curriculum changed over the three decades covered by our interviews, even the experimental three-year program of the early 1970s retained the basic structure of intensive instruction in the basic sciences, followed by immersion in clinical experiences. For 1965 and earlier graduates, the basic science component was taught on the Lawrence campus about 50 miles west of the Medical Center in Kansas City. From the first day in basic science, students were focused on acquiring knowledge and mastering technical skills, but they also had a strong sense of being initiated into an elite profession. Even more than their male classmates, women felt constant pressure to prove themselves worthy of a place in medical school. They were very aware of reports that women were twice as likely to drop out of medical school.[2] As a result, they tolerated a system that was often unfair or even brutal. They sublimated negative experiences as opportunities to prove they *had what it takes* to manage all the duties and challenges of a physician.

The expression "If you can't stand the heat, stay out of the kitchen" originated afterwards, but we understood the principle. We never spent time feeling sorry for ourselves. In fact, we felt lucky to have gotten into medical school at all.

The basic science courses were notorious for the long hours of lecture and the avalanche of information that overwhelmed even the best students. Medical students chafed under the system. They resented being taught by specialists in the scientific disciplines, many of whom they suspected of being focused on the minutiae of their subjects rather than information relevant to medical practice. Medical students struggled to keep up with the pace and volume of information and were obsessed with passing the frequent examinations and obtaining the best possible grades.

"First year 1954: after intensive orientation, subjected to massive inoculations of biochemistry, physiology, anatomy and related subjects in a *very uncomfortable* lecture hall. Constant pressure – only 60% passed first biochem quiz."[3]

DOI: 10.1201/9781003539568-11

The "Boys in White" study of Kansas medical students in the late 1950s describes the first year in Lawrence as a grueling Monday-to-Friday schedule of lectures and laboratory sessions from 8:00 a.m. till 5:00 p.m. with an hour break at noon for lunch. Brief breaks "for a smoke if you think you have time" occurred after some sessions, and the researchers recorded

> "About one-third of the boys went out to see the phenomenon of a girl with a very large bust who goes by the building at ten minutes of eleven every day. They all lined up on the very edge of the sidewalk. Some of them were standing on the stone seats so they could see better, and they were watching students as they came along, laughing and joking somewhat loudly together."[1]

In addition to classwork, smoking, and leering at co-eds, freshmen medical students spent most evening and weekend hours studying, plus regularly returning to laboratories after classroom hours to work on assignments. Overall, the observers calculated a 75- to 80-hour workweek. This continued throughout the decades covered by our interviews and was particularly demanding for women with families. A 1974 graduate recalled, *It was exhausting. For two years, I drove in every day from Leavenworth, dropped the kids off at day care, did classes all day, then drove home. The evenings were for cooking diner, housework, getting the kids to bed, etc., then I studied from about 9:00 p.m. to 1:00 a.m. and got up again at 6:00 a.m.*

Our interviewees confirmed that transfer of the basic science courses to the Medical Center did little to change the intense didactic program, faculty attitudes, or student perceptions. They suspected some faculty members took malicious pleasure in overloading the medical students with inappropriate information.

Felt hostile, hot, uncomfortable, not welcoming.

I didn't like the teaching method. They just threw out the information at you with no indication of what was really important or how to prioritize it. It was impossible, too much.

It was very difficult making it with all this overwhelming information – like an immersion course in a foreign language, a pressure immersion course in a foreign country.

The large classes plus the pace and pressure of the coursework meant students had little opportunity to develop relationships with basic science faculty members or even to ask questions. *No real relationships with them.*

TAs were helpful in basic sciences, but faculty were distant.

The students also perceived that some faculty members regarded teaching the large medical classes as an unwelcome distraction from their research priorities. Many appeared to resent having to teach medical students and regarded them as less competent and of lower priority than graduate students of *pure science*. The goal appeared to be to deliver as much information as quickly as possible with little investment in nurturing learning or understanding of concepts. Many students felt they were barely tolerated and were treated like children.

Some faculty were better than others. Questions were not encouraged. I always found it better not to be noticed. Faculty seemed preoccupied with research or whatever. It seemed like students were just in the way.

The first two years were mostly in the classroom and felt like college.

Early on, I was discouraged by the course structure, everything being organized alphabetically, having to sit there. It felt like grade school, "rinky-dink."

Overall, the descriptions of basic science faculty members from our interviewees match the negative characterizations of the "Boys in White," but some women had more positive recollections. A few individual faculty members were recalled as caring and good teachers.

First two years, faculty good, encouraging, but no real relationships with them.

Gross anatomy was scary. Upperclassmen warned us the professor was out for blood. His second-in-command was the kindest man. He held tutorials in the evening and really explained it, broke it down so we could understand.

The students resented their treatment, but the rapid pace and intense competition meant that most were struggling to survive. *It's only Monday and I'm behind already* was a standard comment. After their success in college and years of work to earn a place, medical school came as a rude awakening and a disappointing surprise. The women were particularly determined not to drop out, regardless of their treatment. For many of our interviewees, the new environment required learning different coping skills and ways of learning.

My father was a physician and tried to prepare me for the pressure of work. He said, "When you walk through the door, you'll be two weeks behind." I expected medical school to be hard as college courses had been, but medical school was not just difficult coursework – it had a hostile environment. The atmosphere and material were difficult and hostile. Miserable experience.

Study habits adopted in college of learning everything thoroughly were inappropriate for the volume and pace of material to be mastered in medical school. In the first exams, I froze and couldn't finish. Failed first exams. Talked to faculty and student services: I had to figure out a different way to study.

In the competitive atmosphere, all students were obsessed with success in the frequent examinations. "Boys in White" describes students as "being very frightened" of testing and going to great lengths to anticipate exam questions and gain any advantage.[1] Faced with an impossible volume of material, students attempted to prioritize studying items that they perceived as important in medical practice and/or high priorities for the basic science faculty. These two criteria did not always match. Faced with the necessity of passing the course, the faculty perspective took priority. The students scrutinized every nuance of faculty comments for indications of what would be asked on the examination. They were bitterly resentful of examinations that focused on what they perceived as *trivia or unimportant details*, but even angrier with faculty members who tested on material that had not been covered or emphasized in lectures, especially if the students felt misled by hints about the significance of specific items.[1] Students sometimes wondered if certain faculty members took malicious pleasure in student failure. The consequences of failure were high. In the lockstep curriculum, each course was only provided once per year. During the three-year curriculum, no summer break was available to remediate coursework. Failing one course could mean having to repeat a year or to drop out altogether.

The testing was intense.

I was preoccupied with keeping my head above water and succeeding academically.

Med school was hard. The hardest was pathology. The professor was a fiery, hot-tempered Italian who prided himself on making it as difficult as possible. Two of our class flunked and had to repeat the course. I had six weeks of tutoring but got through.

So many tests, and everyone was very competitive. Exams every alternate Saturday morning for 16 weeks, so weeks of no sleep on Friday nights. There was one infamous pathology professor who said "nobody passes" his test. It was multiple choice, and I think only about 10% passed. How could that go on year after year? It was wrong, stupid.

As during college, several women reported that their male classmates had advantages through networking with previous students, who coached them on what to expect in different classes and on strategies for success. The male students also had access to examination papers that had been returned with feedback to previous students. The different fraternities guarded their caches of course and examination material tightly and did not share with outsiders – including women. *Most of the boys were in the medical fraternities. They got lots of support, studied together, could get old papers and exams etc. I really missed out on this fraternity support.*

The guys were not friendly. They knew we were there, but they didn't help us. They had information about the tests and shared among themselves, but not with the girls.

Many men were supported by their wives. *The men in fraternities shared information and support – quiz files, exam papers. Their wives typed their lecture notes and reports.*

Throughout the three decades covered by our interviews, the basic science years were perceived by our interviewees as a challenging, almost brutal test of survival required for initiation into clinical training. This perception is also evident in the observations of sociologists studying the medical students of the 1950s, in various memoirs, and most vividly in the class yearbooks of the period.[3-7] Even allowing for the immature (and frequently pornographic) tone of the yearbooks, the resentment and disdain for the basic science faculty are evident. The 1970 Yearbook provides "hints for surviving the freshman year" that include learning how to cheat on tests and focus on minutiae. Anatomy faculty members are described as taking "delight in stumping students, giving lectures like spreading manure, and enjoying the students' difficulty of passing exams."[7] In contrast to the cynical and victimized tone of the yearbooks, some students thrived on the challenges and sought out every opportunity to learn about the practice of medicine, even during the basic science years.

The second-year classes (path, pharmacology, etc.) felt like a more level plane. I was a hard worker and excelled. On Saturday mornings, there were lectures on history of medicine, then clinical-pathological conferences (CPCs). The senior students presented the case, analyzed all the findings, and discussed. All the faculty participated, and the pathologist had the final word. My friends and I LOVED it. We had great admiration for the senior students presenting – so mature, confident. Would current students volunteer to give up Saturday mornings for such activities? I doubt it, but we loved it. Also, often if we didn't have an afternoon class, my friends and I would go to the OR to observe surgery – great experience!

Learning from the Dead

Cadaver dissection is an iconic feature of medical education, often portrayed as a litmus test for students to show "they have what it takes to become physicians."[1] Jokes and anecdotes abound about novice students fainting, vomiting, or otherwise reacting badly to the sights, smells, and requirements of anatomical dissection. An entire subset of medical student cadaver mythology concerns profane remarks and practical jokes directed toward female students. The observers in the "Boys in White" study commented that popular culture accepted medical student "cynical and obscene behavior, including harassing the girls in the class by gags with the sex organs of cadavers." The authors normalized such behavior as a coping mechanism for "the trauma of contact with death."[1] The same authors were surprised and disappointed by the general lack of inappropriate behavior during their observations of anatomy classes, even when students were unsupervised. The observers even tried to provoke the students into conforming to the stereotype, without success. Inappropriate events were "so startlingly rare that we tried to stir things up a bit ourselves by telling dirty jokes, getting little in return except a few smutty stories. Even these were not about medical school."[1]

Like the observers of the "Boys in White," we were surprised that few of our interviewees reported inappropriate behavior during anatomy dissection sessions. An early graduate (1960) commented that the move to the Medical Center could have been associated with more attention to respectful behavior around cadaver dissection.

Things were very different when we started in Lawrence. Nowadays, anatomy begins with ceremony to honor those who donated bodies, and it is all very respectful. NOT

*in our day – they just took us to the basement and pulled cadavers out of a vat. It was
not respectful. Surreal, traumatic.*

Improvements in attitudes and behaviors are more likely due to changing societal
norms and growing attention to professionalism in medical education.[8] Our interviewees volunteered a few anecdotes about misbehavior during dissection but regarded
episodes of gender-based mistreatment and harassment as normal male behavior for
the times. A 1965 graduate told of finding a penis attached to the cadaver of an elderly
woman one morning when she uncovered the body to continue dissection but passed
off the event as *supposed to be funny. . . . they wanted to see if I was shocked.* Similarly, a 1947 graduate stated that *harassment of female members of the class was
never so serious that it couldn't be laughed off,* then gave as an example the story of a
female student having a dissected penis put into her hands when she held them behind
her back while talking to another student. Harassment continued even into the classes
of 1974 and 1975.

*Most male students were collegial, but I felt resistance from my cadaver team. I was
the only woman, and they resented that I had "taken the place" of their male friends
who did not get into medical school. The sexually charged comments directed at
me were unpleasant, especially about my supposed discomfort in dissecting male
anatomy.*

*As we worked down the body into the pelvis, my three male partners started making
crude remarks – not nice. I said, "Enough is enough," but they kept laughing, and
the guys at the next table got involved. The professor came over and asked, "What's
going on?" I said they were driving me nuts with their comments, and asked, "Is there
another body I could work on?" He said lecherously, "Well I have a body you could
work on," and everybody just laughed.*

Despite these anecdotes, many interviewees recalled receiving significant support
from the other four to six students in their cadaver group, and several reported enduring friendships formed in bonding over cadaver dissection. *Did gross anatomy the
old-fashioned way with cadavers, so you became close with your lab partners.*

*Lots of encouragement and support from the three male classmates on my cadaver
team.*

*Having children and being older made it tough. Only two Black men in class. At the
first anatomy session, we "minorities" clustered together, so it was two women and
two Black men on our cadaver. We stayed friends long after medical school.*

Sometimes things did not start out well, but women recounted good outcomes if they
held their own against initial resistance from male classmates – even resulting in a
lifelong partnership!

*I was in the same small alphabetic group of about four for most of the first two years.
I was the only girl in our cadaver group, and the only one who hadn't gone to KU.*

They had all done anatomy so knew what they were doing. I hadn't done anatomy – I did biology – and didn't know what I was doing. One of the guys was upset that I would drag down the group score for dissection. He was pretty gruff and made comments about, "Why are you here?" "Why are you taking up a guy's place?" etc. I told him to get over it. He gruffly offered, "I'll teach you what I know after class. Can't let you mess up our score." After that, we became close friends.

I worked on a cadaver with three guys, all Wichita State grads, so they knew one another. I found it difficult to see the required structures after hours of dissection, but one of my classmates had beautiful illustrations and knew what he was doing, so I asked him to show me. He was very reluctant at first, but we became friends, and I married him after junior year. I always tell people we met over a cadaver.

The Preclinical Experience of Female Medical Students

Our interviewees recalled the basic science years as hectic and stressful. They noted multiple examples of sexism and ways in which they were treated differently from their male classmates. Mostly, they regarded the various "jokes," inappropriate comments, goading, or teasing as tasteless but seldom worthy of complaint or retribution.

Very first lecture, they showed slides of Playboy *pictures, you know, topless. Nothing to do with the topic or context – maybe just to help the guys feel more relaxed?*

It was like M*A*S*H: *off-color jokes, lots of prejudice.*

Sexist attitudes were pervasive nationwide – a faculty member in California commented, "I don't know why you women want to keep coming to medical school: then the men can't tell all the jokes and dirty stories they want to."[5]

Several interviewees commented that they knew what to expect and that the sexist attitudes and behaviors were normal for that time. The women were more visible and held to a higher standard than their male classmates. Being called out in lecture or having their shortcomings made public was common. Most expected this state of affairs, regarded it as normal, and often used it as an incentive to achieve even more. One attempted to hold a tormentor accountable – but only once she had safely completed all her coursework.

A physiology professor singled me out in lecture. Pointed me out. It was inappropriate and made me angry. The guys in the class came to my rescue. They told me to "just get out of it," "never mind," and helped me push past the incident. I confronted the professor after graduation at the big party. He apologized.

I didn't do well on a physiology test and was called in with another woman who also had not done well to talk to the professor. He told us, "If you're going to walk on your hands, you must do it perfectly." His meaning was that medicine was deviant behavior for females, so they were constantly being watched and performance had to be flawless.

Faculty members were almost all male and varied from highly supportive to aggressively misogynistic. One interviewee whose overall recollection was that *women were not treated differently* recounted that her assigned adviser was an exception. *He was a small bitter man – a PhD who had been refused entry to medical school – and his statements included, "How dare you take up a place here! Go home, get married, and have babies."* When the dean called her to task for not completing feedback forms on her adviser, she explained the situation and was promptly assigned a new adviser.

Despite the many challenges of the basic science courses, our interviewees persevered, and their confidence grew. As they approached the end of this first phase of medical education, they felt they had earned the right to advance to the clinical courses. They were excited about finally being involved in clinical medicine but aware that they would need to adjust the habits and skills that had served them in the basic science years in order to survive (and hopefully learn) in the very different clinical environment.

REFERENCES

1. Becker HS, Greer B, Hughes EC, Strauss AL. Boys in white. Chicago (IL): University of Chicago Press;1961.
2. Johnson DG, Hutchins EB. Doctor or dropout. J Med Educ. 1966;41:1107–274.
3. University of Kansas School of Medicine 1958 Yearbook.
4. Morantz RM, Pomerleau CS, Fenichel CH. In her own words: oral histories of women physicians. Westport (CT): Greenwood Press;1982.
5. Martin T. When the personal was political: five women doctors look back. Lincoln (NE): iUniverse;2008.
6. Chin EL, editor. This side of doctoring; reflections form women in medicine. New York (NY): Oxford University Press;2003.
7. University of Kansas School of Medicine 1970 Yearbook.
8. Anon. A brief history of medicine's modern-day professionalism movement. Basicmedical Key. Available from: https://basicmedicalkey.com/a-brief-history-of-medicines-modern-day-professionalism-movement

12

The Clinical Years: Patients, Professors, and Pimping

"The student now enters the clinical years of school. For the first time, the major part of his work consists of direct participation in the care and treatment of medical patients. He works in an institution which is only partly devoted to educational activities – a university medical center in which the care of patients is paramount and in which research also plays a prominent role."[1]

The change to the clinical phase of medical education was abrupt and dramatic. Then as now, clinical education strongly resembled an apprenticeship. The large class was split up into small groups that rotated through the major clinical specialties. Unless assigned to the same small group, students rarely saw classmates during working hours. Didactic teaching continued but took the form of presentations to small groups rather than formal lectures in a large auditorium. Everything was oriented around the clinical conditions of the patients cared for by the clinical team. Students were expected to study these conditions through extensive readings and to demonstrate their understanding of the material during the daily hospital rounds, when the entire team reviewed each patient. *At orientation to internal medicine, students were told to read about 80 pages of* Harrison's *textbook every night. I laughed. It was so unrealistic. Nobody else laughed.*

Instead of spending hours in lectures and laboratories, the students were expected to *learn by doing*. Unlike today's students, for our interviewees, *doing* included a great deal of practical work. The duties required of students varied by specialty and assigned team but generally included conducting and documenting the intake patient history and physical examination, then being responsible for daily reassessment and updating of the clinical record. Students had to be on the wards very early every morning to examine all their patients and update the charts before the interns and residents arrived to prepare for the faculty rounds. In addition, students had to follow up on any overnight developments or orders, ensure that blood was drawn for tests, and check the arrangements made for the day's treatments, tests, or procedures. Unlike modern medical students, those of previous generations performed many routine tasks, such as drawing blood, managing infusions, and even transporting patients for X-rays, tests, or surgeries. These practical tasks, known as *scut work*, feature prominently in medical student culture, with each generation claiming to have had a more brutal experience than their successors.

Students now don't do ANYTHING compared to what we did! WE did anything that had to be done – drawing blood, setting up IVs, taking histories, everything. Medical students had to get there early enough to get everything done.

DOI: 10.1201/9781003539568-12

We looked after all the patients and did all the bloods, IVs, scut work.

The 1964 Yearbook claimed third-year students were "catatonic from overwork and disasters, suffering from 'acute necrotizing scutitis,' for which the only treatment is faith and Dexedrine 10 mg qid!"[2] While this rather immature exaggeration is in keeping with the tone of the yearbooks, medical students did resent the heavy scut work, as it was tiring, time-consuming, and contributed little to their learning. Nevertheless, they performed the many often-menial tasks as the price of being tolerated in the clinical environment – even as *the lowest of the low*. This could include being sent out for food in the middle of the night for hungry residents. *On obstetrics, there was a tradition of sending the student to get BBQ. I refused to go to the REALLY bad area of town on my own in the middle of the night to fetch BBQ. They were NOT happy.*

On some units, especially those at the Veterans Administration (VA) or community hospitals, students had a frightening amount of responsibility for patient care. *It was a different era. Medical students had a lot of responsibility, often unsupervised. We wrote orders and nurses carried them out because everyone else (residents and attendings) was in surgery. I'm not saying the care was bad – we worked hard to give the best care, but we were independent a lot of the time, especially on surgery. On surgery, there was not a lot of teaching. At the VA, I was writing orders on septic burns patients. At the VA, the rule was, anyone in the ER at 4:30 had to be admitted, so we went up to the ward and there was a line of patients to be treated. We did sutures and everything unsupervised because the others had gone home.*

Patients

Students had very close contact with their assigned patients and often developed mutually beneficial relationships. The interviewees consistently reported that many patients were initially surprised to encounter a female student physician but almost all were encouraging and helpful. Indeed, the group expressed a theme that patients preferred female students and made efforts to support them – even ordering the male students to do more of the work!

An elderly lady got upset when I was pushing her on a trolley down to X-ray for a colonoscopy as I was pregnant. She yelled "You shouldn't be pushing me in your condition. Get the men to do the pushing!"

I think they were just surprised and were very kind about it, especially the older men. They were not rude, in fact were helpful. I think occasionally they went easier on the girls. I remember one diabetic older man took a lot of trouble to show me exactly which vein from which to take the blood. I expect he didn't want multiple sticks!

Most patients were very kind. They knew they were in a teaching hospital. As long as we treated them ok and with respect, they were kind and wished us well. The women and a lot of the men were very supportive of the girls and made it easier.

No big issues, occasional little things. I think the patients liked the women, they got more attention, we listened better. We were well received.

The few recollections of negative patient interactions were attributed to embarrassment rather than antipathy from male patients. We did not encounter any recollections of patients being rude, insulting, or threatening toward female medical students.

A lot of patients liked having a woman, especially the female patients. The men were often surprised to have a woman doing the physical. They were embarrassed, not rude.

I don't recall being treated disrespectfully or inappropriately by patients. Maybe some incidents at VA over catheterizing men. Also, guys could be embarrassed by being woken early in the morning by a young woman to draw blood.

Our interviewees overwhelmingly reported that their youthful appearance was more of a concern for patients than their gender. They were regularly teased or patronized as looking too young to be student physicians.

Frequent comments: "You're awfully young to be a doctor."

Mostly, patients were very good, but sometimes problems. More about looking too young than being female. One patient told the attending, "I almost asked for her birth certificate."

Got along pretty well with patients. I looked pretty young and was incredibly naive. Maybe they didn't have confidence in me. Some embarrassment and lack of confidence around male patients and sensitive issues. I had an intention tremor – remember a patient's apprehension when I was shaking getting ready to suture him!

Multiple comments about being just a little girl, but kindly, and they never asked to replace me. I think they were just surprised and were very kind about it.

I was very young and looked even younger so a lot of the time they were astonished, I was not what they expected, sometimes they would question what I was doing. I think it was more about looking young than being a woman.

The only other recurrent issue for female students with patients was being mistaken for a nurse. None of the attendings or colleagues on the health-care team intervened to clarify the female student's role. Our interviewees may have found being mistaken for nurses frustrating, but they took it in stride. Some commented that this assumption had dogged them throughout their long careers.

Patients regularly thought I was a nurse and asked us to do nursing things, like changing the bedpan. We learned to adapt.

Often thought I was a nurse. Nobody corrected them, so I got sent off to do things like fetch a glass of water.

Patients were fine. Still always someone who assumes that if four people walk into a room, the woman is a nurse. That still happens.

Sometimes patients and other people called me a nurse, but I think it was more a mistake than an insult. Most patients were very positive toward female students.

Patients were always surprised by a female physician; we were always assumed to be nurses.

Frequently had to remind them we were MD students. They assumed we were nurses or social work staff.

Clarifying the differences between medical students and nurses had to be done tactfully and with no hint of disrespect for nursing. No matter how frustrated or annoyed, female medical students could not afford to give the impression that they considered themselves superior to nurses or were insulted by being assumed to be nurses. As students were so tightly embedded in the clinical team, nurses played a crucial role in medical student success (even survival) on clinical services.

Nurses

I realized early on it was very important to have good relationships with nurses. They had power and insights. They can help you a lot or make you look terrible. Medical students were pretty low on the totem pole – we got the menial tasks.

Nurses were essential to completing the daily work and could influence how attendings and others perceived the student. In addition to practical help, they could be valuable teachers, pointing out ways to get things done and tactics for medical students to look good to residents and attendings. Many interviewees expressed great appreciation for the nurses they encountered during their training – including some homespun advice! *Some nurses were absolute wonders. I think they realized we were doing our best and it was not easy. One told me when I was having a rotten time, "Honey, just think of medical school as one shit sandwich. Take one bite at a time. Soon, it's all done, and you don't have to do it anymore."*

I generally got on well with nurses. My mother was a nurse, and I have lots of respect for them. I was not treated badly by nurses. They could be tremendously helpful – making suggestions like, "You know this could help," or asking, "Can I help?"

Nurses bailed us out, they knew so much.

Conversely, nurses could be obstructive, difficult, or hostile, making the student experience miserable. Nurses working in operating rooms had a particularly bad reputation for hostility to female medical students. This went beyond the issues over changing rooms and clothing mentioned previously to cover multiple aspects of the surgical environment.

I remember the formidable OR chief nurse roughly teaching us how to behave, giving us the what-for and laying into us about gowns, handwashing, etc.

Scrub nurses hated us. It was a nightmare. Nurses in general treated us lower than bacteria. It was pretty awful.

Students were pre-warned or quickly learned to cultivate good working relationships with nurses. Mutual respect was essential.

Dad told me the secret was to go to the most strict nurse and ask her to show you how to do things. He said, "Win her over and the nurses will not let you fail." So I always went straight to the meanest baddest nurse and asked her directly to show me. I always called her ma'am and was very respectful. No problems with nurses!

I treated them like human beings, and they treated me the same way. I realized early on that nurses did most of the work. They could make you or break you, so I made an effort to be pleasant and complement them, thank them, not to give myself airs.

You got what you gave. If students were friendly and nice, nurses reciprocated; if people were abrasive and rude, they got the same reaction from nurses.

Excellent – always got along very well with nurses. Never any trouble. Some best friends. They were very good and could teach you a lot. I was always eager to learn. I quickly figured out they knew stuff the professors didn't know. I was always talking with the nurses.

Although the majority of our participants recalled nurses as being helpful if treated respectfully, several perceived that male students received deferential treatment. Some attributed this to attitudes that medicine was an inappropriate profession for women, others to romantic competition.

In the 1940s, our earliest interviewee laughingly recalled *the nurses were looking for dates. We girls were competition;* but similar comments were made even by graduates of the 1970s.

Nurses hated the female medical students. They were either old and crotchety or young and looking for a husband. Lots of discrimination against female students. The nurses favored the males in providing equipment, such as needles (no disposables in those days). Good-looking guys were handed the best needles, and we got the old blunt, crooked ones.

If I was called at night to insert an IV, I had to search around and find everything, all the equipment, for myself; but if a guy had to do it, the nurses were all running around to set up for him. The nurses wanted to date the guys.

Nurses were deferential to the men. If one of the guys asked for something, the nurse would fetch it for him; if a girl asked, she would be told to "get it herself."

Residents and Interns: Friends or Foes?

Hard work and subservient behavior were expected to please or placate residents and perhaps motivate them to treat students well – or even provide some teaching! Interns and residents controlled the medical students' daily workload. Our interviewees reported mixed experiences in the use and abuse of this power. Some residents and interns were supportive teachers and positive role models; others appeared committed to perpetuating the cycle of hazing and abuse from which they had suffered as students only a few years earlier. Many were passively hostile. *We tolerated each other.* A certain level of rough treatment was expected and generally interpreted as intended to keep the students in line. *Generally treated students pretty well but liked to harass us at night, play pranks like not telling students about things that needed done till really late or calling at 1:00 a.m., when we were trying to sleep.* The overall impression was that, with few exceptions, a diligent student could expect reasonable treatment. Some specialties, such as surgery and obstetrics, had reputations for being particularly hard on students, but even in these specialties, individual residents or interns could be helpful and supportive. *Residents were generally okay. Surgery could be difficult; I try not to think about it. Some residents in OB treated us like servants, but I had good residents in surgery, pediatrics, internal medicine.*

If you did your work and worked hard, they treated you pretty well, friendly and nice.

Interns and residents were variable – some were serious about instructing, others just wanted students to do jobs, drawing blood, etc.

Some were jerks, but mostly okay. We were not mistreated except by the jerks.

Some units even developed a sense of camaraderie among students, interns, and residents.

I thought it was a good structure working with the residents. We always had help, were in it together, a group effort.

Most were very kind – they remembered suffering through the glories of medical school.

Interns and residents overall were very helpful and supportive. I got along very well. They understood and sympathized with our lowly status. I did get "chewed out" by one surgical resident who criticized me for not paying attention during an informal discussion.

Our interviewees stressed that both male and female students were victimized by some residents and interns. These *jerks* were also likely to behave inappropriately toward nurses, staff, and even patients. Only a few interviewees perceived that female medical students were targeted for verbal or other abuse. *Residents varied a lot – some treated teaching as something they had to do, some were great. I don't think the residents treated the women any differently.*

I thought the OB-GYN residents were not respectful toward women – all women, patients, too.

The residents were pretty rough on everybody. We did what we were told to do to get the work done. Took it in stride. Bloods had to be drawn and patients seen, etc., before the residents came to the wards.

A male resident startled me once by coming up behind me and saying, "Nice legs." I thought that was inappropriate, as I was married.

Female students often found themselves as the only woman in the group of students assigned to a unit. While the majority of our participants did not recall women being treated differently from their male classmates, they conveyed a theme that women were more visible and held to higher standards by residents, almost all of whom were male.

I don't recall any negative experiences with residents. We [women] recognized that we were working harder than the men. We had to do more.

Conversely, a 1971 graduate recalled rampant self-serving sexism by residents.

They wanted us in the hospital every minute of every day. Not good at teaching. Very sexist. Even the married ones flirted heavily with nurses. At that time, a lot of men wanting to be doctors looked for a woman to put them through medical school. They would marry nurses or other women who worked, but after they were through, they divorced them.

In all their recollections of resident and intern interactions with students, our interviewees stressed the very different environment of medical school and hospitals over 40 years ago. At that time, gender-based teasing and hazing were normal behavior and expected by any woman entering a male environment.[3] Institutions were also very different in the period covered by our interviews. Medical centers, especially the clinical units, were strictly hierarchical and dominated by a few powerful and autocratic men.

Overall, residents treated us all right – they treated us better than some of the faculty.

The Faculty: Teachers or Tyrants?

The faculty was a *patriarchy. A lot of male chauvinists, especially the older guys.*

From current perspectives, it is difficult to appreciate the power wielded by senior faculty members during the decades covered by our interviews. Department chairmen and the heads (chiefs) of clinical units had almost unfettered power to ignore, belittle, and abuse learners and staff at will – or encourage, mentor, and advance individuals who secured their approval. Each class yearbook lists the winner of the annual Silver Stallion Award – "to the teacher or administrator who goes out of his way to make life hell for medical students."[4] Throughout the decades covered by our interviews, the yearbooks portray key faculty leaders as powerful and autocratic figures, more feared (even hated) than respected. Cartoons include depictions of faculty members as kings, emperors, generals, dictators, or even the heads on Mount Rushmore. In one yearbook, they are depicted as butchers, gleefully feeding students into a meat grinder.

No women appear as faculty leaders in the archival material or yearbooks during the 30 years covered by our interviews. Some of our participants could not recall any female faculty members. Most remembered a few individuals, but only six female faculty members were mentioned during the 37 interviews, despite specific questions about female faculty members or role models. The few female faculty members mentioned often kept low profiles, but some are remembered as positive influences and role models.

In the 1950s, there was only one woman on faculty, and she was a very good teacher. One other woman came in to give lectures but was not faculty. I had no particular mentors.

Very few female faculty members. Dr. L . . . was wonderful, dynamite. She was a real bright spot.

Very few women on faculty. There were a few good female role models, but nobody thought about mentoring. Looked up to Dr. S. . . . She was a wonderful teacher, did a wonderful job, and later a mentor. One woman in OB was also a very good teacher. There was one woman pathologist who was married and had a family, and another who was "odd" and turned out to be paranoid.

Few female faculty members around. They were amazing women, all so busy and had children. Did not mentor female students unless in her area of interest. Another couple of women who became faculty may have been fellows at that time.

Senior faculty members wielded great power. Student evaluation was based almost entirely on the faculty members' subjective impressions; hence, students were almost totally dependent on key faculty members for grades and the letters of recommendation essential to obtaining a place in a residency or internship program. Our interviewees described the frightening paradox of needing to impress powerful faculty members but risking the awful consequences of being noticed for ignorance, mistakes, or some infraction of the unwritten code of conduct for medical students.

The students came into direct contact with faculty members most frequently during the daily ritual of patient rounds. After frenetic preparation, rounds began each morning when the faculty member (the attending physician) arrived on the unit, expecting to be updated on the status of each of his patients. All other work stopped as the attending, residents, interns, students, senior nurses, and others made a formal procession from patient to patient. At each patient's bedside, the student assigned to the case provided an update and tried to answer questions from the attending and the residents. Attendings were expected to probe student presenters on the diagnosis and management of the case, but also on their understanding of the disease and related medical conditions. This could be a constructive combination of oral examination and teaching from a master clinician; however, some faculty members were notorious for the aggressive questioning and public humiliation of students and junior staff during rounds. Female students frequently found themselves the only woman present and the target of such *pimping* and abuse. Students were powerless to resist bullying by faculty members, and nobody dared intervene on behalf of a victim or criticize an attending, even when he was wrong.

In clinics, lots of bad examples from the faculty. I thought, "There must be a better way to teach!" We were treated like shit. So many bad incidents, for example, being overridden when I had given a correct answer about an organism that had two alternative names. Pimping could be brutal. Another female student was reduced to tears by grilling from a huge group during rounds, but the questioning did not stop. I still feel guilty about not intervening to help her. On another occasion, a male student was being quizzed relentlessly on rounds and was so mad he just walked away. Rounds could also be tedious, non-productive. I recall rounds lasting five hours on infectious diseases and being pimped on minutiae when students were tired and had so much work and so much reading to do.

Questions were not encouraged. I always found it better not to be noticed. I hope women don't feel so oppressed that they can't speak up if they don't understand anything. I am haunted by not speaking up – I saw an attending do something wrong, I looked it all up and it was wrong, but if I said anything, I would have been fired. The patient did okay.

The most extreme pimping occurred during the Saturday noon clinicopathological conference (CPC). This iconic event was held in a large auditorium to accommodate all students, interns, residents, and many attending physicians. One team of students and residents presented a case selected for its diagnostic challenge. They then had to defend their diagnostic and management decisions against a barrage of questioning from the audience, especially the powerful clinical chiefs. All the senior clinicians were present, competing to propose the most obscure diagnoses and demonstrate their knowledge of the latest research and most up-to-date treatments. The entire atmosphere was combative, *like a gladiatorial contest to stay on your feet until the pathologist gave the final blow – the autopsy diagnosis.* Although the CPC was an opportunity to demonstrate clinical acumen before the entire medical community, students were terrified of presenting or of being called out from the audience for a question. The chairman of internal medicine (Dr. D) was notorious for publicly humiliating CPC participants. The medical student ballad in the 1957 Yearbook conveys the students' feelings of helplessness:

"There's a learning experience each Saturday noon
You can feel the tension throughout the whole room

If your number comes up, just give up, nothing helps
Give your soul to the lord 'cuz your rear end is D. . .'s!"[4]

After returning from WWII, Dr. D held several leadership roles in the Medical Center, culminating in chairmanship of the internal medicine department throughout the 1960s. Even in a faculty of strong personalities and competitive male egos, Dr. D dominated the Medical Center like a colossus. A history of the school claims that *his self-discipline, integrity and imposing personal appearance placed him among the most the most inspiring teachers and leaders the School of Medicine has ever produced.*[5] Stories about his dominant personality abounded.

Dr. D had a reputation. He was pretty strict that everything had to be done HIS way. You had to have ALL the information on patients ready for presentation. He was incredibly particular, especially about the history; he was really into the full social history of each patient. He would call you out if things were not right. Everybody was afraid/in awe of him. Someone was stationed at a window to watch for his car (a distinctive black sports car) driving in at 6:30 a.m. and to shout, "He's here!"

On one occasion, a used bedpan was in the patient's room during rounds, and Dr. D asked a cleaner to remove it. When she retorted it was not her job, he threw the bedpan into the corridor and said, "NOW it is your job." Residents and students were aghast.

The autocratic head of medicine had strong opinions about the hierarchy of specialties. Of course, internal medicine was at the top. It was okay for girls to do pediatrics because women like children. Psychiatrists were all crazy, pathologists beyond help. One of the male students in my group was interested in psychiatry, and Dr. D was horrible to him.

Students were afraid of Dr. D, but we were surprised by the contrasting opinions expressed by our interviewees. Several regarded him as the worst bully and most egregious practitioner of the cruel pimping style of teaching. One of our interviewees even reported that he drove her *into clinical depression.* Conversely, a surprising number of our participants remembered him as an outstanding clinician and a tough but worthwhile teacher.

Dr. D was hard on everyone. He wanted to make sure you knew your stuff.

He was a legend. Very reserved – you never knew what he was thinking. Outstanding clinician. He was really nice to me, showed me lots of extra things. He was a very nice man, but very intimidating to some.

Even those who spoke negatively about Dr. D acknowledged that he commanded respect. Fifty or more years later, several women shuddered at the recollections of being on his service. We have noticed that his is the first name mentioned (for good or bad) whenever alumni are asked about faculty members. He certainly dominated the institution and set the tone of medical teaching for generations.

What Was Medical School *Really* Like for Women Prior to 1975?

Terrible and wonderful at the same time.

Our interviewees presented a very mixed picture of how women were treated during medical education in the period 1945–1975. Most described an experience characterized by constant pressure and hard work punctuated by highs and lows. Although several recounted episodes of mistreatment and misery, only one recalled continuous abuse, about which she was still resentful. *Horrible experience. Toxic environment, sexual harassment, especially in the first two years, but some in clinics, on rounds. Males at all levels felt entitled to disrespect women. We were the underdogs. Not valued or appreciated. Constantly embarrassed and humiliated. It was a horrible, horrible experience. Horrible. Faculty acted like students were imposing on them, annoying. Treated us badly. I remember a surgeon screaming at me so loudly I could not hear what he was saying.*

Positive assessments were much more common. *Very busy, a lot to learn, a lot of work, fascinating. I liked medical school, enjoyed it.*

Overall, very positive. Great camaraderie. I wish I could do it again. I really enjoyed medical school. We worked hard together, and all wanted to do well and help each other succeed. It was a very good education. I liked all the classes: LOVED being in clinics.

One participant compared her experience very favorably to that of students attending a Californian medical school, where she was a resident. *My education was superb. I feel lucky, privileged. I really appreciate KU. The medical students got priority. They got a lot of attention and teaching focused on their needs. It was fortunate for me to be a student at KU.*

Several women from the earlier classes commented that they did not believe female students were treated badly, and a few even expressed the belief that women were treated better than their male colleagues. Several related this to the greater visibility of female students. For better or worse, they attracted more attention from the faculty. Some perceived this as unwelcome attention or persecution; others used the situation as motivation to succeed.

Since there were so few women in our class, we could never get lost in the crowd. We were the first ones whose names the teachers learned. Our successes were immediately noted. But so were our deficiencies. The knowledge that there was no possibility of being unnoticed stimulated us to greater effort.

Treated quite well. I have no memory of being disrespected, pointed out, and didn't feel I was subjected to hardships. Quite the opposite – girls kind of standing out. I think an average girl got more credit than an average guy. I never felt any discrimination.

Conversely, some interviewees felt ignored by faculty members and attributed this to either disapproval of women's presence or low expectations.

I have been trying to figure out the attitude of the male faculty – it was kind of different, skeptical. I think they expected women to get married and drop out.

We were not so much mistreated as "overlooked," "not recognized." The worst was surgery. Seemed like we were just retractor holders. It didn't really bother us at that time – it seemed normal.

We encountered several apparent contradictions when an interviewee described her medical education as a wonderful experience and/or stated women were well treated but also provided examples of what is now regarded as blatant discrimination, mistreatment, or even abuse. Such episodes ranged from subtle discouragement to overt sexual harassment.

Faculty were mostly fine. A few didn't take kindly to so many women in the class. It was subtle – facial expressions were different when responding to the guys. Definitely different with the females in tone of voice, curt. We felt the hostility and didn't want to ask questions.

Mostly nice – none I didn't like. The OB-GYN lectures slipped Playboy *pictures into the slides.*

The faculty was terrific. Great in basic sciences, some amazing mentors in the clinical years. My mentors were so kind, especially in surgery. Let me do my first appendectomy – talked me through it. He was an older doc. Did surgery as an early rotation. Loved being in the OR. Loved ortho being able to fix things, make them well. Make things function, work. The orthopedic department was very supportive – helped me get rotations and internship in San Francisco. There was a lot of sexually inappropriate behavior that I really only recognize retrospectively. The worst was in psychiatry. At a diner, the women kept moving away from one man. When I ended up next to him, he was all handsy under the table.

One of the instructors in anatomy brushed his hand on girls' bottoms every single time he walked past. Nobody ever called him out for it.

Treatment was not too bad. They did prefer the men and gave the impression the women were usurping a man's place. We did get sexual harassment from instructors. The male junior faculty were a problem. One of the professors was well-known for wanting to have an affair with every single female going through. He was never called out publicly.

Participants repeatedly cautioned that their experiences must be viewed in context. Almost all forms of gender-based mistreatment were *normal for that time.* What is now regarded as toxic masculinity was not only tolerated but was also condoned, if not encouraged, by colleagues, teachers, classmates, and society in general.[3,6–11]

Some of the behaviors of the old doctors were bad, would be considered unacceptable now, but we shrugged it off: boys will be boys.

I was treated reasonably well, but we tolerated a lot of comments. During lectures, negative comments about women were very prominent, especially in sexualized areas.

In addition, participants frequently reminded us that their male classmates were also subject to the hostile environment and mistreatment. *Didn't treat the women any worse than the guys – but that was pretty badly. Everyone was demeaned, hazed.*

I recall only one male faculty member who made me tear up and said, "If you're going to cry, you shouldn't be in medical school," BUT he made everybody miserable, males as well.

One of our interviewees compared the clinical teaching to Marine boot camp. The same metaphor was used by a female graduate of a Californian medical school in the 1970s.[7] Our interviewees also drew comparisons in the roles and expectations for women portrayed in the television programs *M*A*S*H* and *Mad Men*.

I thought the approach was like the Marines – to break you down then build you back up in the expected image. It was derogatory, verbally abusive. Not just to me or the women – mainly to the men. It was an uncomfortable environment. They placed high value on being aggressive.

Faculty were condescending. I was not easily intimidated. I objected to some of the ridiculousness – they said it was character-building, but my character was already built! I was not treated any differently because female, never any improper sexual advances or anything like that. Lecturers made the occasional sexist joke. Not surprising, maybe a little offensive, but it didn't pay to object. I had so much more on my mind. I felt lucky to be there – impostor syndrome. I was older, no biochemistry in college, admitted because of a change in policy. I didn't want to rock the boat. Derisory comments were usually directed at everyone. I don't think the women were singled out more than the men. Everybody was treated badly on clinics.

Overall, our interviewees recalled their medical school experiences as tough and challenging but worthwhile. The mass of data from 37 participants over a 30-year period includes numerous anecdotes, recollections, and opinions filtered through personal perspectives, biases, and motivations. Generalizations are unwise. Becoming a physician is a complex and very individual experience, but we were struck by the number who recalled the experience fondly – only two interviewees were scathingly critical. The majority expressed a great sense of achievement – they had taken on a huge challenge and succeeded. They realized from the beginning that medical school would be demanding intellectually, physically, and emotionally, and that as women they faced additional challenges. They navigated the process to the best of their abilities, not always successfully. They encountered a great range of experiences and a huge cast of individuals, some good, some bad, and several unfair. The dominant themes were determination and resilience, plus pride and gratitude for their careers as physicians.

They had worked hard to earn a place in medical school and were determined to succeed no matter what was required. The group did not convey a sense of victimization or resentment. Conversely, they stressed that misogyny was prevalent in society at that time and that their male classmates were also abused by the system. Both in our interviews and in published surveys from the 1960s and the 1970s, female medical students appeared to regard challenges and unfair treatment as opportunities to prove they had the robust attitude expected of physicians.[6,11]

No expectation that girls would be any different, and "no quarter" given or expected.

Our interviewees are a select group of women who succeeded in medicine and were willing to share their recollections. The information gathered could be influenced by recall bias or being unwilling to share uncomfortable information. Nevertheless, they openly shared both positive and negative recollections, and consistency was apparent across the interviews. The spectrum of experiences they reported is validated in three surveys of female medical students in the 1960s and the 1970s.[6,11,12] These surveys also report very mixed experiences but draw diametrically different conclusions. A study conducted in 1965 has a surprisingly optimistic tone, reporting that "many women openly admit they enjoy their minority status."[6] Like several of our interviewees, the women in that survey perceived they were more visible and held to higher standards than their male classmates but, also like our interviewees, regarded such treatment as incentives to "work harder and do a better job in order to be accepted."[6] Despite incidents of inappropriate treatment, many felt "it was definitely an advantage to be a woman in medical school."[6] A decade later, a 1975 study involving interviews and a survey of 154 female students and 195 faculty, house staff, and administrators at 11 medical schools described "a complex mixture of inherent and contrived difficulties but lauded the dramatic improvements and encouraging improvements in attitudes toward women students over the last decade."[11] The authors presented a positive picture of the female medical student experience, concluding that although many issues remained to be resolved, the major challenges for women in medicine had moved to residency training.[11] These positive conclusions are in dramatic contrast to the "unremitting recital of Bad Things" reported by a 1973 survey that documented pervasive, multifaceted discrimination and mistreatment based on 47 questionnaires returned from students at 41 medical schools.[12] Despite the highly negative tone of the report, many positive or neutral comments were recorded, and the vast majority of respondents would encourage other women to enter medicine. The author attributed such comments to suppression of negative experiences. "We sometimes deny that knowledge because discrimination is painful to experience," or as a survival strategy.[12] In a later article, she insinuates that women who speak positively of their medical education are traitors to their gender. "Women who defend their own self esteem by 'joining rather than fighting' are, like most proselytes, especially firm in their denial of the existence of medical school discrimination against women."[13]

These very different views emphasize that no writer or researcher, no matter how well intentioned, can be completely objective, especially in a highly charged subject such as discrimination and mistreatment of women. Our interviewees described a complex and multidimensional tapestry of people, places, events, and experiences that were recalled, with a few possible exceptions, as neither completely wonderful nor unremittingly bad. They knew they were intruding on an inflexible male environment and did not expect special treatment or an easy progress. The predominant themes for all interviews were resilience, adaptation, and appreciation of the opportunity to become physicians.

On the wards, there were more problems, interactions that probably would end up in court today, but we/I was so intent on school, learning, taking care of patients, so we/I didn't worry a lot about things that might be said. "Mind your elders and go" – that was the way it was. I was fairly liberated to get there and paid my own way. I didn't do anything to make trouble.

REFERENCES

1. Becker HS, Geer B, Hughes EC, Strauss AL. Boys in white: student culture in medical school. Chicago (IL): University of Chicago Press;1961.
2. University of Kansas School of Medicine Class of 1964 Yearbook.
3. Bourne PG, Wikler NJ. Commitment and the cultural mandate: women in medicine. Soc Probl. 1978;25(4):430–40.
4. University of Kansas School of Medicine of 1957 Yearbook.
5. Friesen SR, Hudson RP. The Kansas School of Medicine eyewitness reflections on its formative years. Kansas City: University of Kansas School of Medicine;1996.
6. Lopate C. Women in medicine. Baltimore (MD): Johns Hopkins Press;1968.
7. Martin T. When the personal was political: five women doctors look back. Lincoln (NE): iUniverse;2008.
8. Walsh MR. Doctors wanted: no women need apply: sexual barriers in the medical profession 1835–1975. New Haven and London: Yale University Press;1977.
9. Morantz RM, Pomerleau CS, Fenichel CH. In her own words: oral histories of women physicians. Westport (CT): Greenwood Press;1982.
10. Chin EL, editor. This side of doctoring; reflections from women in medicine. New York (NY): Oxford University Press;2003.
11. Spieler C, editor. Women in medicine. 1976 Report of a Macy Conference. New York (NY): Josiah Macy Jr, Foundation;1977.
12. Campbell MA. Why would a girl go into medicine? Old Westbury (NY): Feminist Press;1973.
13. Howell MC. Sounding board: what medical schools teach about women. NEJM. 1974;291(6):304–7.

13

Choosing a Specialty and Training Program

"While the surge in the representation of women in medical education in the past decade was welcomed as the dominant development . . . the locus of concern has shifted from the issue of the numbers of women students in medical school to their experiences in the next phase of training – the residency. The consensus of the conference was that personal and professional pressures bear most heavily on women physicians when they serve as house officers in hospitals and that it is during this stage of training that changes are most urgently needed."[1]

(Women in Medicine Conference 1977)

For decades, the struggles to advance women in medicine focused on overcoming barriers to medical school admission and improving the learning environment for female medical students.[1-7] While such efforts continued, by the mid-1970s securing advanced training in medical specialties began to assume greater significance. A 1976 national conference titled, "Women in Medicine," marveled at the increase in female medical students from 9% to 24% of matriculants in a decade and predicted the trend would stabilize around 1985 at about 30%.[1] While acknowledging continuing challenges in medical schools, the experts attending this conference were primarily concerned with securing opportunities for specialist training and improving the conditions for women in the rigid system of postgraduate medical education (GME).[1]

Obtaining specialist training has always been a major challenge for female physicians. Until the 1960s, many US hospitals refused to accept female interns or residents or accepted them "only if a suitable man was not available."[4] Even if positions were officially open to all qualified applicants, many institutions discouraged female physicians, overtly or otherwise, from seeking internships or residency positions.[3,4,7] In particular, the surgical specialties were regarded as hostile to female applicants, a situation that has only relatively recently begun to change.[8,9]

In the decades covered by our interviews, the number of available internship and residency positions greatly outnumbered the number of US medical graduates. Male US graduates had little difficulty finding positions. Conversely, women, non-US graduates, and other minority physicians faced challenges in finding a reputable training program in the desired specialty and geographical location.[3,4,7] Non-teaching hospitals often provided inducements such as apartments for house staff and "more lenient conditions such as one out of three or four nights on duty" to compete with the more prestigious teaching hospitals for interns.[3] Our participants' class yearbooks all include multiple full-page adverts extolling the quality of patient experience, teaching, salary, accommodation, and conditions for house staff at the

DOI: 10.1201/9781003539568-13

large community hospitals in Wichita and Topeka. Nevertheless, a 1947 KUSM graduate describes being refused a position in one of these hospitals because "all interns were required to live in the hospital interns' quarters, which, we were told, had been designed for men *only*."[10] She finally was accepted at the insistence of her husband – a classmate.

> "In this both or none situation, the administrator opted for the package deal. The only adjustments made to accommodate a woman were signs put on the two bathrooms in the interns' quarters, one marked 'Men' and the other marked 'Women.' Since there were only six interns, this didn't produce much crowding, especially as my husband used the women's facility as it was closer to our room."[10]

A couple who graduated in 1944 was less successful in being able to spend their first year of married life together, as she interned in New Orleans and he in Cleveland.[2]

Graduate medical education changed significantly during the three decades covered by our interviews. Until the 1960s, medical school graduates generally completed a one-year internship before either entering general practice or undertaking further training in a medical specialty. In the years following WWII, many physicians who completed internship, including our earliest participant, *just hung out my shingle and waited for patients.* Those preparing for primary care usually completed rotating internships to obtain experience in several areas, such as internal medicine, pediatrics, obstetrics and gynecology, psychiatry, and surgery. Especially in community hospitals, interns were also commonly responsible for the emergency department.[10] During the 1950s and the 1960s, additional training became more routine, and all specialties, including primary care, expanded residency education into three- to five-year organized programs.

Selecting a Specialty – 3P's or 5P's?

A 1986 review characterized the careers of female physicians as dominated by a few specific specialties, all beginning with the letter *P*.

> "Over the years, women physicians have tended to choose anesthesiology and the five "P" specialties more frequently than men physicians – pediatrics, psychiatry, pathology, preventive medicine/public health, and physical medicine/rehabilitation. Women have also chosen certain specialties – essentially surgical fields – less frequently than men."[11]

Our participants reported that students had joked about women being perceived as predestined for one of three "P" specialties since the 1950s – long before the 1986 article.

For a girl, it was thought we should only go into one of the 3Ps – pediatric, psychiatry, or pathology. It was unnatural for a girl to want to do anything except peds.

TABLE 13.1

Specialty Distribution (%) of US Female Resident Physicians by Selected Years and Study Participants

	All US and Canadian Graduates 1968 (n = 1,419)	All US and Canadian Graduates 1970 (n = 1,778)	All US and Canadian Graduates 1974 (n = 2,902)	KUSM Alumnae Study Participants 1948–1975 (n = 37)
Internal medicine	16.8	16.3	18.4	29.7
Pediatrics	17.3	20.0	20.5	18.9
Psychiatry	23.0	23.0	16.6	13.5
Anesthesiology	7.0	4.0	3.7	8.1
Obstetrics and gynecology	5.6	4.3	5.8	5.4
Pathology	8.4	7.8	6.3	2.7
General practice/ Family medicine	0.4	0.4	4.6	2.7
Radiology	5.8	7.7	5.4	2.7
Surgery	4.6	5.3	6.4	2.7
Others	11.0	11.0	12.3	13.5

Source: Spieler C. (ed) Women in Medicine – 1976. Report of a Macy Conference. Josiah Macy Jr, Foundation. New York, NY 1977. Table 1.3 citing data from *JAMA* published in 1969, 1971, and 1975.

In contrast, our participants completed specialty training in 13 different specialties, covering much more of the alphabet.

Four retrained in a second specialty in mid- or late career. Our small sample and the heavy representation of 1974 and 1975 graduates complicate comparisons with national data. The national picture changed over time, with pediatrics becoming less dominant.[11–14] The general pattern of specialty choice of our participants is similar to the national picture, but the representation of pediatrics and psychiatry is lower than the national average for the period. Pathology and physical medicine each had a single representative in our group, and public health was only represented by an obstetrician who retrained late in her career. Conversely, internal medicine was more strongly represented in our interviewees than in the national data. This could reflect a growing interest in internal medicine among female students during the 1970s, and possibly a backlash against the assumption that women should become pediatricians. A study published in 1977 reported that "women believed internal medicine was high-est in status"[14] – a belief that was certainly enforced by the dominant personalities of the internal medicine faculty at KUSM described in the previous chapter. *Never any doubt about doing internal medicine – it was the cat's meow. Very good internists at KU, Dr. D and others.*

When asked why they selected a specific medical specialty, 31/37 (84%) interviewees immediately responded in terms of *I just loved the specialty, the patients.*

TABLE 13.2

Principal Motivations Driving Specialty Training Decisions

Factor	Number (%) of Interviewees Reporting	Illustrative Quotations
Attraction of the specialty, type of patients, scope of practice	31 (84%)	• *I got hooked on caring for sick babies during a neonatal rotation.* • *Chose OB because I thought I can do it all, surgery, general care, and deliver babies.* • *I just got hooked on my psychiatry rotation. I loved the contact with people and the different challenges.*
Role model(s)	10 (27%)	• *Teachers were a huge influence, very good internists at KU.* • *Dr. D, an inspiring endocrinologist. He was my first mentor.* • *Wonderful pediatric rotation. Loved it. ID specialist was very good teacher, encouraging.* • *Some amazing mentors in the clinical years. My mentors were so kind, especially in surgery.* • *The few female faculty members around were amazing women: so busy and had children.*
Lifestyle and control of time	8 (22%)	• *Anesthesiology appeared to offer more control over hours.* • *My first child born during senior year, so I looked for specialty with limited on call.* • *Psychiatry seemed interesting and offered more control over hours.*
Environment, teamwork	6 (16%)	• *I just enjoyed surgery and being in the OR.* • *Really liked the teamwork and activity of the OR, always something going on.* • *Pediatricians seemed more easygoing. I got along with them and felt accepted.*
Technical skills	3 (8%)	• *Always interested in surgery. Liked working with my hands.* • *Always liked sewing.*
Changed program or second residency	11 (30%)	

Note: Each interviewee could mention one or more factor.

They described their decisions as based on instinct, emotion, and intellectual curiosity. Each specialty held a special attraction for its advocates. Most who entered internal medicine cited the intellectual challenge of solving complex problems as a major attraction. *I wanted to help people. LOVED making a diagnosis, working up a patient, so it had to be internal medicine.* Those who became psychiatrists emphasized deep concern for patients and interest in long-term commitment to patient welfare. *I wanted interesting, strong, long-term relationships with patients – so psychiatry.* Several who entered pediatrics stressed that their decisions were based on genuine interest in the specialty and not the prevailing expectations that women should become pediatricians. *Always wanted to do peds, always liked working with kids. It wasn't one of those "women go into pediatrics" things.* Those drawn to surgery or anesthesiology spoke of *loving the atmosphere, the excitement, of the OR* (operating room) and wanting to be part of the surgical team as well as appreciation for technical skills. *Liked working with my hands. Always good at sewing.* Others were attracted by the technical aspects of specific specialties or were fascinated by the underlying science. *I just have this ability to look at something in two dimensions and see it in three. I remember in medical school, looking at a sonogram and "seeing" clearly that she had a posterior placenta previa. The others couldn't see it. I don't know why I could – I just have this ability, so radiology was a natural for me.*

Always loved the science of pathology, the logic of working things out.

Role models and medical school experiences were also influential, usually acting synergistically with an instinctive attraction to a specialty. Interviewees frequently had difficulty deciding which came first – the love of the specialty or the influence of the role model or experience. *A major influence was Dr. R in rehab – he was a real gentleman. Also Dr. K. I fell in love with rehab.*

I was always interested in surgery. I liked working with my hands, and the surgeons seemed so much nicer. Teachers were a huge influence, especially the famous plastic surgeons at KU. Dr. M was so kind. He had great stories. When students were assisting in surgery, he was polite and knew our names.

Very strong mentor in internal medicine – oncology. Had a really good experience on oncology as a medical student and as an intern. All very advanced for oncology at that time. LOVED internal medicine, just loved it. Oncology lets you do everything. I was interested in the whole patient, having serious interaction with them and their families.

Our participants rarely mentioned influential female role models or mentors. *The few female faculty members around (Drs. S and T) were amazing women: so busy and had children. But they did not mentor female students unless in her area of interest.* One female pediatrician, who was married and had a family as well as a successful academic career, was mentioned by several participants as a mentor and influence on their specialty choice. Not all those she influenced entered pediatrics, but she provided a role model, validating that women could achieve success in both their personal and professional lives. *She was a real mentor. I worked two summers in her lab. She welcomed me into her home, took me sailing, etc. I think I was the only one of her students that didn't go into pediatrics. I felt I had disappointed her by not entering pediatrics, but I wanted to work with adult patients and really liked working out the diagnosis so decided on internal medicine.* In the internal medicine department, dominated by powerful male personalities, a single female faculty member provided a more humanistic role model. *Dr. L was wonderful, dynamite, a real bright spot. She was really good. Everyone admired her. An excellent physician. I really admired her care of patients. She was personable and caring.*

Clerkship assignments and electives, including at community hospitals, could be pivotal in decisions. *I really liked surgery but did a rotation with a dermatologist in Topeka. Fantastic experience, all kinds of skin surgeries. Decided on dermatology.* Several of those who participated in the three-year curriculum felt deprived of opportunities to experience different specialties or cultivate relationships with desired residency programs. *Very difficult to decide on specialty as on the three-year curriculum, so no time for electives. Entire clinical experience was only 36 months, so only time for the basic rotations.*

Assignment to a specific unit could have a profound impact on specialty decisions. Some participants talked with a sense of awe about how the random allocation of students to clinical services could almost serendipitously determine entire professional futures. Several ladies described "light bulb" moments when their specialty choice, even vocation, was suddenly clear. *I was allocated to the child psychiatry service and just LOVED it. Suddenly, everything just felt right – felt like I belonged.*

My first rotation on the internship was two months dermatology – I fell into it and thought, "This is IT."

Others found validation of long-standing interests during their clinical experiences. *Always wanted to do internal medicine. Wanted to be the kind of doctor depicted in a Norman Rockwell picture of caring physician. Internal medicine at that time was very exciting.* Several in this group described their specialties in terms such as *something I always wanted to do* or were *just always interested in.* As mentioned in Chapter 3 on motivation, some interviewees were more specific and could even recall ages or events when a specialty became a goal. *I had been interested in psychiatry since aged 12.*

Their commitment to their specialties was clearly emotional. *I got hooked on caring for sick babies.* Many spoke of continuing deep emotional bonds to their specialties and patients. *I chose OB because I thought I can do it all, surgery, general care, and deliver babies.*

Making the Decision

Although our interviewees described their career decisions as predominantly based on positive, often altruistic motives, they were pragmatic in their final choices of specialty and program. Eighteen (49%) described going through a *process of elimination.* This process had two distinct themes. Some participants examined the pros and cons of different specialties, eliminating those that had the most unacceptable or discouraging aspects. This was presented as a positive process, that is, choosing among multiple attractive possibilities rather than selecting the least objectionable alternative. Personal experience remained the most powerful factor in reaching a decision.

Selecting a specialty seemed like a process of elimination – identifying the things I didn't want to do. Electives were influential. Did anesthesia elective and really liked it a lot.

Wanted a career where I could be useful but also have some control over time and decisions. Loved OB but rarely saw the light of day; anesthesia, 99% boredom and 1% terror. Considered internal medicine or family medicine. Radiology seemed a good fit.

Had trouble making up my mind about specialty. Considered psychiatry as I felt really sorry for the patients and their suffering, but it seemed too frustrating. My father thought family doctors were great, so I considered that. Pediatrics at KU was sad and discouraging – the kids were so very sick! But at Children's Mercy, we saw all kinds of kids. Wonderful rotation. Loved it.

Considered pediatrics, but demanding parents drove me nuts. Liked OB, but not the night call. Psychiatry seemed interesting and offered more control over hours. Attracted by interesting, strong, long-term relationships with patients.

Initially considered family medicine but did not care for internal medicine, especially geriatrics. Pediatricians seemed more easygoing.

The second and strongly related theme concerned lifestyle, in particular the challenges of managing both a career and family life. Control over work time, duration of training, and coordination with spousal careers were major considerations.

My first child was born during senior year, so I looked for specialty with limited on call. Chief of neurosurgery tried to recruit me, but I opted for ophthalmology, partly because of interest in neurological system and a (mistaken) perception of call duties.

Really was thinking about plastic surgery but was deterred by length of training and my biological clock. I reckoned I would be 34 or 35 by the time I was finished training.

Initially very interested in pediatrics but realized I didn't want to deal with the emotional strain of serious illness in kids. Psychiatry didn't seem like real medicine. Was very interested in internal medicine and needed to stay in Kansas City, as my husband was a surgery resident.

Loved, LOVED surgery, but my husband was a surgeon and we wanted to live in a small town and have big family. We thought, "It just won't work with two general surgeons." My husband offered to change to another surgical area, but I thought, "Okay, I'll do OB for the surgery." Considered anesthesia but wanted to DO surgery, and I couldn't bear being at the head, watching someone else do it. I loved OB.

We were surprised that no participants mentioned being actively discouraged from surgical specialties. Conversely, three participants volunteered experiences of being encouraged to enter highly competitive surgical specialties (orthopedics, neurosurgery, plastic surgery) and of faculty members actively recruiting them or making personal recommendations to program directors in other institutions. In the environment of that time, active discouragement may have been unnecessary, as the male-dominated surgical specialties were universally assumed to be hostile to women. In 1968, a female resident in plastic surgery was quoted as saying:

> "If you decide to become a surgeon, you'd better be sure you can carry through without having to ask for any dispensations for your feminine needs. It's the only field where you can be 30 years old and still get spanked every day."[3]

At least two participants decided applying to surgical subspecialties was unwise or not worth the effort. *Seriously considered pediatric surgery or pediatric orthopedics but deterred by length of training and prospect of a tough road for women at that time. Not a good field for women, and I didn't want to fight those battles.*

Really was thinking about plastic surgery but deterred by length of training and my biological clock. This participant channeled her love of surgery into a dermatology practice, with emphasis on procedures. Others who had an interest in surgery entered specialties that incorporated procedures and required manual dexterity, such as anesthesia, radiology, or obstetrics and gynecology. These women conveyed their decisions as positive choices. None of our participants described being refused or overtly discouraged from a specialty choice. Even when asked about what they would change if given the opportunity, those who had initially considered surgery stressed that they were very satisfied with their professional choices and had experienced rich and fulfilling careers.

Finding a Training Program

Unlike the modern, complicated national computerized system, the National Residency Matching Program (NRMP), our participants secured their internships or residency positions through personal contacts with program directors. These directors had almost unfettered power to select house staff. In making decisions, they relied on personal experiences and perceptions of the applicant plus letters of recommendation from medical school faculty members. The personal views of the residency director on women in medicine were of critical importance. Directors of surgical programs had an especially bad reputation for hostility to female applicants.

> "In order to enter a specialty, one must win the approval of the head of the residency program and it is here that women have sometimes faced an unconquerable barrier. . . . Department heads in the surgical specialties feel they would rather pick from the best male candidates than take a chance on a woman. . . . Their higher rate of mobility and even their temporary withdrawal to bear children can create difficulties in the administration of the department."[3]

In academic programs, an autocratic department chair or division chief could interfere with the program director's recruitment decisions. The entire system was highly subjective and vulnerable to the biases and wishes of a few individuals – almost all of whom were senior male physicians. This is vividly illustrated by the experience of one of our interviewees, who graduated at the top of her class.

I was sabotaged by the chair of internal medicine at KU. He was a new chair and wanted to keep all the best students in the class in his program, which he did. I was at the top of my class and a member of AOA. Although I received superior honors for every one of my internal medicine rotations, including the subspecialities, he would not write a letter of recommendation. He said he didn't know me well enough because he was new. I interviewed at East Coast schools and did very well, but he didn't send letters of recommendation, so I had to take the KU position.

Overall, 17 (46%) of our interviewees began postgraduate training in a KUMC program. An additional 7 (19%) participants entered programs in the Kansas City area. Individuals transferred across programs for various reasons, including advancing to fellowship positions. In total, 23 (62%) of our participants did some or all their postgraduate medical education in a KUMC program. Those who left the state volunteered reasons that clustered around characteristics of the training programs, family issues, and a desire to head for more exciting areas than Kansas. *It was the 1960s – time to get out of Dodge!* Most who left headed for cities on the East or West Coasts. For a liberated young woman without family ties, residency offered great possibilities to move to a new city and start her first real job in a completely fresh environment.

I went to University of Washington because the internal medicine program was one of the best in the country.

I was young, and everyone wanted to go to San Francisco. Incredibly difficult program to get into. I was only the fourth woman admitted to orthopedics at UCSF.

First did rotating internship and selected Portland, Oregon. Wanted out of Kansas. Wanted to live somewhere with more liberal politics. Looked at East and West Coast programs. Considered Philadelphia, but neighborhood felt unsafe. After internship, started a two-year family medicine residency in Salinas, California.

University of Maryland. Program was great, outstanding. I had attended college in Virginia and wanted to get back to the East Coast.

I wanted to get out of Kansas and go to the East Coast. I started a rotating internship in New Haven, Connecticut, in a hospital affiliated with Yale. Then did residency at New England Deaconess Hospital in Boston.

Did my first-year residency at KU, then went to Downtown VA in New York City. Very exciting city before they cleaned it up. Worked on Fifth Avenue and could walk on lunch break to Macy's and through the Garment District. There was SO much to do!

Several interviewees remained in the Kansas City area as their husbands were in residency, graduate school, or employed in the area. Three couples managed to match together to out-of-state programs – two in California, and the other in Michigan – largely driven by the husband's preferences. *My husband wanted to match in surgery at Michigan – managed to match together into great programs.*

We did rotating internships in Los Angeles County Hospital. We wanted to train in the same place, and my husband had attended college in Los Angeles.

Although husbands' careers appear to have taken priority for most couples, one interviewee's husband moved across the country to accommodate her residency training. *My specialty interest was encouraged by a very thoughtful KU faculty member from Boston who encouraged me to go out of Kansas for residency. We were interested in the East Coast, so my husband took a position in Providence, Rhode Island, and I started internship there. Halfway through the internship year, I took an opportunity to transfer to residency at Beth Israel in Boston.*

The most extreme challenges in finding training programs were faced by women whose husbands had military obligations during the Vietnam War. They went to great lengths, including soliciting political favors, to secure residency positions close to military bases. They were often unsure where their husbands would be assigned and had little opportunity to cultivate contacts with potential programs. Despite the stress and effort involved, two commented that they serendipitously secured outstanding residency experiences.

I could not plan ahead as my husband was drafted as a doctor in the Navy in the Vietnam War, and we did not know where he would be assigned following basic training. He requested San Diego but got Norfolk, VA. It worked out great – could not have been better! We needed to live within range of base, so I wrote letters to every medical program in the Washington, DC and Virginia area – must have been over 30. Mostly got ignored and multiple rejections. Finally got a call from the chief at Johns Hopkins offering a position on condition I would be a seven-day-a-week resident and NOT a five-day-a-week resident and a two-day-a-week housewife!

The Vietnam War was just ending, but my husband had deferred his draft to finish residency training so he had Air Force obligation. We searched for a city with an Air Force base and good obstetrics programs. Phoenix had two bases and three obstetrics residencies. One of my husband's attendings had been President Truman's doctor, and he offered to help secure his posting to Phoenix. The residency considered itself very progressive by having one female resident at a time (one in all three years combined, not one per year). I replaced someone who left, so the program had an unprecedented two female residents!

With these few exceptions, none of our interviewees across the three decades covered by their experiences recalled great difficulty in securing an internship or residency position – in fact, several commented on how easy their experience had been compared to that of current medical graduates. *The process of getting a residency was very different from now. I called up the chair and asked for an appointment. Discussed becoming a resident, and he said to show up July 1 – that was it!*

We didn't do match (NRMP) or anything, just negotiated directly with the program.

The head of ophthalmology was eager to have a female resident – only prior had been one during WWII.

No trouble getting a residency position.

Most of the women I knew managed to get into residencies they wanted.

The application process for most programs consisted of personal letters or discussions with the program directors. For non-KUMC programs, the personal letter was usually supplemented by letters of recommendation requested from selected KUSM faculty members. Faculty members who would make a personal contact with an out-of-state program director were especially valuable. We heard several accounts of faculty members making calls through *the old boys' network* to colleagues in other institutions to advocate for an applicant.

Local graduates had an advantage in securing a position at KUMC or an affiliated institution, as they were known to the faculty and familiar with the workings of the institution. In some specialties, especially pediatrics, local programs were not highly competitive. During the 1950s, a major teaching affiliate, Children's Mercy Hospital, was threatened with losing accreditation and underwent many years of substantial reforms. This damaged the reputation of the region in pediatric training for decades.

In those days, it was pretty easy to get into residency at KU, as the institution struggled to attract US grads. Lots of foreign graduates among the residents. Pediatrics welcomed us (KU grads) with open arms.

My husband was in law school in Kansas City. No problem finding a residency position at Children's Mercy. I think I was the only US grad.

The informal and highly personal process for obtaining positions extended to more advanced training, such as fellowships.

I put off decisions till last months of residency and thought I was going to have to work shifts in the emergency department, but I went to my oncology mentor, and he said, "Sign this and you are an oncology fellow!"

Comparisons and Reflections

We were surprised that our participants reported so few difficulties in securing GME positions in the specialty of their choice. About midway through the 37 interviews, we began directly asking about difficulties for women in obtaining internship or residency positions. Even direct questions did not elicit additional evidence of major problems for our interviewees or their female classmates. Conversely, the literature of that time insists that accessing advanced training was a major challenge for women and that positions were only readily available to women in "specialties that do not attract adequate numbers of men."[14] Specialties such as pediatrics and psychiatry were perceived as "suited to feminine nurturing attributes of tenderness, patience, understanding, sympathy, and maternal interest which are womanhood"[5,15] – strange priorities at a time that considered "toughness of character was the first prerequisite for women applying to medical school."[1] The masculine environment of medical schools at that time seems unlikely to nurture a transformation into the softer image of female physicians portrayed by the author. Perhaps he had been unduly influenced by the dilettante lady physician myth. By the end of medical school, our participants were experienced and pragmatic in navigating medical education and clinical situations but remained enthusiastic and altruistic about medicine. They conveyed that they made specialty choices primarily on their personal convictions and aspirations. We did not encounter any mention of being discouraged or mocked for considering a surgical career. Conversely, at least three participants described being encouraged to enter a surgical field, and one recalled being aggressively recruited by both neurosurgery and ophthalmology during the 1960s. Another described extensive support from surgical faculty to facilitate securing highly competitive places in orthopedic surgery in San Francisco for both herself and her husband. Those interviewees who considered surgery but chose another specialty clearly conveyed that this was a personal decision based on practical issues, mainly the duration of training, and not attributable to hostility from surgeons or others. We certainly did not perceive the avoidance and possible self-deception described in the 1966 Conference on Women in Medicine.

> "Being skillful at their own protection, few contemporary women actually come face to face with a door locked against them. Most veer off into the more acceptable and accepting specialties, without even a wistful look at those fields which might have spurned them. There is little of the suffragette attitude which once inspired women physicians to enter a specialty simply because their sex was not represented."[3]

Our interviewees, including those from the 1960s, were courageous and feisty women, quite accustomed to fighting or negotiating for desired positions. Even when asked directly about decisions they would do differently if given the opportunity, none expressed regret over being denied or discouraged from entering a specialty. All were positive about their specialty choices, and many spoke enthusiastically about experiences and new developments in their areas of interest.

Apart from the one chairman who refused to recommend an applicant to another program, we did not encounter any mention of difficulty in obtaining letters of recommendation or of faculty providing inappropriate recommendations for female applicants. Differences between letters for male and female applicants have been noted for decades. Letters for female applicants have been shown to frequently have inappropriate content, language, and style and to be less positive than those for male applicants. In particular, letters for female applicants have been shown to more frequently comment on appearance and personal life and personal attributes as opposed to work ethic, intelligence, or profession attributes and achievements.[16] None of this was evident in the recollections of our interviewees.

Our findings about selection of specialty and ease of obtaining positions are in stark contrast to a survey conducted prior to the 1976 Women in Medicine conference that reported that "the majority of female faculty members interviewed said they would have entered specialties other than those they were in if the opportunities had existed when they chose their internships."[1] Positions could have been easier to secure in the Midwest region, but as half of our participants entered out-of-state programs, this cannot fully explain the differences between our findings and other reports. The discrepancy could be due to many factors or combinations of factors. The informant groups could not be comparable; interviewees could have suffered from recall bias or have been unwilling to reveal sensitive personal information; interviewers could have used leading questions, conveyed an expected or "right" answer to participants, or even interpreted data in light of preconceived perceptions. Nevertheless, there is a striking lack of objective information about the specialty choice of women during the decades 1950–75. Much of the literature is based on anecdotes and opinion. Our findings are the recollections of a small group of female graduates of one Midwestern institution, but they cast doubt on the prevailing narrative that women faced universal exclusion and difficulty in finding GME positions, especially in traditionally male-dominated specialties.

REFERENCES

1. Spieler C, editor. Women in medicine. 1976 Report of a Macy Conference. New York (NY): Josiah Macy Jr, Foundation;1977.
2. Morantz RM, Pomerleau CS, Fenichel CH. In her own words: oral histories of women physicians. Westport (CT): Greenwood Press;1982.
3. Lopate C. Women in medicine. Baltimore (MD): Johns Hopkins Press;1968.
4. Walsh MR. Doctors wanted: no women need apply: sexual barriers in the medical profession 1835–1975. New Haven and London: Yale University Press;1977.
5. Bowers JZ. Special problems of women medical students. J Med Educ. 1968 May;43(5):532–7.
6. Braslow JB, Heins M. Women in medical education: a decade of change. N Engl J Med. 1981 May 7;304(19):1129–35.
7. More ES. Restoring the balance women physicians and the profession of medicine 1950–1995. Cambridge (MA): Harvard University Press;1999.
8. Lautenberger DM, Dandar VM. The state of women in academic medicine 2023–2024; progressing towards equity. Washington (DC): AAMC;2024.
9. West MA, Hwang S, Maier RV, Ahuja N, Angelos P, Bass BL, et al. Ensuring equity, diversity, and inclusion in academic surgery: an American Surgical Association white paper. Ann Surg. 2018 Sep;268(3):403–7.
10. North DG. From house calls to high-tech, memoirs of a 20th century woman doctor. Xlibris Corp;2002.
11. Bowman M, Gross ML. Overview of research on women in medicine – issues for public policymakers. Public Health Rep. 1986 Sep–Oct;101(5):513–21.
12. Martin SC, Parker RM, Arnold RM. Careers of women physicians: choices and constraints. West J Med. 1988 Dec;149(6):758–60.
13. Powers L, Parmelle RD, Wiesenfelder H. Practice patterns of women and men physicians. J Med Educ. 1969 Jun;44(6):481–91.

14. McGrath E, Zimet CN. Female and male medical students: differences in specialty choice selection and personality. J Med Educ. 1977 Apr;52(4):293–300.
15. Bowers JZ. Women in medicine: an international study. N Engl J Med. 1966 Aug 18; 275(7):362–5.
16. Khan S, Kirubarajan A, Shamsheri T, Clayton A, Mehta G. Gender bias in reference letters for residency and academic medicine: a systematic review. Postgrad Med J. 2021 Jun 2;99. Available from: https://10.1136/postgradmedj-2021-140045

14

Internship and Residency

Following medical school, graduate medical education (GME) traditionally comprised a one-year internship followed by three to five years of residency. Beginning in the 1960s, most US internships were merged into residency training; but first-year residents are still commonly called interns. Eighteen (49%) interviewees described completing internship before moving on to residency. In addition, 17 (46%) followed residency with fellowship training. For all interviewees, GME was challenging but critical to the transition from learner to practitioner, from tentative novice to full member of the profession.

At first, I thought I would die. My first rotation was tough, trial by fire.

In the three decades covered by our interviews, internship and residency had well-deserved reputations as tests of stamina and commitment to medicine. House staff positions were the ultimate tests to determine if a graduate

> "had what it takes to finally be admitted to the profession of medicine. The aura attached to the internship, like a puberty rite through which all boys must pass to achieve their manhood, medical students look forward with pride and fear to the internship."[1]

Internship and residency were robustly male environments, usually described with aggressive metaphors, such "battlefield," "front line," "war zone," and "Darwinian – survival of the fittest."[1–3] The training made unreasonable demands on all participants, but conditions were especially arduous for women.

> "Residency is still perceived to be a war zone, notoriously stressful for both male and female doctors. But over and above the usual stressors – chiefly the lack of sleep and the 'sink or swim' quality of many residency programs – gender discrimination was reported by many."[2]

"Women trainees were often treated as intrusive. Male physicians sometimes expressed their resentment in the form of remarks that women who received specialty training would probably never put it to any valuable use in the profession."[3]

For our interviewees, internship and residency were dominated by work rather than learning. Graduate medical education was characterized as a "time commitment rather than a learning commitment and the hundred hour week was not unusual for trainees."[4] The long hours, responsibility for patients, sleep deprivation, and stress

DOI: 10.1201/9781003539568-14

were justified as necessary experiences to prepare trainees for the harsh realities of practice; but house staff spent much of their time and energy providing services that often had little educational benefit.[1,3-5] A well-known saying quipped that "education is a by-product of residency training."

When our participants were interns and residents, they usually lived in the hospital and were expected to be available at all times. This tradition is reflected in junior hospital physicians still being called house staff or house officers. "The operating ethic for everyone is duty; a great deal of time is spent in the hospital in case an emergency should arise."[1] Although house officers had an official on-call requirement, such as every other night or every third or fourth night, many felt obligated to remain in the hospital even when technically off-duty. "This paralysis which keeps so many physicians in the hospital when they are free to leave"[1] can largely be explained by the heavy responsibility placed on trainees for assigned patients. Interns and residents remained responsible for their patients at all times; they had to know every detail of their patients' care and progress. The fear of missing some development was intense. Attending physicians could be merciless toward the trainee who was not fully informed. Not being on call or having been out of the hospital was not an acceptable excuse. While much of the pressure to remain on duty was imposed by supervisors, much was also generated by the house staff culture and personal competitive drives to succeed, or at least survive, this brutal stage of training. Residents regularly competed for boasting rights about their toughness. A male surgical intern is cited as saying, "In order to impress the department head, I spent 18 days straight without leaving the hospital, going several times for 72 hours at a stretch without sleep – at the time I thought it was great!"[1]

Trainees were terrified of being labeled as unreliable or lacking in dedication to medicine or commitment to the specialty. For women, this situation was intensified by the three major recurrent challenges to women in medicine, namely, the long-standing myth of the dilettante female physician who lacked the physical and/or emotional stamina for the tough world of medicine, the repeated reports of female physicians not being as productive as their male colleagues and much more likely to drop out of training, and the seemingly impossible task of succeeding simultaneously as a professional, wife, and mother. For many women, these challenges acted synergistically to make internship and residency a particularly demanding stage of their lives.[1,6,7]

"I practically killed myself never to let anybody down because I was a woman. I was always keenly aware that whatever behavior I displayed had the potential of reflecting on all women. I HAD to deliver the goods."[7]

I worked harder than the men – I was afraid of being branded a slough-off.

Married women, in particular those with children, were especially vulnerable to suspicion of lacking commitment or the potential to succeed as physicians.

"Women physicians were not expected to marry and if they did, it was assumed they were less devoted, less committed, less serious, that for them medicine had the status of a hobby."[7]

Our 37 interviewees completed training in 13 different specialties and participated in very different programs across the country. Despite this wide variety of experiences, several themes emerged from their recollections of GME experiences (Table 14.1). The strongest and most consistent themes concerned arduous work, long hours, responsibility, supervision and teaching, and issues related to gender. Additional themes focused on relationship with nurses, collegiality, and family issues. Despite the many challenges, our participants expressed a surprisingly positive overall picture of their GME experiences.

Fabulous experience. It was challenging, but amazing and a great experience.

TABLE 14.1

Graduate Medical Education: Major Themes

Theme (Number, % Reporting)	Illustrative Quotations (Specialty)
Workload (26, 70%)	• *Internship was a nightmare. It was a tough program.* (Surgery) • *It was hard. Big hospital, very busy.* (Pediatrics) • *Tons of patients. Just had to work and take care of all these patients.* (Pediatrics) • *We were always working – we did all our own bloods and things.* (Pediatrics) • *It was tough, heavy workload.* (Psychiatry) • *Backbreaking work. Medical school had been hard, but NOTHING like residency.* (Obstetrics/Gynecology) • *As an intern, I worked SO hard. I thought about changing to pathology.* (Medicine) • *The staff expected you to do everything.* (Anesthesiology)
Hours (22, 60%)	• *We worked 137 hours a week. We had every other Sunday afternoon off – that was it.* (Surgery) • *Very busy, hard work, on call every other night.* (Radiology) • *We were on call 1/3 nights and had lots of sick kids in ER every night.* (Pediatrics) • *I rarely had a full night's sleep – we were on call continuously for our patients.* (Medicine) • *Intense. Call every other night. Exhausted, but you just made it through.* (Medicine) • *On call 1 in 3 nights. Exhausting.* (Psychiatry)
Responsibility (15, 41%)	• *I felt cast adrift to take care of patients, often without knowing what I was doing. As interns, we had little supervision from residents. I really felt alone.* (Pediatrics) • *We learned pretty fast, but we were short-staffed, and supervision was inadequate.* (Pediatrics) • *Learning by doing. Just had to go to work and take care of all these patients.* (Pediatrics) • *Thrown into everything with minimal supervision. We were on call on our own at night in that big hospital.* (Medicine)

TABLE 14.1 (*Continued*)

Graduate Medical Education: Major Themes

Theme (Number, % Reporting)	Illustrative Quotations (Specialty)
Teaching and mentoring (31, 84%; 21, 57%, positive; 10, 32%, negative)	• *General surgery faculty were often quite abusive; the orthopedic attendings were actually supportive.* (Orthopedic Surgery) • *The chair was NOT a mentor to me; I am not sure he supported any women.* • *Tons of patients, but not strong on teaching.* (Pediatrics) • *Very good experiences: good rapport with professors.* (Medicine) • *Wonderful teachers on faculty. Great people.* (Psychiatry) • *Program was great, outstanding. Attendings were wonderful.* (Psychiatry) • *Residency was good experience. I totally appreciated it. The program was strong on teaching.* (Pediatrics) • *Experience was incredible. We saw everything. Top people, great experience.* (Pediatrics)
Accommodations (10, 32%)	• *When on ER call, we slept on the floor.* (Physical Medicine) • *I was supposed to share the call room, but the senior resident refused, so I slept on a gurney in the hall.* (Radiology) • *We lived in the hospital dormitory.* (Medicine) • *No issues over changing rooms or call rooms except when one guy wanted to sleep in his boxers and was told that was not appropriate.* (Anesthesiology)
Nurses (13, 35%)	• *Got on very well with nurses – we went out together, partied together. How they treated you depended on how you treated them. You had to carry your load and not dismiss them.* (Pediatrics) • *Got on well with nurses. I think the nurses kind of liked female residents.* (Medicine) • *Learned a lot from the nurses.* (Psychiatry) • *Nurses were very supportive.* (Pediatrics) • *Nurses were very nice to me.* (Medicine) • *Nurses were somewhat confrontational. Didn't like "orders" from females.* (Surgery) • *They were flirtatious with the male residents.* (Anesthesia)

Hours and Workload

The training was really rigorous, and call was brutal.

All participants mentioned the long hours and heavy workload required of trainees in "the senseless endurance test of residency."[8] Around 70% elaborated on aspects of the physically and emotionally draining experience. Interns lived in the hospital and were expected to be available almost continuously for their patients. A rotating intern at a Wichita community hospital described her hours and duties in 1947:

> "My duties included the history and examination of newly admitted patients and making rounds with the attending physicians of all patients. I was also expected to give intravenous injections, do spinal taps and other procedures, and be on call for the hospital patients and emergency room patients during every day and every other night. On the obstetric service I was on call for deliveries every day and two out of three nights."[9]

Thirty years later, little had changed. A 1974 surgery resident in a Californian teaching hospital recalled, *It was a tough program. We worked 137 hours a week. We had every other Sunday afternoon off – that was it. If we looked tired holding retractors, one attending told the nurses to pour alcohol down the back of our gowns to wake us up.*

The excessive work hours were justified as preparation for the real world of private practice but sometimes had the opposite effect. One participant decided on a sub-specialty with little inpatient work because of her grueling experience as an internal medicine resident.

We lived in the hospital dormitory and were on call continuously for our own clinic patients. I rarely had a full night's sleep for eight months. It was to prepare us for the reality of full responsibility for patients in practice but convinced me that I could not do general internal medicine.

House staff were responsible for all aspects of the management of hospitalized patients, from the comprehensive admitting history and physical examination to the detailed discharge summary. They conducted daily assessments and updates, managed all diagnostic tests and treatments, and maintained all medical records and communications with the attending physician, other specialists, nursing staff, patients, and families. Those in teaching hospitals supervised medical students and were required to participate in teaching both at the bedside and in presentations, conferences, or lectures. These residents had to prepare for and participate in the teaching rounds that dominated each working day (see Chapter 12). Interns and residents were subject to similar or even worse pimping than that endured by medical students. They could be publicly blamed for setbacks in a patient's progress. This included being shamed and scapegoated for bad outcomes.

We always felt like we were on trial.

One interviewee described a morning conference after she and a male intern had worked hard all night on a challenging patient – *you didn't call anyone for help in those days.* The patient was doing well, but their care was criticized in retrospect by the attending physician. Asked what he would do to the intern over the management of the case, the professor said: *"I would castrate him."* He said that, to an intern, in front of the entire team!

Teaching rounds inevitably generated demands for new diagnostic tests and changes to treatment. House staff spent hours updating orders; changing medications; negotiating with nurses, laboratories, and others to expedite diagnostic tests and treatments; conducting procedures; and doing everything necessary to ensure the changes ordered by the attending physician were promptly and correctly implemented and documented. House staff and students did almost all the basic work of patient care, such as drawing blood for tests, managing intravenous infusions, and even moving patients to radiology and other departments. House staff in community hospitals did not face the ordeal of formal teaching rounds but had to accompany the different attending physicians whenever they came to the hospital to see their patients, so the working day could be unpredictably disrupted. Just as their peers in teaching hospitals, they had to be prepared to update the attending physician on the progress of every patient and to ensure all follow-up orders were implemented. Whether in community or teaching hospitals, our interviewees described the daily work of internship and residency in terms such as *backbreaking, demanding, tough, unrelenting,* and *exhausting.* (For additional quotations, see Table 14.1.)

Regardless of specialty or institution, the working day began early for house staff and regularly continued into the evening or overnight. In addition to long tiring days, they worked at night to take care of any concerns arising in assigned patients as well as managing new admissions or patients arriving at the emergency department. It was not uncommon for house staff to work all day, throughout the night, and all of the next day without sleep or with only naps snatched between calls to patients. As interns or first-year residents, our interviewees described official "on-call" duties of between every other night and one night in four. More senior residents typically had less-frequent night call, but many remembered being on duty every third or fourth night even as third- or fourth-year residents. An intern or resident could be called to the hospital even if not officially on duty. The call schedule was frequently overridden for emergencies or an influx of admissions.

In the first month, we had a major outbreak of Reye's syndrome. It was a baptism of fire – lots of blood infusions and night call in ICU with very sick kids. All hands on deck.

In the 1957 Asian flu epidemic, there were lots of young adult cases. One of the other pediatric interns died. I was on call every other night.

Excessive hours and sleep deprivation were the norm and generally accepted by leaders of the profession as necessary for quality specialist training, as expressed by the chairman of a leading academic department of obstetrics and gynecology in 1976:

> "Shorter hours, fewer nights on call, more time at home are all fine and desirable, but they can't be made available within the present time frame of most residency training programs without compromising the quality of the experience. It takes a certain amount of time to acquire information, develop the skills, and to learn to apply them to the practice of a medical or surgical specialty. I have no interest in training incompetent specialists."[4]

Responsibility, Supervision, and Teaching

Our interviewees described their GME experiences as *learning by doing – and doing came first!* Their primary concerns were to take care of the patients to the best of their abilities and to satisfy, if not impress, the attending physicians and service chiefs. This came down to *get the work done, stay out of trouble, and try to get some sleep.* Compared to current trainees, our interviewees described a frightening degree of responsibility. Interns were commonly *thrown in at the deep end.* Especially at night and on weekends, they could find themselves responsible for large numbers of hospitalized patients or faced with triaging all emergency room attendees. They made critical decisions about patient care, often with little support from supervisors.

I, fresh from medical school, was called to give emergency treatment to whomever came to the ER, whether with a heart attack, a gunshot wound, or whatever. (For additional quotations, see Table 14.1.)

Although senior physicians were theoretically available to support the house staff, the unwritten code prohibited trainees from calling for help, except in the most extreme circumstances – or for an especially important patient, such as a local politician, established physician, or personal friend or family member of an attending physician. Even if called, attendings could refuse to come to the hospital to assist struggling house staff.

The supervision was inadequate. I remember a child dying from a congenital heart condition. The cardiologist wouldn't talk with the parents. I did it all by myself.

Program did not have sufficient supervision/support. Many of the attendings even lived in another town! I remember, a woman came to the ER in premature labor with twins. I was the only one there, and the attending said he would not get there in time, so he didn't come in. The babies died.

The resident or intern who called for help risked gaining the reputation of lacking the knowledge or courage to manage clinical situations. Women already felt under suspicion of being unreliable or lacking the stamina to *cut it* in medicine so felt especially reluctant to call for assistance or advice.

We were scrutinized!

Residency was competitive, intense pressure to do well, but nobody went out of their way to support me. I learned a lot in taking care of my patients, but overall, not a great time from a personal standpoint.

They agonized over the potential benefits for patients versus the consequences for their professional reputations of calling an attending or more senior resident for help. Trainees were completely dependent on the principal attending physicians and unit leaders for the letters of recommendation essential to advance to fellowship training, be accepted by a community practice, be admitted to the staff of a hospital, or be granted membership of professional organizations. Evaluations were almost completely subjective and based on the personal interactions between trainees and attendings – everything depended on the attending physician's perception of the intern or resident. While some attending physicians took their responsibilities to supervise, teach, or mentor trainees seriously, others were remote or even hostile. Our interviewees reported a huge range of experiences with GME faculty, from frank abuse to outstanding teaching and mentoring. The chances of a good experience seemed completely serendipitous. We could not detect a pattern by specialty, region of the country, or year of residency. The amount and quality of teaching appeared to depend on the interests or whims of individual faculty members and the atmosphere fostered by departmental leadership. *Some attendings were academic and taught, but others didn't.* Even in the residency programs of prestigious teaching hospitals, our interviewees' recollections of teaching covered the gamut from negligible or inappropriate to outstanding. One interviewee described the dramatic contrasts within the same program.

I did two years internal medicine and two years cardiology. The medicine chief drove me into severe clinical depression in my first year. Cardiology faculty were admirable.

The teaching hospital attendings were very difficult and pretentious – and the VA attendings were rarely seen.

They taught by intimidation.

In contrast to the reports of negligent or bullying supervisors, many attendings and faculty were recalled as supportive and knowledgeable teachers. Overall, positive comments about faculty teaching and support were twice as common as negatives (21 versus 10). For additional quotations, see Table 14.1.

Residency was incredible: We saw everything. We had top people, great experience.

There were three full-time professors and three residents (one per year) in this new department. We were a tight-knit group and studied and worked together well.

The residency program was great, outstanding. Attendings were wonderful.

Expectations for teaching were generally lower for interns and residents in community hospitals. *The program was not academically rigorous. Had to study on my own and go to review courses for boards.* Nevertheless, outstanding teaching could be provided by individuals in both community and university hospitals. *Dr. J was a genius and Renaissance Man. He had a large consulting practice in the community. In spite of many preoccupations, he found time to teach the interns and was a frequent resource for curbside consultations.*

Our interviewees were sometimes the only women in their residency programs or in the institution. *Very few other female residents around – a couple in OB, some in peds, and anesthesia.* A few were the first female residents accepted by the program. Only in the final graduating classes did four participants find themselves in programs in which at least one-third of the residents were women. One of these programs was in New England, and the other in California. The majority of our interviewees had few female colleagues among residents or faculty. *One other female resident when I started, but I was the only woman for about two years, then a couple of others showed up. One female staff member. Very nice lady who did pediatric anesthesia. But she left.* Very few encountered female faculty members. Not all female faculty members were helpful. *Even the older women were not very welcoming – almost like*

I was competition. Those interviewees who worked in the Kansas City area repeatedly mentioned the same handful of female faculty and role models. *Few women on faculty, but Dr. L was definitely a mentor. I had mostly male role models and mentors even in pediatrics.*

One wonderful female faculty during residency, and another during fellowship in child psychiatry.

One other woman in residency. Dr. L was very good and really helpful. Did several papers and presentations with her. Don't recall any other female faculty.

Gender-Based Issues and Collegiality

> "The young woman of today (1977) may face minimal barriers in medical school, a different experience than our counterpart ten years ago, but she may be poorly prepared to cope with unwelcoming attitudes during her postgraduate years."[4]

The major finding of the 1976 Macy Women in Medicine conference was that progress had been made for women in medical school but that much remained to be done to improve conditions in residency. Many of our interviewees expressed the sense that they had become skilled in navigating issues for women in medical school but felt *thrown back into the bad old days* upon entering internship and residency. In 1947, a new intern at a large community hospital was greeted with "We don't like women doctors" by the first two senior physicians she met. "Now that's a conversation stopper. I let those 'greetings' pass because the doctors who made them outranked me professionally – what doctor doesn't outrank an intern?"[9] Things improved somewhat over the 30 years covered by our interviews, but a 1974 graduate was also made very aware of persisting negativity toward women joining the residency program. *Some of the older doctors were chauvinistic, surprised I got the position, but overall, they treated me fine. I had learned to be my own advocate and did a lot for myself.* Similarly, a 1975 graduate struggled against bias in a department of obstetrics and gynecology. *Attitudes were very belittling, patronizing to women. I was miserable.*

Sometimes, even a well-meaning attending could display inappropriate underlying attitudes toward female physicians. A 1972 graduate reported, *Some overt hazing, but overall, just a totally different atmosphere for women. When I and another resident were pregnant, an attending said, "What am I to do with you two invalids?" – and he thought he was one of the liberated men!*

Others encountered more subtle discrimination from colleagues and their wives.

Lots of discrimination, for example, a prominent, distinguished cardiologist gave party every year but only invited males. They said it was because they served mountain oysters, but it was just discrimination.

It was a very masculine environment. Had one female resident per year, sometimes none. Morning report was all guy talk – football and things. Also, little things, for example, when the chair's wife sent invites to a party, it was addressed to "MISS" not "Doctor" for my invitation, but the men had "Doctor" on their invites.

Not all our interviewees agreed with the picture of widespread mistreatment and discrimination against female residents generally portrayed by the literature.[1–3,10] Some reported adverse incidents in an otherwise-positive experience, but ten specifically volunteered comments such as, *Didn't have any trouble. Had prestige and respect from the others.*

Only woman in residency, but no differences. I was treated the same as the men.

Did not feel treated differently from the guys.

They stressed that internship and residency were tough for everyone. *Don't think it was any different for the women residents.* With a few exceptions, they felt supported by their male colleagues and spoke warmly of the collegiality among residents. *We were a tight-knit group, as we never left the hospital – it was a bit like* Grey's Anatomy.

Residency was a good time, fun, good group of residents. Women were better accepted than in medical school. Good group of people.

We were a tight-knit group and studied and worked together well. We were very supportive of each other.

We noted a general trend for improvement over time, and for women in pediatrics and psychiatry to report a more positive experience, but the small number of interviewees limits drawing conclusions about the overall treatment of women in different specialties or institutions. Attitudes and behaviors toward women varied enormously by program, even within the same specialty. The traditionally male-dominated specialist areas, such as surgery, are generally portrayed as more hostile to women, but the information from our interviewees suggests the environment was determined predominantly by the culture and leadership of individual programs. One interviewee thrived on being the *only woman in a surgery program* and went on to fellowship, whereas another left surgery after a *nightmare internship; the male/female thing was SO nasty.*

As women became more senior in residency programs, they sometimes encountered new challenges. *Everyone got along fairly well, except one guy in the year behind us. It really bugged him to have a woman technically ahead of him and giving him orders. He would ignore or cancel my orders – he just couldn't stand having women in charge. It was against his strict Mormon code.*

Challenges for female interns and residents were not limited to the workplace. As in medical school (Chapters 9 and 10), issues arose over accommodation. Interns and many residents lived in the hospital. A 1947 graduate recalled receiving room, board, laundry, uniform, and $75 a month as an intern – a sum that rose to "a munificent salary of $300 a month" upon becoming a resident at the county hospital.[9] In 1957, an intern at KUMC received $40 per month plus uniform, accommodation in the nurses' home, and meal tickets for the cafeteria. As noted previously, hospitals had commonly cited lack of accommodation for women as a justification for refusing female interns and residents. A 1960 graduate found herself improvising a solution to a "Catch-22" situation. *Interns lived in quarters in the hospital, but married interns got a stipend to subsidize nearly accommodation. Women were not allowed in the interns' quarters, and as an unmarried person, I was not deemed eligible for a stipend. No call rooms were available, so I made up a bed on a couch in the library. One day after rounds, my supervisor decided to discuss cases with the team in the library. He was horrified to discover my sleeping arrangements! He went through the roof and demanded administration do something to accommodate me. Administration said, "We will never have another woman intern, so we can't create a call room just for her!"*

Even our 1974 and 1975 graduates frequently found themselves allocated accommodation in the nurses' home rather than in the residents' quarters. They were expected to abide by the house rules but were exempt from curfew – they were granted the luxury of a key to avoid rousing the housemother throughout the night!

Those who lived off campus or needed to be closer to the wards when on call faced the same issues as in medical school over shared sleeping arrangements. Call rooms were designed to allow two to six members of the house staff to rest. The single or bunk beds, some basic furniture, and a bathroom with shower offered little comfort and even less privacy. Several women opted not to use the call rooms and slept where they could in the wards, emergency department, or labor and delivery rooms. *There was a call room with six bunk beds, but only for the guys. A woman had to find a gurney. One night, I was woken by a janitor wanting to mop the floor* (for additional quotations, see Table 14.1).

Relationships with Nurses

Nurses were an important influence on the daily lives of interns and residents. They were essential in getting orders implemented and the work done. An experienced nurse not only knew how to most efficiently navigate institutional systems but could also provide insights on the preferences of individual attending physicians – often even anticipate the orders or questions the attendings would demand of house staff. A good nurse could keep an inexperienced house officer out of trouble. Facing her first ER shift, a 1947 graduate was advised, *If you have no idea what's wrong with the patient, just hold out your hand. The ER nurse will put the right instrument in it. This advice proved invaluable. As advertised, she would tactfully let me know what I should be doing without making me look stupid in front of patients.*

Interns and residents frequently *learned a lot from the nurses.*

They were very good and could teach you a lot. I was always eager to learn. I quickly figured out they knew stuff the professors didn't know.

Learning from nurses and productive teamwork were contingent upon mutual respect. Several interviewees spoke of taking care to be considerate toward nurses and appreciative of their efforts. *I never had any conflicts with nurses, but I tried hard to never act superior to nurses.*

How they treated you depended on how you treated them. You had to carry your load and not dismiss them.

Most of our participants provided highly positive comments about nurses. *I always got along very well with nurses. Never any trouble. Some became my best friends.*

A few of the earlier graduates spoke of encountering older nurses who didn't think women should be doctors and balked at women taking charge of a patient's care. *The nurses were somewhat confrontational, didn't like things being called "orders."* Throughout the three decades covered by our interviews, female house staff in every specialty encountered nurses who acted deferentially to male physicians – and many who flirted or pursued the young men romantically.

Nurses were not as bad as in medical school. Women physicians were still competition – it was galling.

They were okay with us, but more flirtatious with the male residents.

Nurses were very deferential to the men but didn't say much to the women. They would get whatever the men needed, but if I asked for something, like a pair of gloves or an instrument, they said it's in the storage room. I was expected to get it myself.

For additional quotations about nurses, see Table 14.1.

Family and Personal Issues: Mothers in Residency

"The years of residency – normally served when a doctor is between the ages of twenty-six and thirty – are regarded as a woman's optimal childbearing years. The pressures on married women physicians are therefore often greatest precisely at the time when the professional demands on them are least manageable."[4]

Pregnancy

Despite the increasing numbers of women graduating from medical school and the obvious biological imperative of their age group, the institutions attended by our participants showed no awareness that female physicians might become pregnant. This appears to have been a blind spot even for reformers and advocates for women in medicine. Surprisingly, the 1976 Macy Conference on Women in Medicine devoted substantial attention to childcare and issues of family life for female physicians and trainees but made no mention of their needs during pregnancy and the puerperium.[4] Perhaps conference participants assumed that the "superwoman accepting the double burden of full responsibility for a medical career and marriage and motherhood"[4] represented all female physicians. She certainly is portrayed as capable of managing a pregnancy during her hundred-hour workweek and returning immediately to work after the uncomplicated delivery of a robust, healthy baby.

In reality, our interviewees typically found they had to fend for themselves in programs that were unprepared for, or even unwilling to acknowledge, the possibility of pregnancy. At an internal medicine program, a 1974 graduate reported, *When I asked about maternity leave, I was told we don't have a policy. We've never had a pregnant resident. My contract had nothing about maternity leave or pregnancy. I took vacation and sick leave and hoped I wouldn't get sick.*

Even a program in obstetrics and gynecology did not appear to have considered the possibility of pregnancy in female residents. *I arrived for residency visibly pregnant, but nobody said anything directly to me. About six weeks before delivery, an attending asked, "When are you due?" I was told that there was great consternation – everyone was flabbergasted. It caused a fluster, but this was all behind my back. Nobody would talk about it, and I figured I would not bring it up. I took three weeks off – all my vacation.*

In contrast to this "don't ask, don't tell" approach, a participant in an ophthalmology program with an unusually supportive director had a good experience. *My second child was born during residency. The chief was excited, like he was the grandfather. He promised the program would "bend like the willows in the wind" to accommodate the pregnancy. I took six weeks off after birth.*

A woman whose husband was drafted into the Navy during her residency training found great support from colleagues and others when her pregnancies ended tragically. *I had a miscarriage, followed by a stillbirth – terrible experiences. We knew for two weeks that the baby was dead. I had lots of support. Wonderful support from nurses, colleagues, and from other Navy wives.*

Childcare Issues

I did nothing except work and home. Was completely focused on work and home. I had two little kids and a new baby and a surgeon husband – it was nuts.

Managing the demands of internship and residency was especially challenging for women with children. Our interviewees knew they were under suspicion of being unreliable or causing problems for the program in scheduling rotations and call duties by requesting time for family responsibilities.[1,4] They were on their own and under great pressure to find absolutely reliable childcare close to the hospital that could cope with the long hours and unpredictability of the resident's role. Physician mothers relied on a network of other women plus their own ingenuity to find childcare. They did not expect their husbands (several of whom were also residents) to provide substantial support, or for institutions to provide resources for working mothers.

Men brought up in the 1950s had a lot of trouble adjusting to women working. I had a new baby at the start of residency. Finding good babysitters was essential. Got names of babysitters from other women (students, nurse anesthetists, etc.). Had to be prepared for emergencies.

Most relied on babysitters, neighbors, or family members. Several spoke of long-term helpers *who became part of the family*, but with limited incomes, few residents could afford live-in help.

Extremely difficult and stressful to get childcare. I was lucky to find great daytime childcare – a grandmotherly neighbor who was available long hours whenever I needed and was wonderful. For weekends and overnights, I depended on neighbors. Stay-at-home mothers in the neighborhood where my kids could go.

Our interviewees spoke of using all possible resources in childcare and of requiring at least one contingency plan for the inevitable breakdowns in the system. For one participant, the breakdown started on her first day.

During my interview, we discussed "on call," as I had a young child and my husband was a surgery resident. I was told 1 in 7 overnight call in the hospital, but upon arrival, I found it was 1 in 3!

Night calls were unpredictable and difficult to manage, especially for more senior residents, who were called less frequently, so could not predict when nocturnal childcare was needed. Several women described taking sleepy children with them when responding to emergencies at night.

Psychiatry residency was tough. I had not mastered juggling childcare with being a resident. If I got called in, I took the baby. There was a room for residents to sleep. Told the staff, "I got to bring the baby. Help me out. You can hold it together for two hours."

Being on call was a problem. No call rooms for women – we were all together. At times I took my children with me, and they spent the night in the call rooms (aged about 8 and 10), then I took them to school and went back to work.

Even the most carefully prepared plan could break down, leaving a resident literally holding the baby while trying to cope with a medical emergency. An anesthesiologist told a complicated story of trying to locate childcare late at night when her overnight babysitter was called away for a family medical emergency. After multiple unsuccessful phone calls, she located a substitute babysitter in an unfamiliar area of the city. *I got someone to cover me while I rushed out to pick up the baby, transfer to the new sitter, and find the location – all this without cell phones or GPS. I was stopped for speeding in the middle of the night, but when the traffic cop heard this tale of woe, he let me off. I was very flustered – I think I cried!"*

Childcare arrangements also had to adapt to the changing needs of growing children. A single mother recalled things getting more complicated as her daughter grew.

We were on call 1 in 3 nights and had lots of ER calls every night. It was exciting, but hard. Especially difficult as a single mom with a young child at home. I had a young woman come to my house to care for her when she was a baby. Childcare got more difficult when my daughter started preschool, as schools close at regular hours and I needed flexible childcare.

Three interviewees described divorces during residency. One attributed the end of the marriage to her workload. *Residency did cause my divorce. I attribute it to so much time away and always being tired. Have some guilt about it, as the kids were affected, but my husband stayed close and involved. Seemed like I was always not doing any-thing to the full extent – lots of trade-offs.* The three divorcees plus one interviewee who had divorced prior to medical school managed all the demands of residency and motherhood as single parents. Some of the married residents discovered they actu-ally had a third job as the spouse of a physician, businessman, or other professional. *My husband was a pastor, so I was expected to do a lot of church activities on top of everything else. Sometimes old ladies commented I was not at Sunday service. "Little wife not coming today?" I was either in the hospital or asleep!*

Summary and Reflection: The Best of Times *or* the Worst of Times?

Our interviewees validated many of the notorious aspects of internship and residency during the period – the long hours, demanding work, physical and emotional stress, and sometimes abusive system. They described being totally immersed in their respon-sibilities. A resident in 1969 described, *I went to do pre-op checks on patients who were watching the moon landing – I didn't even know we were going to the moon – that's how focused I was!* They were hypervigilant for changes in the condition of their patients and felt unable to detach from their responsibilities even when officially off duty. Many felt vulnerable to criticism, public reprimand, or verbal abuse, against which they had no recourse – except to leave the program and, hence, reinforce the reputation of women being unreliable or unfit for the tough world of medicine. Most tried to navigate this experience with few female colleagues and few, if any, female role models, but they often found support in the collegiality of other residents and nursing staff.

Graduate medical education for our interviewees was drastically different from cur-rent programs, especially in the lack of attention to patient safety and trainee well-ness. Interviewees spoke of harrowing episodes and periods of self-doubt and stress. Nevertheless, they also spoke of fun, camaraderie, and pride in work well done. The predominant themes of the GME training period from the interviews are of challenges met, difficulties overcome, and personal growth achieved. Our interviewees were proud of their achievements during internship, residency, and fellowship – specifically in the care they provided to thousands of patients despite often difficult circumstances. They may have been battered by the challenges of training, but they proved themselves worthy to take their places in the profession of medicine.

Worked hard for four years but would not trade it for anything.

Loved the scope and variety of work having access to the whole hospital.

Fabulous experience. It was challenging but amazing and a great experience.

Lots of patients and got lots of experience with common conditions.

Worked hard, interacting together, teamwork.

REFERENCES

1. Lopate C. Women in medicine. Baltimore (MD): Johns Hopkins Press;1968.
2. More ES. Restoring the balance: women physicians and the profession of medicine, 1850–1995. Cambridge (MA): Harvard University Press;1999.
3. Anon. Women in health care and pediatrics: women medical students and pediatric residents. Pediatrics. 1983 Apr; 71(4):681–7.
4. Spieler C, editor. Women in medicine. 1976 Report of a Macy Conference. New York (NY): Josiah Macy Jr, Foundation;1977.
5. Mills JS. A rational public policy for medical education and its financing. New York (NY): National Fund for Medical Education;1971.
6. Walsh MR. Doctors wanted: no women need apply: sexual barriers in the medical profession 1835–1975. New Haven and London: Yale University Press;1977.
7. Morantz RM, Pomerleau CS, Fenichel CH. In her own words: oral histories of women physicians. Westport (CT): Greenwood Press;1982.
8. Assefi N. Life in the trenches: how I survived residency. In: Lo Chinn E, editor. This side of doctoring. New York (NY): Oxford University Press;2003.
9. North DG. From house calls to high-tech: memoirs of a 20th century woman doctor. Xlibris Corp;2002.
10. Campbell MA. Why would a girl go into medicine? Medical education in the United States: a guide for women. Old Westbury (NY): Feminist Press;1973.

15

Practice: Getting Started

Where to Practice?

As each of our interviewees finished residency or fellowship, she faced the major decision about where to seek her first practice. For all physicians, the first appointment is crucial in building confidence, developing networks and support systems, and beginning the process of establishing professional credibility, reputation, and success. Our interviewees had to consider more than their own professional needs and aspirations. By this time, most were married, and several had children; finding a suitable first practice was an important decision with multiple implications.

Our participants described several factors that influenced their decisions about selecting their first practices. These factors clustered into five themes (Table 15.1). Most interviewees reported more than one of the principal themes.

Staying on Familiar Ground

About half of the group (18/37, 48.7%) began practice in the community where they had completed graduate medical education. Eight accepted faculty positions in their training institutions. Remaining in the training institution or a nearby affiliated community hospital or practice offered many advantages. The new physician was familiar with the environment, culture, expectations, and work patterns of the institution. Although changing roles, she *knew the system and the people – how everything worked.* Even those who entered private practices in the community had usually worked with those practices during their time as residents and/or fellows and were familiar with the working environment.

I was offered a partnership within a good local private practice. One member had been a faculty member, and we knew the practice well. Great advantage to be with a well-established partner to build my own practice.

Residency programs often encouraged graduates to practice locally in hopes of increasing the referral base for the institution. *Residency programs helped graduates find positions.*

Outside the work environment, remaining in the community reduced disruptions and distractions for the young female physician as she set out to establish her career. She

DOI: 10.1201/9781003539568-15

TABLE 15.1

Factors in Location of First Practice

Factor Number (%) Reporting	Illustrative Quotations
Remained in training institution or community 18 (49%)	• *Stayed on as faculty – more controllable hours and close to home.* • *Stayed on but moved to VA for better hours and conditions.* • *Moved to a suburban community hospital where I could be part-time while I had small children.*
Training program experiences or contacts 7 (19%)	• *I had done moonlighting shifts in the community during residency and liked the ER and community.* • *I was recruited by guys I had known in residency to join their practice.*
Husband's education or employment 9 (24%)	• *Stayed on and worked at VA while husband finished residency.* • *My husband was an academic and worked all the time, plus I had two stepchildren, so stayed in the area.* • *Returned to Kansas for husband to set up practice.*
Proximity to family members/return to hometown 8 (22%)	• *Returned to Wichita mainly for family and friends.* • *Practice in my hometown offered me a job. Community docs made no objections to an incoming female physician. They were much nicer than my classmates had been!*
Public service commitment 3 (8%)	• *Had a Public Health Service commitment to pay off loans.*

Notes:
1. Individuals could mention more than one factor.
2. Eight who remained in the same community accepted faculty positions.
3. Interviewee self-identified as "trailing spouse" in four couples who moved for husband's education; five couples made joint career moves to the same institution or community.

could usually retain her personal and social networks, decide to remain in the same home, utilize the same childcare and other support systems, and did not have to learn how to live in new community – she was already practiced in navigating all the local resources, such as grocery stores, schools, transportation systems, and all the other practical essentials of daily life.

Experiences or personal contacts during residency or fellowship were also important for many of those who moved away from their training cities. Three participants relocated to join practices they had experienced as rotations during training. One opted for the lifestyle endorsed by student preceptorship and residency rotations in rural areas.

I had experience at the community mental health center during residency and really liked the center, the people, and the area. I was offered a position following fellowship, so I moved to the town.

I spent the first couple of years doing locums through the state medical association. Did 1–4 weeks, mostly in rural towns, staying in physicians' homes and doing all the expectations of a rural physician, including attending football games.

Two were recruited to faculty positions in other states by alumni of their residency programs. *I was recruited by two alumni of the KU Peds residency to a new medical school. They wanted specialists to teach medical students, plus great need. I was the first full-time female physician in the group. Welcomed with open arms.*

One was encouraged to apply to a prestigious clinic by a residency faculty member who facilitated her acceptance as the only female physician. *I had a really good residency experience on an oncology rotation where I spent a lot of time with a female faculty member. We talked shop a lot, and she was very encouraging. She suggested I apply. She thought it would be a good match for me.*

Husbands and Family

About one-quarter of the interviewees (9/37, 24%) cited their husband's training or occupation as crucial in decisions about where to start their careers. For five of these women, their husbands' situations contributed to staying in the community in which they had finished training. Four were married to physicians and reported that negotiating two appointments in the same institution was much easier in a familiar environment. One interviewee was married to a local businessman and had strong family ties to the community. Conversely, four interviewees moved substantial distances, including one from coast to coast, when their husbands entered postdoctoral training or practice in another city.

After residency, moved to Washington, DC, for my husband's doctoral studies, and I worked for Group Health.

A husband's career decision brought one participant back to Kansas following fellowship in New York State.

My husband wanted to do a second residency and go on to do research, so he returned to KU. I joined a multispecialty group in Kansas City.

Five of the nine interviewees who cited husbands' careers as factors in selecting initial practices presented the decisions as joint career moves, that is, both husband and wife negotiated positions in the same institution or community. In the remaining four couples, the interviewee identified herself as the *trailing spouse*, that is, following her husband's career opportunity. These interviewees described the familiar pattern at that time of a wife's career taking second place to that of her husband. They were familiar with managing the turmoil of family relocation, then *finding a job* in whatever community the family had located because of the husband's career needs. *I moved to Kansas with a 4-day-old baby and three other kids! I was so naïve!*

In contrast, one participant recalled with relish that her surgeon husband followed her to a Kansas community – a highly unusual situation in the Midwest of the 1970s.

It was a very prestigious multispecialty clinic, and I was overjoyed to be accepted. We liked small towns. I was the only woman in internal medicine, and my husband was recruited "on my coattails" to surgery. He thought it was funny that they really wanted me and recruited him as well.

Eight (22%) interviewees described family considerations as important in decisions about their first practices. Seven returned to Kansas upon completing residency or fellowship out of the state in order to live close to family members. This group included four who had completed training in institutions on the East Coast. *Always wanted to get back to Kansas.* These four interviewees were all married to physicians, and both families lived in Kansas. Being close to family had multiple professional and personal advantages. For two participants, their physician fathers facilitated entry into the local medical community. *My father had been a family doc for over 40 years, so my name was known – in the community. Maybe that helped.*

I had several good offers of positions, but Dad wanted me to join his clinic.

Everyone who began her medical career close to family members appreciated the availability of additional support and practical assistance, especially with childcare.

We returned to Wichita mainly for family and friends. I had one son and was pregnant with my daughter.

When I had babies, my mother was close by. She was a pediatric nurse and loved babies. She would always help out.

Family support was crucial for our oldest participant, whose husband was sent to join the Army in Korea soon after she completed internship. She was left *holding the baby* and faced with beginning practice alone. She found herself welcomed into a community practice in her hometown and supported by her parents and relatives through this stressful transition.

Student Loan Commitments

Three interviewees began their careers in the Public Health Service to repay student loans. They found themselves in very different environments, one in inner-city Baltimore and one in rural New Mexico. *Who had ever heard of that place? It was so small and 17 miles from the nearest town – even that was small.*

Another participant and her husband were less dismayed by a posting to a remote area with the Indian Health Service.

After residency we returned to the Indian Health Service in Northern Arizona for three years. About eight young doctors out in the middle of nowhere. We ran a small hospital and did all the outpatients. Good unit, good experience. Civil service, so good hours. A good time.

Recruitment Experiences

Almost all our interviewees began their careers working in institutions or large practice groups. For some specialties, such as anesthesiology, this was the only practical decision for a young woman with family commitments and limited resources.

I was concerned about the hours, and at that time, insurance rates went sky-high, so you had to be part of a group.

For most interviewees, the available initial practice opportunities were limited to teaching hospitals, private practice, or employment with an organization such as the Veterans Administration or Public Health Service. This differed from the situation described for 1976 graduates entering the workforce in the Bay Area of California.

> "The choices for non-academic physicians were public clinics, private practice or a staff model health maintenance organization (HMO). The HMO was the largest employer of physicians in Northern California. The jobs at the public clinics paid about half of an HMO salary so appealed only to the most dedicated political types, or those with enough family money to ease worry about real estate prices."[1]

Managed care did not become prevalent in Kansas until the 1980s. The only interviewee who started out in a managed care practice had moved to Washington, DC, because of her husband's graduate studies. *I worked for Group Health from 1976– 1979 and then spent almost my entire career working for some form of managed care. Always a fair number of women in managed care, regular hours.*

The decades covered by our interviews were dominated by concern about an escalating national shortage of physicians.[2-6] During the 1960s and the 1970s, the number of accredited medical schools increased by 50%, and the number of physician graduates doubled.[4] At the same time, as described in previous chapters, societal and legal changes made it somewhat easier for women to enter medical training. As a result of all these factors, more women began entering the medical workforce during the mid-1970s.

The medical manpower crisis of the 1960s and the 1970s meant that young physicians completing residency or fellowship training were in high demand. Several participants described being *welcomed with open arms*, well treated, and mentored. Others encountered difficulties in being accepted on equitable terms with their male colleagues. *Women were not allowed to be partners at the clinic. They thought, "Your husband's a doctor, he'll take care of you, you don't need the money."*

Some of the resistance to recruiting a young female physician was attributed to the universal acceptance of reports that female physicians were significantly less committed and productive than their male colleagues – and less likely to fit in with the workplace culture. The belief that female physicians were a poor investment was deeply entrenched.[7] Even articles by female authors confidently stated "it has been estimated that female physicians practice an average of 40 percent fewer hours over their lifetimes compared to their male counterparts."[8] Potential employers or partners could also harbor suspicions that women would seek special treatment and cause disruption due to pregnancy, childcare issues, or female ailments – or even leave the practice completely to care for children or if the family moved because of their husbands' careers. The unreliable, dilettante female physician image of the 1890s continued to cast a long shadow over young women seeking their first professional appointments in the 20th century. Other common objections to hiring female physicians included that staff would have difficulty working with a female physician, and that women would have difficulty displaying leadership or exerting appropriate authority – more bluntly stated that staff would resist taking orders from a woman. Finally, some claimed that patients would be reluctant to consult female physicians and that male patients would be uncomfortable, especially in disclosing sensitive information or undergoing intimate examinations.

I do not recall any overt gender-related difficulties, negative statements, or behaviors, but many older male colleagues had their views. Women physicians were unusual. I found out later that the front desk staff were instructed to ask all patients, "Do you object to a female physician?"

I wanted to do occupational medicine. Finding a job as a plant doctor in the industry was difficult. Lots of discrimination. I was told men wouldn't like a woman examining them for hernia.

Reluctant potential employers or partners could find plenty of studies and anecdotes supporting the belief that women were bad investments for a practice or institution.[9-13] Some did not trouble with such justifications. Several of our interviewees encountered overt discrimination, and many others referred to more muted and less-obvious mistreatment. *The environment was paranoid and an "old boys' club."*

For some, discrimination and mistreatment by professional colleagues came as a shock. Entering practice in the early 1970s after years of interacting with community physicians during her training, one interviewee was stunned by the attitudes of many whom she considered established colleagues.

My first serious encounter with discrimination occurred when I was seeking to join practices. Most were solo or small groups. I was repeatedly turned down and told it might not work to have a female partner. I eventually set up my own practice – it was wonderful! I was solo for ten years, then took on a partner. I was totally unprepared for exclusion, discrimination by fellow specialists and other physicians. They would not send me referrals and never reciprocated professional courtesies, except the academic centers. It was a rude awakening.

Even individuals who were actively recruited by a practice could learn later that not all the partners supported the appointment. *My father wanted me to join his clinic, but not everyone was on board. They had several meetings before agreeing to offer me a position. My father was upset that a friend, a man he had brought into the clinic, voted against having me. Some said they were opposed to bringing in family members of partners, but some older physicians were opposed to having female colleagues – worried about how to handle pregnancies, and whether I would quit working, etc.*

Some of the most virulent objections were voiced by the physicians' wives.

Later, I was told by one of the group that everyone had advised against recruiting a female physician – even the wives of the partners. "All the wives told us we were foolish to hire a woman. Only one wife stood up for you – she was a professional woman, a lawyer."

In one situation, the objectors put a brave face on being overruled by reframing the recruitment of women as an indication of how modern and progressive the organization had become by accepting token female physicians in the late 1970s.

I joined a multispecialty clinic. There was only one other woman in the clinic when I joined. The older physicians were patronizing – made a huge deal of how progressive they were because of installing a women's restroom in the physicians' lounge. "Aren't you proud of us? Now we have two female physicians!" Previously they never expected to have female doctors. The younger guys were totally okay with it and were used to having female physicians.

Summary and Reflections

The recollections of our interviewees illustrate many of the themes in the history of women in medicine since WWII described in Chapter 2. Those entering practice in the early years competed with the influx of male physicians returning from military duty or navigated around husbands being deployed. Some of our oldest participants described their good fortune to be accepted into an established practice through personal or professional personal contacts, usually having a father or uncle in the medical community. Otherwise, starting in community practice could be an uncertain proposition, even in the community where the young physician had trained. The autobiography of a 1947 KUMC graduate describes setting up practice in 1949 and her decision to delay joining her husband in practice in Wichita.

> "My husband hung out his shingle and purchased the office furniture and equipment from the widow of a recently deceased physician, then waited for patients to trickle in. That's how doctors started then. There were no private clinics where doctors could get jobs with guaranteed salaries. It was unethical to advertise. A new physician could visit other physicians and leave his card, hoping they would refer patients to him when they vacationed or became too busy. Otherwise, he could drink coffee in the physicians' lounges of the hospitals and hope his presence would remind other doctors of his availability. For me to have started practice at the same time would not have helped the family finances. I would just have been competing with him for his first few patients. He estimated he made 50 cents an hour during the first year!"[14]

The earlier graduates also experienced many negative aspects of the return to the cult of domesticity described in Chapter 2 that discouraged women from aspiring to work outside the home and disapproved of those who sought to make careers in the professions. The virulent criticism experienced from physicians' wives is sad, but not unexpected. The biography of an earlier distinguished female physician recounts, "Physicians' wives really resent female doctors. I have really been insulted – at times really badly."[15] A physician's wife in the decades covered by our interviews had a prominent role in many communities. In addition to high social status, she was expected to undertake leadership roles in civic organizations and volunteer activities, especially those connected to health or health services. Every local medical society (to which all community physicians belonged) had an active women's auxiliary organization, through which physicians' wives vigorously undertook fundraising for the hospital and volunteered for other worthy causes. Many physicians of that time worked excessive hours. Outside of office hours, calls came directly to the physician's home, requiring wives to be responsible for taking and relaying messages – even giving patients instructions in emergency situations. A physician's wife was a full-time occupation in managing the household, raising children, and supporting her husband both professionally and socially. For a young woman to establish herself without such support was an inherent criticism of the accepted role of the physician's spouse. Female physicians were a threat not only in potentially causing disruption within the practice but also in negating the necessity for a full-time supportive spouse. As late as 1980, the author was chastised by the president of the medical society's auxiliary association for practicing because "You're vocation is to be a doctor's wife – to support your husband. I feel sorry for the poor man!"

The experiences of our married interviewees also illustrate the trends described in the literature regarding how decisions in dual-career families evolved from priority being assumed for the husband's career to a more balanced approach. As late as 1983, the conventional wisdom held that "a woman who is married will generally modify her career choices to the consideration of her husband's career in location, permanency, and hours."[16] This was true for some of our group, especially among the older participants, but even these interviewees conveyed a strong sense of shared decision making. The wife's considerations were especially likely to be prioritized among those for whom proximity to family was important and in the alumnae of the 1970s.

The participants' recollections of their recruitment and entry into practice illustrate the evolution of attitudes among male physicians toward women as colleagues. Earlier graduates were more likely to recall resistance and hostility from older male physicians, along with a strong sense of being closely monitored for weakness or potential failure. Later graduates also reported more intense scrutiny and less mentoring and support than their male contemporaries, but this was mostly limited to older physicians in the group or community. Several participants from 1974 and 1975 spoke of being recruited by and practicing collegially with male physicians in the same age group.

Only three interviewees spoke of difficulty in finding an initial practice. Two were entering practice in the 1950s, when resistance to female physicians, especially those with little experience, was unusually high. The third specialized in occupational medicine and found the male-dominated industrial environment very suspicious of a female physician. As described earlier, our participants considered multiple factors in deciding on their initial career position. As described in the following chapter, some settled immediately into the environments in which they spent their entire professional careers, some encountered nasty surprises and disappointments that necessitated finding new practices, and some adapted over the years to challenges and opportunities to make moves of location or even careers in order to fulfill their professional aspirations.

REFERENCES

1. Martin T. When the personal was political: five women doctors look back. Lincoln (NE): iUniverse;2008.
2. Lopate C. Women in medicine. Baltimore (MD): Johns Hopkins Press;1968.
3. Bornemeier WC. The physician shortage, 1972. JAMA. 1973;224(7):1033–4.
4. Mallon WT. Medical school expansion: déjà vu all over again? Acad Med. 2007;82(12):1121–5.
5. Surgeon General's Consultant Group on Medical Education. Physicians for a growing America. Washington (DC): Public Health Service, U.S. Department of Health, Education, and Welfare;1959.
6. Carnegie Commission on Higher Education. Higher education and the nation's health: policies for medical and dental education. New York (NY): McGraw-Hill;1970.
7. Jussim J, Muller C. Medical education for women: how good an investment? J Med Educ. 1975;50(6):571–80.
8. Lanska MJ, Lanska DJ, Rimm AA. Effect of rising percentage of female physicians on projections of physician supply. J Med Educ. 1984;59(11 Part 1):849–55.
9. Powers L, Parmelle RD, Wiesenfelder H. Practice patterns of women and men physicians. J Med Educ. 1969 Jun;44(6):481–91.
10. Dykman RA, Stalneker JM. Survey of women physicians graduating from medical school 1925–1940. J Med Educ. 1957;32:3–28.
11. Bobula JD. Work patterns, practice characteristics, and incomes of male and female physicians. J Med Educ. 1980;55(10):826–33.
12. Heins M, Smock S, Martindale L, Jacobs J, Stein M. Comparison of the productivity of women and men physicians. JAMA. 1977 Jun 6;237(23):2514–7.
13. Pepitone-Rockwell F, Rockwell DA. Women in medicine: myths and realities. West J Med. 1981 Jun;134(6):559–60.
14. North DG. From house calls to high-tech; memoirs of a 20th century woman doctor. Xlibris Corp;2002.
15. Morantz RM, Pomerleau CS, Fenichel CH. In her own words: oral histories of women physicians. Westport (CT): Greenwood Press;1982.
16. Anon. Women in health care and pediatrics: women in pediatric practice. Pediatrics. 1983;71(4):699–705.

16

Career Changes and Transitions

The last of our interviewees entered practice in the mid-1970s, when the United States was struggling with multiple internal controversies, including the women's movement and the related backlash. Amid all the public noise about women's roles, individuals and families made their own decisions as the era of domesticity of the postwar years faded.[1,2] By 1974, about half of women of working age were employed outside the home, and women comprised 40% of the US labor force. In health services, women held 75% of jobs.[3] Nevertheless, less than 10% of US physicians were women.[3] Female physicians were clustered in specialties perceived "suitable to women's nurturing natures and special capacities."[4] Even in such specialties, women represented only 22% of pediatricians and 14% of psychiatrists, anesthesiologists, and pathologists.[2–6] Their overrepresentation in salaried positions probably reflected practical issues, such as more predictable schedules and less out-of-hours call.[2,3]

Our interviewees entered a profession where the ideal young physician was assumed to be a White male, well-informed, technically skillful, and possessing many other positive qualities. Nevertheless, his success depended on demonstrating complete dedication to the profession. This required putting medicine first, regardless of the impact on the physician and everyone else, including family members. Young physicians were expected to be hungry for success and to aggressively build practices and reputation through long hours of grueling work and careful navigation of the maze of organizational politics using the old boys' network. The physician's spouse had a defined role, dedicated to supporting her husband and minimizing the demands of family on his pursuit of professional success. Fee-driven private practice was the norm, and physicians dominated hospital management through powerful staff committees. Whether in academia, private practice, or a salaried position, the career prospects of a young physician depended on decisions made by a few powerful senior individuals – almost certainly older White male physicians who had been accultured during a period when women were rare in the profession. Even those patriarchs who were supportive of female physicians had little experience of interacting with women as colleagues or trainees. They were unlikely to have developed a concept of a successful female physician, let alone encountered an appropriate role model. As our interviewees built their careers in medicine, they often encountered senior colleagues who *sometimes were not really opposed to women physicians; they just didn't know what to do with us!*

Our interviewees initially described their practice careers in terms of the chronological succession of professional appointments or jobs. Career changes featured prominently in these narratives. Undertaking a career change was a serious business for a female physician. If she was also a wife and a mother, a move required re-establishing the services and support systems necessary to ensure childcare, housekeeping, food

DOI: 10.1201/9781003539568-16

preparation, and all the other myriad responsibilities of managing a household in addition to developing new personal and professional networks – plus attending to the relocation needs of children, spouse, and other family members.[2,3,6–10] Sometimes, even a tempting offer entailed just too many complications and hard work. Conversely, remaining in an unsatisfactory situation could be increasingly stressful. Because of family commitments, a female physician could do little to negotiate improvements in her salary or working conditions. A 1968 report describes the frustration commonly experienced by married female physicians seeking such enhancements:

> "The woman knows that even if she demanded it, her request would carry little weight: because of her husband's job and her children's school, she is tied to this particular locale, and cannot threaten her superiors with leaving for an institution somewhere else."[2]

Early Experiences

Eleven (30%) interviewees remained in their initial practices for their entire careers. Six (13%) made only one career move. Two and three moves were each reported by seven interviewees, five reported four moves, and one individual described five work-related moves during her long career. Moves were more common early in their careers as they attempted to settle into communities and practices. The transition from training to practice did not always go smoothly. Promising institutions or practices could turn out to be unwelcoming or even hostile environments, and recruitment promises were not always honored. Several participants recalled feeling that they had no choice except to leave difficult professional situations. These were very painful decisions, especially for single mothers, and reached only after struggling to exhaust all possibilities of improving the situation.

Many participants were the first women in the practice or academic unit. Often, they were the only female physician, at least for the first years of their careers. *I was asked to join the staff at KUMC. I was the only female staff member. A few others came and went.*

As with other women of their generation, almost all interviewees recalled feeling great responsibility to succeed in their own careers and to *clear the path* for women in the future.[4,8] Many felt they were under constant scrutiny and were afraid that any missteps would be cited as justification for not recruiting female physicians in the future. Those individuals who had opposed the appointment were eager to seize on anything that vindicated their objections to female physicians. Even if the environment became highly uncomfortable for a female physician, resigning risked being labeled as a failure, thus providing further evidence that women were unreliable and *couldn't cut it in the real world* of medical practice. One participant recounted a harrowing story of her reception in her first practice.

I was about four months pregnant when I arrived in the group, and some of the men, especially the older guys, threw a fit! They all descended on me. "Why are you pregnant? Who will take care of the baby?" It was 20 questions, personal questions. It was humiliating and intrusive. They were NOT happy. I explained we wanted to start a family. I told them, "Don't worry." I was looking for a nanny and would take care of everything. I came home in tears. In the end, I had stillbirth, a terrible experience requiring a C-section to remove the dead baby. I took two weeks off and returned to work. Not much support or sympathy.

Several interviewees described being treated in their initial appointments *like second-class citizens* or *handmaidens* who did a disproportionate share of the work, especially the unpopular jobs, but received little recognition or reward. For women in academic positions, this demoralizing situation limited time and energy for the research essential for advancement. Women were further disadvantaged in the male-dominated system of mentoring and sponsorship.[11–16] Both in academia and private practice, those in authority did little to intervene. Women generally avoided raising objections about unfair treatment, partly because they regarded the effort as futile, and partly out of fear of being labeled as a discontent, troublemaker, or failure. As during medical school and residency, they felt an absolute imperative to prove they were *tough enough to cut it in practice.*

My "partner" had the attitude of "she will do it." He didn't give the lectures he had agreed to do and passed on other things – then he upped and left! I was left on call 24/7 and responsible for supervising two fellows.

It was a horrible experience. I was supposed to work in a team with two male colleagues covering a busy clinical service and doing research and teaching. It was very demanding in time and emotionally; plus, we had a lot of critically ill patients. I was expecting to rotate duties and share the work, but it didn't work out. Somehow the two guys were never there, and I ended up doing all the work – taking care of everything, clinic, the whole unit, a huge job. I have never talked about it, but turned out they were doing other things that they shouldn't have been doing. I have never discussed it, and the few people who knew were not receptive to doing anything. It was bad. KU wanted to know why I was not getting research done. It was the most miserable time of my life. I realized very early that I just did not fit in.

In private practice, the overworked and underrecognized handmaiden was vulnerable to financial exploitation. She was likely to be patronized, denied a voice in the management of the group, and ultimately refused partnership.

I was told, "Don't you worry your pretty little head about money. Your husband's a doctor – he'll take care of you."

I joined a clinic with one other obstetrician. He was not thrilled to have me, so he never shared call. I was the only female OB-GYN and very popular with patients. I worked very hard – over 80 hours/week. I had been promised partnership after one year, plus bonus based on any earnings over $50,000 salary. I earned $150,000 the first year, but their billing and collection systems were so antiquated they wouldn't pay my bonus. They argued it was based on collections, NOT earnings. They also *declined to make me a partner. I left, resigned, and told them, "You guys are just out to bilk me."*

I was so naïve. I assumed I would share call, and the other two OBs would mentor/assist me getting established in practice. But I ended up being solo and always responsible for my own patients. The other two offered NO mentorship or support. I was very popular with patients – overwhelmingly busy. I was on call 24/7. My patients did not like seeing the others, even if I was out of town. The first thing I had to do was always to call the hospital, even if I got back to town after midnight. If one of my patients was in labor, I had to go in. I lasted three years.

My partner/colleague treated me like a superfellow. He didn't think I should have money or time to go to meetings. I did his work, saw his patients, but he billed under his name. The situation was brought to light by the practice bookkeeper. She told me, "You see the patients, but he changes the bills to get the credit." They had this weird equation – the ones with the highest billings paid the lowest overhead, so he benefitted twice. There was no way of working like that – it was so dishonest. It was not very civilized. However, I needed to prove myself and not just quit. If I left, I didn't want the partners to make up a story and say that they wanted to get rid of me or that I couldn't cut it. I waited until they offered me partnership, and then I started looking for something else. I wanted to tell them, "Thanks, but no thanks to your partnership."

Early-Career Moves

Almost all the women who felt they had been deceived in recruitment and/or mistreated in their initial practices moved on within a few years. Some were fortunate to find perfect situations immediately, sometimes almost by accident. One interviewee who had realized very early that she just did not fit in moved from the most miserable time of her life to an almost ideal practice on the advice of a family member.

My uncle practiced in a small town for 40–50 years. He said, "Come on down and see what it is like." It was about 30 miles from an Oklahoma college town, and I arrived in football season, when everything was football-mad! He loved medicine. We talked about his interesting cases. He was a mentor, took me under his wing, helped me set up a full internal medicine practice. He referred cases to me, and word spread. I quickly learned I needed more phone lines. Within a year, I had more than I could get done. Fantastic practice. I saw everything – clinic and hospital practice. The hospital had 120 beds, so plenty of backup in the community, plus that available from the cities. I was my own boss. I was the only woman on hospital staff for years, then a female OB-GYN joined. I got on well with colleagues. My uncle and I were independent, but most of the others were in this big group. It was the best of the best. I loved every minute of it.

Another interviewee, who recognized almost immediately that she did not share the values of the group, worked to gain their respect before moving to an academic position. *The group focused on business and finances. We met every month at the country club for dinner and went over all the finances. It was a complete switch from fellowship in priorities from patients and giving the best possible quality of care to a focus on money. Not scholarly. I missed the intellectual stimulation and scholarship. I eventually won respect – even the older guys liked me in the end – but it was a painful two years. I moved to a faculty position where I stayed for 19 happy years.*

About one-third of the early moves were to accommodate a husband's career. This is in keeping with descriptions of dual-professional marriages from the 1950s to the 1970s as "asymmetrical – a consistent pattern in which the professional wife gave preference – often willingly to her husband's career advancement."[9,10]

Some of these moves were across huge distances and required the young physician wife to be very adaptable to start over in different communities.

My husband was from Georgia, and I had promised when I married him that we would move to the South. When he returned from the Korean War, we opened an office in Athens, GA, looking to practice together, but there was lots of racial trouble and unrest at that time. It was pretty uncomfortable. After about a year, my husband realized he needed additional training to provide full-scope rural family practice, so we moved to a training program in North Carolina for a year. Then we settled in rural Appalachia and practiced together for over 60 years. To start in practice, I just put out a sign that I was taking patients.

I worked for the VA in San Francisco for 2–3 years. Then my husband did a vascular fellowship in Chicago. We wanted to return to the Midwest. There were too many people, too many doctors, on the West Coast. Unexpectedly, I received multiple faculty offers from medical schools in Chicago. I thought, "Wow this is unbelievable!"

We started in Washington, DC, for my husband's doctoral studies, and I worked for an HMO. Then we moved to Houston for his first appointment. Almost my entire career, I worked for managed care.

It was daunting. My husband was recruited by a group in a small town, but I had to set up on my own. I had a lot to learn, but nice fellows in the community showed me how to do things like hiring and how to run a practice.

Sometimes an interviewee attributed an early career change to her desire to settle down after testing different locations. In the restless 1970s, a young single female physician could feel unwilling to be tied to a single community until she was sure of making a long-term commitment.

I saw lots of communities but felt at home in a little German town in Texas. Very friendly people, never a lack of babysitters, and good help for a single mom. I had a single-handed practice but a great nurse and plenty of help. I could take my child with me if necessary. I LOVED the town. Built a house on a hill in the country. Lots of friends and group activities – cycling, walking, lunching, etc. My best friend introduced me to the nicest man in town, who became my second husband. I was very happy there for 30 years.

Evolving Careers

The majority of the 11 interviewees who spent their entire careers in the same practice or institution reported being well received but were aware of initial misgivings among older male colleagues and patients.

Some of the old docs had, like, an attitude, but most people were fine.

Some of the old-fashioned guys were a bit dubious, but I held my own, protected my turf.

I recall a male patient who said he was uncomfortable and skeptical when he first started seeing me. But when I was closing out my practice, he said it had been a good experience and that actually it was the best encounter he ever had with a medical doctor. That made my career. I felt like I had really become a good doctor.

Conversely, 4 of the 11 shared that they had decided to *stick it out*. They committed to building their careers in difficult environments rather than moving despite significant challenges and mistreatment. All four were in dual-career marriages with children and were well-established in the community – any move would have been highly disruptive. They did not regret their decisions, and all were proud of the success they achieved. Indeed, the adverse treatment acted as a spur to greater achievement. *I just thought, "I'll show them!"* – a sentiment that we heard from multiple interviewees at various stages of their lives, starting in grade school.

Two interviewees who remained in initially challenging situations were in academia. They both experienced the common reality for female faculty members of professional isolation, overwork, and undersupport. Most importantly, they were excluded from the mentoring, sponsorship, and networking systems essential to flourish in academia and develop the credentials necessary for advancement.[12–17]

I built the center, cared for the patients, wrote grants, did research. I became chief of the division. It was a really good section. Administration generally very good for things to benefit patients, but not supportive of me academically. At my annual review with the dean, I mentioned that I didn't have time to write all the potential papers from my research grants as I was doing so much clinical work. He took the hard-core attitude of "publish or perish" and did not offer any help.

I stayed on as faculty in academia for 20 years. It was difficult. The attitude was, "Just go away (more like just be quiet and keep your head down), we don't want any trouble." There were a lot of dark days. They didn't want to promote me. I finally hired an attorney and got promoted in 1.5 hours. I specialized, so I worked with a small group, including several women. We were very close; we took care of one another.

Two women who discussed persisting in their initial private practices focused on financial challenges. They were acutely aware of the stigma of low productivity attached to female physicians and the universal doubt that they could contribute appropriately to the practice finances. Even after almost 50 years, they conveyed the grim determination of their younger selves to prove their worth in full-bore competitive private practice. In retrospect, both recognized that the issues had been as much about respect and equality as money. Each of these women had to fight, not only for salary equity, but also for the resources to practice to her full potential and to be recognized as a full and valued partner in the organization.

I was aware of the negative doctors, the doubts that I could hold up the income. I had to prove myself. I was very well received by patients. I listened to them, spent lots of time with my patients. Initially, I was not paid as well as the men or offered joining incentives or resources like remodeled rooms or new equipment. I practiced with that clinic for 35+ years. I built my specialty department from nothing. Initially, I practiced in ordinary internal medicine exam rooms. As my practice became more sophisticated and involved more surgery, I struggled to do complex procedures in medicine exam rooms. I complained, but the clinic, especially the surgical department, resisted providing more suitable space for my procedures. I had to educate them about how much the specialty had changed. Finally, I put my foot down and threatened to leave. The clinic then remodeled an area for my own surgical suite. I recruited two other specialists, and we were gradually provided with very adequate space in a new building, including larger exam rooms with better lighting and two large surgical suites plus specialized consultation rooms. We had good production and proved our department was important financially for the clinic. I was very busy, but maybe oblivious to being treated differently as a woman.

I was still refused partnership after six years of successful practice, but an incoming male physician was offered and loaned the money for partnership after only six months. Partners said, "He has a family to support," BUT his wife was a lawyer! There was one older female partner who had been there for ages and was very timid. To everyone's surprise, she threatened a lawsuit if I wasn't made a partner. It was the only time she stuck up for me – I think the only time she ever raised her voice! The attitude of the male partners was, "Honey, don't bother your pretty little head about business." I outlasted them all. Now it is MY clinic. I will never retire.

Moves in mid- and late career were serious undertakings. A female physician had to calculate if the benefits of the new position would more than compensate for the inevitable disruption of established family and professional lives and the challenges of relocation.

The 26 women who each reported between one and five moves over their long careers identified multiple factors that clustered into six principal themes.

TABLE 16.1

Factors in Career Changes

Factor	Number (%) of Participants Reporting	Illustrative Quotations
Opportunity	18 (49%)	• *Offered to make me a professor, head of my own unit, and double the salary – sounded pretty good, so I moved.* • *I was recruited for a faculty position. It was a better option than private practice, as greater flexibility: more controllable hours, mostly in clinic, and night call was mostly covering residents.* • *I received a good offer – no call, six weeks' vacation, good salary! What's not to like?*
Problems in practice environment	18 (49%)	• *The hospital politics were horrendous, so I phased out practice and focused on long-term care.* • *I joined a private group practice close to home so avoided a bad daily commute, but it was a bad experience.* • *The chief of the department turned out to be a bad actor. He was using questionable practices, was out of control. It was bad care, and I was very uncomfortable.* • *Initially, we had four specialists in the department, but two left. Excessive workload seeing patients and teaching. It was not sustainable. The dean was not interested in recruiting or helping me out – so I moved.*
Changes in health-care systems	13 (35%)	• *Medicare changed policies in the middle of my practice, and I had no cash flow for three months before it finally was straightened out.* • *All the billing codes and regulations! All the hoops to jump through, the obstacles. I wasn't trained in business! I was tipped over the edge by excessive demands from Medicare – always being asked to prove you are honest.*
Career change	8 (22%)	• *I decided to shut down my office and do public health.* • *Aged 50, I decided to do fellowship in geriatrics for two years. Best thing I ever did was the geriatric fellowship – really found my niche.* • *I developed an interest in addiction and was invited to direct the impaired physician program. Really enjoyed the work. Good program. Fascinating to see the doctors get well.*
Family issues	13 (35%)	• *My husband wasn't getting enough specialist work, and a friend from residency persuaded him to relocate.* • *We were concerned about the quality of schools in our rural area.* • *Returned to Kansas to support our parents as they aged.*

TABLE 16.1 (*Continued*)

Factors in Career Changes

Factor	Number (%) of Participants Reporting	Illustrative Quotations
Personal health	5 (14%)	• *I had multiple medical problems and surgeries. Decided ER practice is killing me! I enjoyed the career change to urgent care. It was nice to work regular hours and have less stress. Emergency medicine is a young person's job!* • *My hands were in bad shape from arthritis, so procedures were difficult – I decided to make a career change.* • *I suffered a serious intracranial bleed, then worked part-time, then did independent medical exams and consulting.*

Note: Individuals reported 1–5 career moves and could implicate more than one factor in each move.

Moves rarely had a single motivation; most resulted from a combination of factors, some positive and some negative, some circumstance over which the woman had control, and others in which she had to react to unfavorable events or take the least objectionable course.

Opportunities and Changes

The two leading reasons given for moves were new opportunities and problems in the current position. Interviewees frequently linked these two reasons, that is, a woman was increasingly uncomfortable with her current working environment and was recruited to a new position through professional networks and/or personal contacts, sometimes before she had made a firm decision to leave.

I was happy in my situation for nearly 20 years. Problems started with the new dean in 1999. Also, my position and activities were becoming stale. I was losing interest and was at a point in my life for a change. At a conference, I met a colleague who was enthusiastic about a new National Cancer Institute (NCI) designated Comprehensive Cancer Center, very prestigious, so growing and hiring faculty. They made me a very impressive offer financially, and I would be able to focus on my areas of interest, plus I had family connections in the area. Good move all round!

I was extremely busy, working 80–100 hours per week. There was a great scarcity of mental health professionals in the area. Only two psychiatrists to cover 20 counties. By 1992, I was exhausted, then a once-in-a-blue-moon opportunity came up, so I moved. (For additional quotations, see Table 16.1.)

Changes in Health-Care Systems

In about one-third of moves, changes in health-care systems were cited as major factors. This was most apparent in psychiatry, when the shift from inpatient to outpatient care that began in the 1980s coincided with significant reductions in payments for psychiatric services. These changes had devastating impact on psychiatrists both on hospital staff and in private practice.

I had a great practice with three other psychiatrists plus social workers, psychologists, different types of staff. Also had a day center, but was always worried about funding from the state.

Expenses became too heavy, plus managed care suddenly halved the fees.

It was a county hospital psychiatric department. It was a good job, primarily outpatient child and some adult, but began to obviously look like it was running into financial and other problems. They started not renewing contracts, so looked like the unit was going to fold. I started looking for another position.

After over 20 years in practice, one psychiatrist adapted by subspecializing and found fulfillment in her new role. *The biggest change was 1987–1997, getting into Jungian analysis and the international association of Jungian therapists. Many great friends in Jungian groups – local and nationally.*

The perception that *psychiatry has always been stigmatized* and vulnerable to budget cuts was echoed in pediatrics, another specialty that suffered financially and lost prestige during the last decades of the 20th century. *Pediatrics being low in the hierarchy of hospital and clinic and being a woman was the double whammy. Constant pressure to see more patients, generate greater income, work harder! I was told I "spent too much time with patients." It seemed time to leave.*

Beginning in the 1980s, physicians in all specialties were impacted by the takeover of solo or small group practices by large staff-model health systems or the buyouts of local hospitals and clinics by national organizations.

Occupational medicine was changing, with health care increasingly outsourced to national chains. I felt I was losing my identity as the plant doctor.

Changes in medical practice and payment arrangements impacted almost all specialties and communities. When a rural community hospital closed, one interviewee found her internal medicine practice became financially unsustainable, and she sought a salaried position in a nearby city. Similar experiences were reported by specialists in rehabilitation medicine and in pathology.

Even in specialties that were less severely impacted by the changes in health services during the period, the majority of interviewees cited the increasing administrative burdens and commercialization of medical practice as contributing to moves or retirement decisions. *The paperwork! Even when computers came in – forget it! Also, the administrative politics. Medicine changed. I had a hard transition when the physician-owned clinic sold to a commercial entity.* These experiences drove several interviewees to join larger groups or accept salaried positions during the 1990s.

When the practice was bought out by a national company, I moved. (For additional quotations, see Table 16.1.)

Career Changes

Eight interviewees (22%) decided to make complete career changes after 10–15 years in practice. One described her change as a *counterattack* to the impact of managed care on psychiatry.

I decided to enter the cave of the enemy and became medical director for a managed care company. Mostly reviewing charts, nagging doctors, and supervising nurses. The nurses really taught me what to do. The secret was to balance what the doctors wanted and what the company required. I enjoyed the big game of "How much care can I give away today without incurring your wrath?"

More commonly, an interviewee made a career change because she felt she had *outgrown the job or just wanted a change.*

After seven years as internist, I started getting bored. I took care of the full gamut of conditions, but in a multispecialty clinic, cases were passed on to subspecialists. My remaining practice was too routine and just boring. I felt I was no longer learning, being curious. Internal medicine (IM) was grueling. I worked very hard. I increasingly wanted to help and spend more time with patients who had unmet needs. Lots of patients had problems whose source was not medical. Considered doing endocrinology or another subspecialty, but I believed psychiatry would give me more time to help patients. I was not sure where it would lead, but my youngest child was starting kindergarten, so it seemed a good time to make a change. Gave myself permission to take a year off, and I loved it – it was great! During my interview for psychiatry residency, a resident (much younger than me) was concerned about my having children and asked how I would handle the call. After years of IM call for in-hospital, outpatient, and ER coverage, this was amusing!

Then I thought, "I'm tired of all this," and quit. Worked for the Department of Defense in Europe for three years, then back to academia for seven years, then retired. It's been a very interesting career! (For additional quotations, see Table 16.1.)

Although dissatisfaction with current position or a need to adjust to health or personal issues contributed to many career moves, several interviewees described aspirational motivations. These women wanted to prioritize caring for patients or *making a difference* amid the increasing commercialization of medical practice.

I decided to go back to West Virginia and give back to the people there. It had been a wonderful experience when I was in high school, and I wanted to go back. I started a private practice from scratch in a small town in West Virginia, internal medicine plus endocrinology, especially diabetes. Very hard work and stressful, but proud to make a go of it.

For the last 16 years, I have been working in program to provide indigent care that includes precepting medical students. Patients really seem to like me. I have generations of the same family coming to me.

The company was bought out, and the new one was too hard to please. I thought, "I can't do this anymore." I was feeling guilty. I looked around for a way to help sick people out. A church group had a grant to help homeless people with mental problems, so I started talking to people on the porch. Word got around. We had groups, individual discussions. Enjoyed it so much. Helped a lot of people.

Some interviewees conveyed a sense of giving themselves permission to take on interesting opportunities or follow some long-standing interest in the final years of their careers. These changes often opened up entirely new careers for women, some of whom were over 60 when they made the change.

I decided to shut down my office and do public health. My hands were in a bad shape from arthritis, and I was interested in bridging the gap between people who worked with populations and those who worked with individuals. Public health training in the United States was two years and expensive. In the UK, I could train in one year and it cost less. I went to Liverpool, and I loved it! As part of training, in 2001, I did a project in South Africa, driving to rural villages for fieldwork on prenatal care. Very interesting. Hung around UK, looking for a job, but too old and too American. They implied I should be looking to retire, not start over. Returned to United States and worked for Doctors of the World writing programs and grants, looked for money. Foreign development is a young person's game. I was too cynical and too salty, so I quit aged about 64. I was offered a job in New York investigating maternal mortality, and I investigated these deaths till I was 70.

Some women described seeking adventure after decades in practice.

Maybe we had some sort of mid-life crisis! A friend worked for the State Department and went all over the world – sounded like fun to travel the world and have the government pay for it. The State Department only recruited primary care physicians, so my surgeon husband was the trailing spouse! I was responsible for US citizens in 17–18 countries of former USSR and eastern Europe and traveled 50% of the time while my husband volunteered as surgeon. My family supported the adventure!

I had a taste for overseas work from working in 1990s in Project Hope. I went to Pristina, Kosovo, right after the bombing as a volunteer for Doctors of the World. It was a war zone. You had to be very careful.

Family Issues

Several different family issues factored into career moves for our interviewees. The early careers of married women were commonly influenced by the professional needs of their husbands. This priority was much less apparent in later career moves. In the mid- and later careers of dual-professional couples, our participants reported that the wife was just as likely as her husband to initiate a move – one interviewee even described her physician husband as *the trailing spouse* in her late career change. These reports correlate with studies of dual-career marriages, as married women became more common in the professions during the last decades of the 20th century. A 1982 study concluded that career decisions reached by dual-physician couples had become much more mutual and that marriages between professionals "had become more egalitarian although there was still a long way to go."[9,10,18]

In some mid-career moves, interviewees were influenced by family concerns, such as availability of good schools for their children. This was conveyed as an additional factor for physicians who were already uncomfortable with their practices and considering a move, rather than the direct cause of a family relocation. Conversely, four participants cited the need to care for elderly parents, spouses, or other family members as the principal cause of mid- to late career moves. In one case, this opened up an entirely new career.

I would have stayed longer in that practice, but my mother and sister both got breast cancer, and Mother was not doing well. This was 1983. Women with breast cancer metastases usually didn't last. I was the only backup, so I packed up and drove 300 miles to Texas. I moved to be with family and didn't care if I had a job, but a cousin was a surgery intern and said, "Surgery needs an ER doc, and they want to interview you – think about it." I had taken care of ER patients at KU, so I thought, "Sure," and went over like an idiot. It was fairly slow (thank God). I grew up in this new specialty, and ER flourished with me. It was exciting, thinking on your feet. I fell on my feet in the ER, and I loved it. A thrill a minute. Wonderful time in my life. (Mother and sister both did well. Mother lived to 93, and sister 30 years out from diagnosis – with lots of bumps in between!) (For additional quotations, see Table 16.1.)

Personal Health

Interviewees reported a variety of personal health issues contributing to career change decisions. Stress and medical conditions were much more important factors in decisions to reduce workload or retire than in decisions to move or change careers. Some participants attributed their health problems directly to their work.

All the stress, I believe, culminated in my having cardiovascular disease that necessitated a quadruple bypass at age 58. It was a wake-up call: I needed to reduce my workload.

I was very stressed and had poorly controlled hypertension. My nurses told me, "You can't go on," so I decided to make a change. (For additional quotations, see Table 16.1.)

To Retire or Not to Retire?

Although our participants were all over 70 years of age when interviewed during the winter of 2020–2021, 11 (30%) reported working full- or part-time. Work was very important for these participants, even during the pandemic and lockdowns. They conveyed enthusiasm and pride in being practicing physicians. A strong sense of service was evident.

We see patients from all over the world with all types of conditions. I learn something new every day. I truly like what I do. There is always new information. Now, getting into prevention and evaluation of patients at high risk. We have research retreats to develop/share/bounce ideas around with colleagues from widely different areas. People ask me about retiring or slowing down, but having too much fun – too interesting. I told my chair I would quit if he ever thought I was not pulling my weight, but I am going strong and feel productive, supported, and valued.

Not sure the end is in sight! I enjoy working. This year in the pandemic, I am working more, as I can't travel or do other things. Medicine is a calling, an honor, extremely rewarding. We are given the privilege to be with people at the most stressful times of their lives. It is an honor and a privilege. Medicine enables us to be constantly learning, continue to be curious, to expand our knowledge. I really like teaching and patient care. I like helping the learners develop professionally and become excited about the field.

Aged 88, I am still practicing – always said I would retire when I was 90!

Rather than slowing down, two interviewees described important projects they had initiated within the last three years. Both projects were challenging but obviously very fulfilling capstone professional experiences.

Still working in my 70s – so much for the concerns of that interviewer on the med school admissions committee! I am currently working with the VA to develop breast cancer screening for female vets – women are now 59% of new vets, and the numbers keep increasing. There is a tremendous need nationally for health promotion and screening for female vets. They are so neglected, so vulnerable. I love what I do! It is a real opportunity to train fellows and residents and to give back.

I retired in 2015. I have now become an interfaith chaplain, and currently, I am taking a course in clinical pastoral education. I intend to become an interfaith chaplain for retirement communities and establish a chaplain consultancy service with my partner, specializing in serving long-term care facilities.

One retired participant was seriously considering returning to full-time work and had an offer of a new appointment once the pandemic restrictions were lifted. Conversely, another interviewee was considering retirement, mainly due to telemedicine and other changes in medical practice resulting from the COVID-19 pandemic.

For the last 16 years, I have been working in a medical school program to provide indigent care. It includes precepting medical students. Since March 2020, working via telemedicine, but it is not the same. I have always worked full-time. Worked hard. Now I am thinking about retiring.

Reasons for Retirement

Family considerations and issues in the local and national practice of medicine were important in decisions to retire. Personal health issues or serious health problems in a family member also factored into many retirement decisions. Several participants were current or recent caretakers for family members suffering from long-term or terminal illnesses. Again, decisions were seldom based on a single issue or event; retirement was generally described as a decision that evolved from growing frustration with the administrative burden of practice plus increasing need to manage personal or family health problems. Being a physician and service to others were important components of the identities of our participants. They described struggling with the decision to retire, especially if they perceived unmet need in their specialties.

I hung on as there was a great shortage of child psychiatrists.

I had an exceptional career. It was a bit less fun at the end – medical records, etc., were less rewarding, more stressful, time-demanding. It was a good time to retire but makes me a little sad. I still miss some things.

I retired at 62 in 2003 mainly due to changes in practice. Pressure to see more patients, generate greater income – seemed time to leave.

I retired 2013. Tipped over the edge by excessive demands from Medicare, always being asked to prove you are honest.

I worked until I was 70. It was fine, but I fell badly a couple of times and decided to retire. I had several health problems, including breast cancer and spinal stenosis.

Retired at 60. Husband had retired, and after my cardiac surgery, I realized that I couldn't tolerate the lifestyle I had adopted.

I moved to part-time in 2008 following hip replacement and retired in 2012 in part because practice was selling the lab to a national group, but also because of increasing paperwork and the challenges of keeping up with molecular biology and other advances.

Several interviewees found the transition to retirement difficult, and some remained involved in professional activities.

I do consulting in my field and chart reviews for a large federal program, plus intensive COVID-19 education for the community where I live.

I volunteer in the community. Important to give back. After retirement, I volunteered in a clinic for those without insurance.

When I retired in 2018, I felt done, but patients still call, and I talk with them.

I retired about two years ago, but I keep up my continuing education requirement and love to read and keep up. Sill in touch with many ex-patients – they call or drop in for advice.

One interviewee reflected that her demanding career had inhibited building up support networks for retirement and that she had found the transition difficult. *Career probably detracted from relationships – didn't have time to build up social networks, play bridge, have lunches, etc. Felt this at retirement. The lack of diverse outside interests probably stunts growth.*

Others embraced retirement with the same energy they had brought to building their professional lives.

I loved practice, but this retirement is SO much fun.

I retired to assist my mother with Alzheimer's, but I am very busy with multiple activities – sports, gardening, friends, hobbies, traveling.

Summary and Reflections

Each of the 37 interviewees spent more than 50 years in medical practice. They cared for patients in diverse locations and types of practice in 13 different medical specialties. As expected from national statistics, their most common careers were in internal medicine, pediatrics, psychiatry, and anesthesiology (Table 13.1), but our group had a high number of internal medicine specialists (30%). This may reflect the dominant roles of that department and its charismatic teachers on their training, as described in Chapter 12. Across all specialties, their firsthand accounts of practice illustrate the enormous variety of experiences for individual female physicians since the 1950s. Each alumna described a unique career pattern; nevertheless, their stories resonate with several key issues in the literature about women in medicine over this period.

The most striking theme is of *going it alone*. Although not the first women in medicine or sometimes even in their personal practice situations, our interviewees expressed a sense of having to continually work out their own pathways or adapt within systems designed for men. They repeatedly had to clear obstacles and navigate difficulties that were not encountered by their male colleagues. These ranged from the oldest woman's difficulties in securing premed courses to fighting for academic recognition and promotion to full professor. One senior academic commented that this was a lifelong process – even the services for the transition to retirement were entirely male-oriented. Her comment that, even at the end of a very long career, the system had not caught up with the concept that some physicians were female led us to investigate the scanty literature on senior female physicians.[19] The only study we found that looked at retirement issues for women in medicine confirmed that female and male faculty members had multiple significant differences in the factors influencing retirement decisions and their priorities for resources and services in the retirement transition and beyond.[20] Nevertheless, we have been unable to identify any programs or other studies concerning the final career stages and retirement transitions of female physicians. As one of our participants expressed, *despite the numbers, the saga of acting as if all physicians are guys continues.*

This sense of always breaking new ground is not new or unique to our interviewees. One of the first female deans of a medical school (and a KUMC 1944 graduate) commented, "Every step of the way is a way in which I had to work it out myself."[7] A 1968 report concluded that

> "present women physicians are in many ways guinea pigs for future generations, sometimes performing this function happily, and at other times grudgingly. Many are trying to find out for themselves whether it is possible to combine the satisfactions that are traditionally feminine with the fulfillments of an engrossing, all-encompassing profession like medicine."[4]

A more belligerent metaphor was used by Californian graduates in the early 1970s who described themselves as "shock troops storming the beaches of enemy territory."[8] Given the large numbers of women in the classes after 1975, a better metaphor might be of surfers riding the waves in advance of a tsunami. We prefer the concept advocated by several writers that women are no longer outsiders struggling against the norms of the profession but are improving the culture of medicine from within.[4,5]

Some of the lack of a clear career pathway for women in medicine related to confusion and controversy over an appropriate ideal (or even tolerable) female physician. Was she supposed to demonstrate all the attitudes and behaviors of her male colleagues and be *one of the boys*, or was there some unique way of being both a full-fledged physician and a woman? The older literature offered two contrasting stereotypes to a woman trying to develop a professional identity – the defeminized, unattractive "hen medic," who aggressively tried to "outman the men" and had no interests or life outside of medicine, and the demure, attractive "dilettante lady physician," who was content to dabble in medicine, accepting part-time and low-prestige positions that posed no threat to her male colleagues.[2,4] As they built their careers, our interviewees recognized both as grotesque caricatures, but they encountered few role models of female physicians who were successful both personally and professionally. Many reported struggling with the more daunting and equally unrealistic third stereotype of the superwoman who could do it all that developed during the 1960s and the 1970s.[1,5,8]

When asked about female role models, the entire group could only name about five individuals over the decades covered. Several mentioned encountering senior female physicians who were *distant, difficult, unhelpful,* or even *odd.* One interviewee described a senior woman who discriminated against female trainees as acting as a *queen bee who only mentored guys.* Overall, the group did not perceive they had received adequate support and mentoring as trainees compared to their male peers; only four reported mentoring and guidance from male faculty members. Similarly, in practice, they often contrasted their own experiences with those of male newcomers, who were welcomed into the professional and social milieux with practical assistance and colleagues willing to *show them the ropes.*

The lack of female role models, the discrimination in career development, and the professional isolation described by our participants are strong themes in the literature on women in medicine.[2–17] Until recently, relatively few women attained leadership roles or high academic rank, and those who do are commonly overburdened with administrative responsibilities, such as the token woman on committees. Even if available, senior women have not always been helpful mentors or provided useful role models for other female physicians. Senior women may have doubted their ability to mentor or had misgivings about being regarded as positive role models; others felt just too overwhelmed by the multiple demands of their personal and professional lives to devote appropriate time and energy to mentoring.[21,22] Ironically, successful women have sometimes been unsympathetic to struggling juniors. Especially in older reports, friction was evident between women who had achieved success through complete personal dedication to the profession and those who sought to combine medicine with marriage and family. As one unsympathetic senior female physician remarked, "this modern quest for fulfillment seems crazy. . . . Few persons, doctors included, have everything as they dreamed it."[4] The perspective that women who were not sufficiently dedicated would damage the credibility of other women was learned early. A 1968 survey reported that the majority of female medical students opposed increasing the numbers of women in medical schools on the grounds that only those with the dedication and emotional preparation should be admitted. "The stringent process of natural selection is necessary, they feel, to ensure that those girls who reach medical school are prepared to give what the training demands."[4]

Almost all the literature related to career development and mentoring concerns of women in academic medicine. The vast majority of female physicians have been on their own as they sought to build their careers in private practice or salaried positions. Only relatively recently have health-care organizations, specialty societies, and other groups recognized the importance of support and career development for female physicians outside of academic centers.

Given the consensus on the lack of career guidance and support for women of that time, the recurrent theme of chance or serendipity in career moves is not surprising. This was the underlying factor or tipping point behind many of the reasons for moves listed in Table 16.1. Interviewees repeatedly described how conversations with colleagues, relatives, or others resulted in decisions to make significant career changes. Some of these contacts were portrayed as casual comments or lighthearted suggestions; others occurred during collegial networking. Several interviewees referred to *corridor conversations* as the impetus for exploring or being offered new positions. Nevertheless, almost all moves involved multiple factors. Opportunities that appeared serendipitous only resulted in a move if the female physician was already primed to take up the opportunity – for example, beginning to feel restless or unhappy with her current position or considering relocating for other reasons. Whatever the circumstances, multiple references were made to unexpected opportunities, often encountered seemingly by chance, that resulted in pivotal career changes.

Across all specialties and working environments, our interviewees revealed a major theme of openness to change and adaptability to new circumstances. The relative lack of role models or clear expectations for female physicians could have contributed to them feeling less constrained by stereotypes and more open to new opportunities than their male colleagues. Conversely, years of experience of adapting to adverse circumstances could have equipped them to deal with unanticipated changes in family circumstances or organizational changes in medicine. Several commented that they had continued to enjoy practice, relish contact with patients, and even flourish professionally in their senior years, whereas many of their male colleagues were bitter, disillusioned, and burned out.

I suspect the women enjoy it more than the men, especially as we get older. Men seem to turn into grumpy old men, complaining especially about being called at night.

The interviewees certainly seemed to grow in confidence and self-determination with age. We were reminded of the "pioneer pride" term used in a study reporting higher career satisfaction in older female physicians compared to their younger colleagues.[23] Other studies of career satisfaction by age and gender provide mixed results.[24,25] Several studies reporting greater career satisfaction among older physicians attribute this to the older groups containing those who had learned to adapt and flourish within the system.[23–26]

Career satisfaction clearly relates to multiple factors, including personal characteristics, sense of control over time and work, collegiality, support and respect, and importantly, a sense of meaningful work – *making a difference.* Our interviewees conveyed continuing enthusiasm for medicine, curiosity about life, and deep interest in people, balanced with a pragmatic understanding of the many challenges and difficulties involved in life as a physician. We explored this further by inviting them to tell us more about their years in practice and specifically asking them to talk about the best and worst aspects, including if they had ever felt burned out or considered giving up medicine.

REFERENCES

1. Douglas SJ. Where the girls are: growing up female with the mass media. New York (NY): Times Books;1994.
2. Lopate C. Women in medicine. Baltimore (MD): Johns Hopkins Press;1968.
3. Spieler C, editor. Women in medicine. 1976 Report of a Macy Conference. New York (NY): Josiah Macy Jr., Foundation;1977.
4. Morantz-Sanchez R. Sympathy & science: women physicians in American medicine. New York (NY): Oxford University Press;1985.
5. More ES. Restoring the balance: women physicians and the profession of medicine 1985–1995. Cambridge (MA): Harvard University Press;1999.
6. Anon. Women in health care and pediatrics: women in pediatric practice. Pediatrics. 1983;71(4):699–705.
7. Morantz RM, Pomerleau CS, Fenichel CH. In her own words: oral histories of women physicians. Westport (CT): Greenwood Press;1982.
8. Martin T. When the personal was political: five women doctors look back. Lincoln (NE): iUniverse;2008.
9. Eisenberg C. Women as physicians. J Med Educ. 1983;58:534–41.

10. Marwell G, Rosenfeld R, Spilerman S. Geographic constraints on women's careers in academia. Science. 1979;205:1225–31.

11. Bowman M, Gross ML. Overview of research on women in medicine – issues for public policymakers. Public Health Rep. 1986 Sep–Oct;101(5):513–21.

12. Levinson W, Kaufman K, Clark B, Tolle SW. Mentors and role models for women in academic medicine. West J Med. 1991 Apr;154(4):423–6.

13. AAMC Project Committee on Increasing Women's Leadership in Academic Medicine. Increasing women's leadership in academic medicine. Acad Med. 1996;71:800–10.

14. Ochberg RL, Barton GM, West AN. Women physicians and their mentors. J Am Med Womens Assoc (1972). 1989 Jul–Aug;44(4):123–6.

15. Bates C, Gordon L, Travis E, Chatterjee A, Chaudron L, Fivush B, et al. Striving for gender equity in academic medicine careers: a call to action. Acad Med. 2016 Aug;91(8):1050–2.

16. Bickel J. Women in academic medicine. J Am Med Womens Assoc (1972). 2000 Winter;55(1):10–2.

17. Tesch BJ, Wood HM, Helwig AL, Nattinger AB. Promotion of women physicians in academic medicine: glass ceiling or sticky floor? JAMA. 1995 Apr 5;273(13):1022–5.

18. Lorber J. How physician spouses influence each other's careers. J Am Med Wom Assoc. 982;37:21–6.

19. Templeton K, Nilsen KM, Walling A. Issues faced by senior women physicians: a national survey. J Womens Health (Larchmt). 2020 Jul;29(7):980–8.

20. Levine RB, Walling A, Chatterjee A, Skarupski KA. Factors influencing retirement decisions of senior faculty at U.S. medical schools: are there gender-based differences? J Womens Health (Larchmt). 2022 Jul;31(7):974–82.

21. Shen MR, Tzioumis E, Andersen E, Wouk K, McCall R, Li W, et al. Impact of mentoring on academic career success for women in medicine: a systematic review. Acad Med. 2022 Mar 1;97(3):444–58.

22. Levinson W, Kaufman K, Clark B, Tolle SW. Mentors and role models for women in academic medicine. West J Med. 1991 Apr;154(4):423–6.

23. Frank E, McMurray JE, Linzer M, Elon L. Career satisfaction of US women physicians: results from the Women Physicians' Health Study: Society of General Internal Medicine career satisfaction study group. Arch Intern Med. 1999 Jul 12;159(13):1417–26.

24. Wetterneck TB, Linzer M, McMurray JE, Douglas J, Schwartz MD, Bigby J, et al. Worklife and satisfaction of general internists. Arch Intern Med. 2002;162(6):649–56.

25. McMurray JE, Linzer M, Konrad TR, Douglas J, Shugerman R, Nelson K. The work lives of women physicians results from the physician work life study: the SGIM career satisfaction study group. J Gen Intern Med. 2000 Jun;15(6):372–80.

26. Haas JS, Cleary PD, Puopolo AL, Burstin HR, Cook EF, Brennan TA. Differences in the professional satisfaction of general internists in academically affiliated practices in the greater-Boston area: ambulatory medicine quality improvement project investigators. J Gen Intern Med. 1998 Feb;13(2):127–30.

17

Practice Realities: The Good, the Bad, and the Intolerable

By the early 1980s, all our interviewees had joined the approximately 51,000 active female physicians in the United States. Women represented about 12% of active physicians – roughly double the percentage of earlier decades. The percentages of residents (23%), medical graduates (26.7%), and matriculants (33%) were at historical peaks and accelerating.[1] Nevertheless, women continued to be clustered in allegedly female appropriate specialties. They represented 30% of pediatricians, 26.5% of physicians in physical medicine/rehabilitation, and 21% in public health. With the exception of obstetrics and gynecology (13.7%), less than 6% of physicians in all surgical specialties were women.[1]

Women had momentum to advance in medicine, but attitudes and the realities of daily work changed slowly, especially in private practice. Surprisingly, little information is available about the collective personal experience of women physicians practicing during the second half of the 20th century.[2–7] Until the Women Physicians' Health Study (WPHS), studies of physicians had few female participants.[8]

During the latter decades of the 20th century, the sparse literature on women in medical practice was dominated by concerns about their low productivity. Increasing the numbers of female physicians was perceived as counterproductive to addressing the "medical *man*power crisis."[9,10] A 1968 report conveyed the sense of national emergency. "With such a shortage of physicians, we have to get the optimum amount of service out of every one we train."[11] Training women was regarded as a poor investment – even an unpatriotic waste of resources. Throughout their decades in practice, our interviewees encountered this belief that female physicians were less productive than their male colleagues and were best employed as adjuncts or handmaidens in "appropriate roles in specialties that do not attract adequate numbers of men."[12]

The WPHS data demonstrated that over the final decades of the 20th century, female physicians were outgrowing stereotypes and becoming a highly heterogenous group. They gained representation in specialties other than the 5Ps (pediatrics, psychiatry, pathology, public health, physical medicine/rehabilitation) and were increasingly unwilling to accept adjunctive roles or any available position in practice. The WPHS and other studies documented differences between women who entered medical school during and after the 1970s and earlier cohorts of female physicians in hours worked and types of clinical practice.[1–4,8] As women expanded their hours and scope of practice, their male colleagues were generally decreasing hours and increasingly selecting salaried positions. The practice patterns of male and female physicians were

DOI: 10.1201/9781003539568-17

already converging when all physicians were faced with adjusting to the massive changes of the late 20th century in financing health care, rise of large health systems, and decline in traditional fees for service in private practice.[13]

The WPHS generated several articles about the practice characteristics of female physicians, their personal health, and even domestic responsibilities.[8,14–17] As described in Chapter 1, however, insights on their personal experiences can only be gleaned from essays, biographies, autobiographies, and a few oral history collections.

Every woman physician has a unique life experience and perspective on her career. A 1968 review abandoned the attempt to "communicate what it is like to be a woman in medicine in the United States, as summarizing the contradictory and ambiguous impressions of women physicians would be an impossible task."[11] This sobering warning that lifetimes of diverse experiences in practice could not be reduced to a few adjectives, phrases, or even a single book chapter became very real as we considered how to encourage our participants to speak freely about their experiences of practice and document what they revealed. As described in the introduction, we used a combination of open questions to invite their overall recollections of practice, with follow-up prompts to address key areas. The interviewee controlled the conversation. Some participants made sweeping generalizations about their professional lives; others described key aspects in detail. Most interviewees illustrated their recollections with anecdotes about patients, colleagues, family members, and others. The amount of attention to any single area varied enormously. Most responded spontaneously to the open prompts ("Tell me about your practice" or "What was practice like for you?") with multiple positive comments. We followed up on these immediate responses with questions to clarify both positive and negative experiences. We used the discussion of negative experiences to transition to any experiences of burnout or thoughts of giving up medicine. This chapter covers these three aspects of practice, namely, best aspects, worst aspects, and any periods of burnout or wanting to quit medicine. Other unique aspects of life as a female physician are discussed in the following chapters.

The Best Aspects of Practice

All participants were quick to identify the best aspects of practice as female physicians. In response to the single prompt question "What was the best thing about being in practice?" they spoke enthusiastically about their professional lives, generating approximately 100 positive comments that clustered into seven major themes (Table 17.1). Almost all participants identified several themes and conveyed a strong sense of synergy across themes.

The dual concepts of enjoying patient care (relationships, helping people, making a difference) and appreciation for the personal fulfillment they found in meaningful work (intellectual and technical challenges, teamwork, sense of accomplishment, leadership) were apparent in all descriptions of the positive aspects of their lives as female physicians.

Relationships with patients. Being able to do good work, be helpful. Also work relationships with other professionals.

I enjoyed the prestige, the intellectual challenge. It felt good to do work that helped people, occasionally even saving their lives.

The very best times were late 1980s and into 1990s. I had the rigors and satisfaction of a full practice, plus a range of related other activities that were very worthwhile and interesting – Board of Healing Arts, committees for my specialty national society, question-writing for board exams, etc. I felt I brought a long experience to bear on these things.

The interviewees spoke candidly about core issues that physicians sometimes find difficult or embarrassing to articulate, such as the paradoxical combination of humility and pride in being able to serve others, and the challenges and delights of wrestling with intellectual challenges in solving complex problems. They conveyed genuine and enduring enthusiasm for medicine but had a pragmatic understanding of the arduous physical and emotional demands of their profession.

I LOVE making diagnoses. LOVE making people better, healthier. Learning something new every day, contributing to society. Always exciting, new knowledge, sparking ideas off colleagues. The WOW! Where else in a profession can people be so honest and open with you? People tell doctors everything. The patient stories, every one is different, unique. I have learned so much and am still learning about human nature, life, and I am in awe of the strength of people to survive and endure struggle and hardship.

(For additional quotations, see Table 17.1.)

TABLE 17.1

Best Aspects of Practice

Theme Number (%) of Interviewees	Illustrative Quotations
Patient relationships 32 (87%)	• *Interacting with patients, easily the best part.* • *I am sold on understanding and listening to people.* • *Working with people one-on-one.* • *Relationships with patients. They are dealing with major disruptions in their lives. They are so resilient.* • *The kids! I love taking care of kids.* • *I loved being with the patients, watching them grow up, treating the children of children you had treated. I loved dealing with parents.* • *I appreciated cultivating long-term relationships with patients and their families.* • *Relationships with patients. Trust. I have generations of the same family coming to me – I really like that.* • *Taking care of patients. It is about the people. Seeing the same people over 43 years, taking care of families.*

(Continued)

TABLE 17.1 (*Continued*)

Best Aspects of Practice

Theme Number (%) of Interviewees	Illustrative Quotations
Helping others/ Making a difference 25 (68%)	• *Being able to make a difference in the care of women. Women deserve respectful service, help understanding their self-worth and ability to make decisions.* • *Working with kids early in life to make things better, to get them on a healthy developmental course, to watch them blossom, go on to do well.* • *I loved getting graduation announcements from kids – "You go, kid, you did it!" Lovely to get thank-you notes from patients, families, students.* • *Watching children grow up and succeed. Seeing them go from not functioning to their full capacity. Getting them on the right track. Seeing them succeed.* • *There is nothing like being with a patient and family. GREAT when that door closes and just you and the patient and the family to figure out what is going on – it's just great. Knowing your knowledge is going to make a difference. Making people more comfortable.* • *Having the knowledge and ability to make a difference in other people's lives.*
Professional activities 21 (57%)	• *ER was exciting, to think on your feet. I loved it. A thrill a minute. Wonderful time in my life.* • *I enjoyed being an anesthesiologist. Always a lot going on in OR. On your toes all the time. Enjoyed the action.* • *Worked with many different bright, curious, intelligent colleagues with broad interests, always fascinating. Challenging me to move to learn more, to learn how to do better.* • *Rewarding. I love psychiatry and worked in a wonderful facility. Advocating for training therapists, nurses, and support staff to help kids with trauma.* • *Really like teamwork, great respect for teamwork and for really smart nurses and social workers. I liked staff meetings – everyone working together for the patient.* • *Relationships with staff and colleagues. Everything goes down to the team. I always valued the opinions of nurses, therapists, others.* • *Friends and colleagues on the faculty – they are the best!* • *Worked with an exceptionally nice group of people, wonderful colleagues. Really dedicated and supportive.* • *My colleagues were wonderful.*
Learning, problem-solving 19 (51%)	• *Constantly learning, being curious, constantly expanding knowledge.* • *Always learning new things – I love to learn.* • *We confronted issues and challenged traditions such as the Freudian approach. We made a difference to the specialty.* • *The challenge. I loved helping sick babies. I really, really loved working all night at the bedside, trying different things to work out how to help them.* • *I really enjoyed the thought processes of diagnoses, like solving detective stories.* • *Love the intellectual challenge to figure it all out.*

TABLE 17.1 (*Continued*)

Best Aspects of Practice

Theme Number (%) of Interviewees	Illustrative Quotations
Sense of accomplishment 12 (32%)	• *The work is increasingly recognized in the field. I felt fortunate to be part of the change in treatment.* • *Great sense of accomplishment about building a small-town practice from scratch and learning all the business things, etc.* • *I think I had the reputation as a person who really took care of patients. Colleagues and trainees asked my advice. The department named the Patient Advocacy Award for me. I worked a lot of cases and was treated with respect. Proud of my expertise.* • *Women doctors get tremendous admiration from society for what you have done – that is lovely. "Wow, you are a doctor?" It's nice. It's a privilege.*
Leadership, national/ international activities 7 (19%)	• *Many great friends in professional groups – local and nationally, even internationally.* • *Active nationally. Lots of committee service, and I was the first female president of our specialty society.* • *Very active in state medical society and national academy. Lots of traveling for the politics.* • *Being very active in my professional organizations, nationally and locally. I was the second woman president of our national group.* • *Really enjoyed my national activities, especially service on FDA and National Cancer Institute review panels – fascinating groups and good people.* • *Most fun from being very active nationally, especially with national academy. Very active for many years. Participated and/or led national high-level committees and task forces. Got to work with so many wonderful people, from all kinds of areas – government, clinicians, researchers, big corporations. All SO smart. Doing something really important. Trying to make this technological age work for patients and docs.*
Teaching 3 (8%)	• *Teaching is very rewarding. It's exciting when they see something like an eardrum, or you gather them around so they can hear the heart murmur.*

Patient-Related Themes

Relationships with Patients

All interviewees conveyed that interacting with patients was the best aspect of practicing medicine, and 32 (87%) elaborated with specific comments. They expressed genuine interest in people and appreciation for the personal interactions that medicine enabled them to have with individuals. They spoke with deep respect and admiration for the endurance and resilience of patients and families, even in the face of serious medical problems.

I am in awe of the strength of people to survive and endure struggle and hardship.

Long-term relationships with patients and families were important. The interviewees felt this represented patient trust in their professional expertise and validated the quality of the care they provided. They were humbled by long-term patient relationships and proud of years of service to individuals, families, and communities. Above all, they were still enthusiastic about medicine.

Privilege to be entrusted, good life – I had a great time.

Pride in caring for individuals over decades or several generations of one family was not limited to primary care specialties. Ophthalmologists, dermatologists, and even anesthesiologists spoke movingly of being repeatedly sought out for care by individuals or family members. Some of these professional relationships lasted for decades.

The best part? Definitely the patients. Delightful, wonderful, made life fun. I had patients I cared for over 40 years. I had four generations of some families.

Further evidence of the importance of continuity of care and trust was found in stories of patients who remained in touch or traveled to consult interviewees after they had closed practices or left the community. Our interviewees enjoyed their patients and felt honored to be trusted with their care.

Helping Others, Making a Difference

Interwoven with descriptions of relationships with patients was a strong theme of appreciation for *having meaningful work* and *opportunities to make a difference* in the lives of patients, families, and communities. The interviewees conveyed an enthusiastic yet vocational approach to medicine characterized by a sense of service, humility, and personal dedication. They expressed a sense of being in the optimum profession. *Medicine was absolutely the right thing for me to do.* Two-thirds of the interviewees specifically identified helping others or making a difference as the *best thing about being a female physician.*

We are given the privilege to be with people at the most stressful times of their lives. It is an honor and a privilege – extremely rewarding.

Several interviewees expressed delight when patients did well. While proud of their efforts to help others, they tended to credit good outcomes more to the courage and tenacity of patients and families than to their efforts as physicians.

Lovely to see patients "graduate" from care. Someone who came in really depressed, for example, needing inpatient or suicidal, we worked with them, they got better and I wasn't needed anymore – SUPER!

(For additional quotations, see Table 17.1.)

Professional and Intellectual Themes

Enjoyment of Practice

All interviewees conveyed that they enjoyed or even *loved* practicing medicine. *Got up in the morning looking forward to it.* Just over half (57%) provided specific comments articulating this view. Several appreciated the variety of medicine and how their opportunities and experiences evolved over time. *Lots of good experiences. Each thing seemed to fit my stage of life.*

Enthusiasm for medicine was especially apparent in those who continued to practice into their 70s and 80s (approximately 30% of the group). A 1974 graduate explained why she relished continuing her full-time work as a physician and researcher.

I learn something new every day. I truly like what I do. There is always new information. Great colleagues and opportunities to develop/share/bounce ideas around with colleagues from widely different areas. Conversations can spark ideas that could become significant advances. People ask me about retiring or slowing down, but I'm having too much fun. It's just too interesting to quit.

While much of the enjoyment of practice was based in the relationships with patients described earlier, interviewees also found technical aspects of practice interesting and rewarding. In particular, anesthesiologists, neonatologists, obstetricians, and emergency medicine specialists described enjoying the excitement of managing urgent or life-threatening situations. Terms such as *exciting* and *always being on your toes* were also frequently used by women in other specialties to describe practice during a period of rapid innovations and advances in medicine. This was especially noticeable among the psychiatrists as they had experienced the revolutionary changes in psychiatric care during their decades in practice. Similar comments about the thrill of keeping up with medical advances and being able to use innovative treatments to benefit patients were made by oncologists and those who had cared for patients infected with HIV. The appreciation of being able to take part in dramatically improved treatments was not limited to the care of seriously ill patients. Several pediatricians spoke movingly of being involved in establishing services for handicapped or developmentally delayed children or those suffering from abuse or mental illness. *When I started, there was nothing for these kids. When I was treating a sick kid, I noticed his sister sitting in the corner. She was a mongol (per M-W), and nobody paid any attention to her. She just sat there.*

Teamwork was a major component of the enjoyment of practice. The interviewees valued collegiality and took great pleasure in *working with really smart, dedicated people.* They appreciated the expertise and dedication of their colleagues, especially the non-physician members of the health-care teams in which they worked. Long before the current emphasis on teamwork and interprofessional practice, they developed styles of practice that promoted mutual support and synergy among diverse health-care professionals.

I viewed us working as a team, with everyone making a contribution in caring for the patient. In the stress of the moment, it is easy to make a mistake, so I wanted the people working along with me to feel comfortable offering their opinions.

Positive comments about colleagues and team members were not limited to interviews with pediatricians and psychiatrists, whose practices usually involve teams of nurses, therapists, and other professionals; interviewees from all specialties credited interacting with colleagues as one of the best aspects of practice. Even a pathologist noted, *I worked with good colleagues. I wanted to make a contribution to the group.*

Intellectual Challenges, Opportunities to Learn

About half of interviewees identified the intellectual aspects of medicine as among the best aspects of practice. Intellectual activity was strongly linked to benefiting patients. *Having the knowledge and ability to make a difference in other people's lives.* Taking pleasure and pride in *always using my brain* was frequently articulated by internists and emergency medicine specialists in terms of working through problems to reach the correct diagnosis and provide the most appropriate treatment. Similarly, a pathologist described, *I like solving puzzles, coming up with the answers. I enjoyed solving the cases.* Nevertheless, several interviewees relished learning for its own sake. Many actively kept up with developments in medicine and conveyed continuing delight in *always learning. I would love to live for another 100 years – so many new things. I love to learn.*

One interviewee articulated how intellectual activity, patient relationships, and serving others came together in the intimacy of consultation with anxious patients and families.

There is nothing like being with the patient and their family. GREAT when that door closes and just you and the patient and the family to figure out what is going on – it's just great. Knowing your knowledge is going to make a difference. Making people more comfortable.

Sense of Accomplishment

In keeping with the strong theme of serving others and making a difference for patients, almost all interviewees described satisfaction or even pride in their professional achievements. Mostly, this focused on care of individuals, families, or even communities – they conveyed a sense of accomplishment and being appreciated by the people they served. This was expressed as personal satisfaction in *doing a good job* or being recognized for their expertise and high-quality patient care.

Several interviewees also identified the sense of accomplishment in building practices or contributing to raising the standards of care in their specialties. Their roles in developing new entities ranged from *building a small-town practice from scratch* or developing new services for communities to creating innovative academic units that introduced new patient care services, fellowship and training programs, and research enterprises.

I was always my own boss, always trying to build, doing lots of consults. The practice grew gradually until the hospital built a new facility for my specialty. It made a good asset for our community.

Initially, I was the only pediatric oncologist in the state. Easier to take care of these kids by myself, so the families had my phone number. We knew all the patients and families. Had partners only in the later years. I felt respected and supported by the organization.

I built the center, developed the fellowship, did research. I was chief of a really good section. Really worked to develop the team. I am proud of the improvements in patient care. I was running programs, writing grants, doing research. Ended up being busy all the time.

The sense of accomplishment was enmeshed with other themes, especially enjoyment of practice, love of learning, and the emphasis on teamwork and support of colleagues and trainees.

Being the director was amazing, satisfying. Always taking courses, adding new therapies and courses for staff.

Leadership and National Recognition

As indicated earlier, many interviewees achieved respect in their local communities and among their colleagues. Several mentioned being elected chief of hospital staff or holding important committee positions or administrative roles in their practice groups, health service organization, or academic unit.

I was president of the medical staff twice so had a lot of support from the men. I had very good references from colleagues when I applied for the fellowship. I think I was well respected.

In addition to local leadership roles, seven (19%) interviewees identified national activities as among the best aspects of their professional lives. This included service on federal and other committees and task forces developing policies, reviewing grants, or making national recommendations for standards of care. Many interviewees were active in the professional organizations for their specialty and used these organizations for networking as well as keeping up-to-date with clinical and other developments. Professional organizations were especially important to women who had few local female colleagues. Working at the regional, national, and even international level provided personal and professional support for women who were otherwise professionally isolated. Three interviewees mentioned becoming president of their national specialty organizations, usually the first or one of the first women to hold this office.

Other Factors

The initial responses to the question about best aspects of practice always focused on patient care and/or the intellectual and technical aspects of practice. Additional factors were only mentioned by a few participants, and always after the interviewee had elaborated on the factors discussed earlier. They were presented as adjuncts to the principal themes rather than leading sources of enjoyment or satisfaction in practice. Three interviewees included teaching as one of the best aspects of their professional experiences. The other additional comments concerned aspects of personal independence.

The flexibility of working for myself.

Being able to take the time to talk to patients, to get them comfortable.

Having control of your life, financial control. The power to live where you want and do what you want.

The Worst Aspects of Practice

Interviewees were slower to respond to the question about the worst aspects of their careers. A few immediately blurted out, *The paperwork!* or a similar comment, but even these women then took some time to reflect before speaking slowly and carefully about negative aspects of their lives in practice. The thoughtful, rather somber tone of the narratives was in stark contrast to the spontaneous and upbeat responses to questions about the positive aspects of their careers. One interviewee even responded to the question about negatives with an emphatic, *None!*

Despite this overall reluctance or difficulty in speaking about the negative aspects of their careers, the interviewees provided 101 comments that generated 12 themes. These themes clustered in three areas, namely, administrative and organizational problems, practice-related issues, and personal and family challenges (Table 17.2). Themes were often interrelated, especially concerning the consequences of changes in health services and the impact of practice demands on personal and family life.

TABLE 17.2

Worst Aspects of Practice as a Female Physician

Theme Number (%) Mentioning	Illustrative Quotations
Health-Care System Issues	
Documentation, administration 15 (41%)	• *Regulations: all the billing codes and regulations! All the hoops to jump through, the obstacles. I wasn't trained in business.* • *Dealing with the complexities of insurance reimbursement.* • *Like everyone else: the worst was the paperwork! Even when computers came in – forget it! Also, the administrative politics.* • *Absolutely the computer! Seems like I try so hard to learn things, then a few months later, they change it all again. Frustrates the heck out of me. The changes that salary is based on the number of patients. I was never big on billing.* • *The electronic medical record. It's designed for billing. Takes enormous amount of time for no clinical advantage. I hate it!* • *The EMR! All the documentation – you can do an entire visit and hardly look at the patient's face. Now, data are always coming in. Medicine is more intrusive.*
Organizational changes 5 (14%)	• *Hard transition when physician-owned clinic sold to commercial entity.* • *The worst time for stress and anger was when the hospital was considering eliminating psychiatry. Felt devalued, stigmatized – as well as the practical issues of losing my job. Communication was poor. We didn't know what was going on.* • *Changes in practice. The pressure to see more patients, generate greater income, being told I spent too much time with patients.*
Medical Practice Issues	
Bad patient outcomes 8 (22%)	• *One patient who successfully suicided. She didn't call for help in time. It was awful. We couldn't pull her back from the overdose.* • *Mostly when surgery has complications. When you have to put on your "big girl" suit and talk to families about bad outcomes, etc.* • *When things go badly obstetrics is the worst thing, the saddest. When you get a stillbirth at 36 weeks or a girl with her fourth miscarriage. You make close personal relationships. I remember a husband crying in the post-op room over a baby who died after in utero surgery for spina bifida. They went on to have five children but still grieve that lost child.*
Self-doubt, lack of confidence 7 (19%)	• *Women constantly have to promote themselves, and they don't do it well. They don't talk about their good qualities and accomplishments. Women continually need to promote themselves.* • *Learning to set limits – took a lot to get over my upbringing. Work was overvalued. I was raised to do it all yourself, had to work through that, from my stoical family.* • *I regret not having the confidence to go back into academia, to teach.* • *I struggled continuously with low self-confidence.*
Long hours 8 (22%)	• *Having to work nights. I don't tolerate nights well.* • *The hours could be tedious.* • *Being on call. Could be away from home day, night, and into the next day, so I missed my children.*

(Continued)

TABLE 17.2 (*Continued*)

Worst Aspects of Practice as a Female Physician

Theme Number (%) Mentioning	Illustrative Quotations
Professional conflicts 5 (14%)	• *The practice was just not safe. Absolutely couldn't continue. Forced me to make my closest friend/partner and husband extremely unhappy. It was absolutely horrible. Took years to recover relationship with friend/partner.* • *Conflict in operating rooms, really stressed me out. I couldn't do my job, please everybody.*
Disrespect 8 (22%)	• *In my administrative positions, being underestimated. Myth of the angry Black woman if I snapped back too strongly. I knew what I was doing. I had to work twice as hard and know three times as much.* • *People being patriarchal, discounting what I say, really got to me.* • *Recently, dealing with COVID, the antivaxxers, conspiracy theories. Very discouraging. Physicians are not valued as they were previously.* • *Probably pediatrics being low in the hierarchy of hospital and clinic. The double whammy of disrespect.* • *The aggressive attitudes of the male doctors when I worked overseas.*
Discrimination 5 (14%)	• *Constantly fighting for my freedom and self-respect. I'm pretty obstinate. I'm motivated by being told "no."* • *The discrimination by my colleagues.* • *Being paid less than the men. Always too busy to resent it.* • *I didn't like being forced or pressured to do things.*
Professional isolation 3 (8%)	• *I was always very isolated.* • *Guys were bonded, close-knit. They had groups – I was never asked to join.* • *Men have the "boys' club" – where they party and socialize with one another and their wives more than women physicians do. It is especially difficult for single women physicians.*
Personal and Family Issues	
Fatigue, stress 8 (22%)	• *The tension in having to be a "triple threat." I felt constantly that I could not keep up with all I had to do.* • *All this stress.* • *I was so busy trying to keep all the balls in the air. Constantly too much to do. More than 500 times a day dealing with big and small questions and making all those decisions. When I retired, I was exhausted.* • *The physical stress. Dealing with unhappy, disgruntled people.* • *Always being very TIRED.*
Lack of personal time 8 (22%)	• *I was always working hard – would have liked more activities with friends.* • *Other people didn't understand. No time for social life. Lost friends as no time for socializing. Couldn't keep up with college friends.* • *Career probably detracted from relationships – didn't have time to build up social networks, play bridge, have lunches, etc. Felt this at retirement. Lack of diverse outside interests probably stunts growth.* • *Didn't always take time to take care of myself. My diet was terrible in internship – working all day and night, then grabbing a candy bar. I often missed eating well, trying to stay heathy, because of working all the time.*

TABLE 17.2 (*Continued*)

Worst Aspects of Practice as a Female Physician

Theme Number (%) Mentioning	Illustrative Quotations
Strain on family 24 (65%)	• *Marriage did not last.* • *Terrible time around divorce.* • *Took a toll on marriage – physical and emotional.* • *Wish I had had more time with my kids.* • *Trying to balance career with children was challenging and stressful. Very hard. There were assumptions about care of house and children being the woman's responsibility.* • *Hard to be two people at once, doctor-on-call vs. mom. Sometimes I brought it home with me. Difficult to be 100% mom when worried about patients.* • *Being a single parent, how to constantly juggle job and child. Worried about if she got sick, what would I do? Lots of conflicts, last-minute things. I could get called anytime.* • *Separation from my family. Long hours and hard work away from my kids.* • *I missed a lot of my kids growing up, like doing a delivery while my son sang a solo at the church Christmas concert.* • *Trying to do justice to your children and work at the same time.*

Health-Care Systems: Documentation and Administration

Almost every participant made negative comments about the administrative aspects of practice during her interview, and 15 (41%) identified *the awful paperwork, regulations, etc.* as *the worst* aspect of their lives as female physicians. If an interviewee identified more than one worst aspect, an issue concerning documentation and paperwork was always identified first.

The biggest issues concerned documenting patient encounters to meet the requirements of organizational policies and obtain payment from insurance companies or other payors. When these women entered practice, a physician's notes were personal, confidential records of patient interactions designed to assist physicians to provide continuity of care and facilitate communication of important clinical information to other physicians. As the US health-care system changed, the medical record became less important as an aid to ensuring continuity of care and more significant as the basis of payment systems. How much a physician or clinic was paid for a patient visit – or even if the services merited any payment at all – became completely dependent on what was recorded in the notes.

I worked hard, and in the last few years, the paperwork demands were stressful, but I didn't realize till I quit how tired I was. I did old-style notes. Very time-consuming but valuable to me and other physicians who might take care of my patient. New systems don't value in-depth information and insights.

The stress and time required to ensure patient care services would be paid for drove some women to modify their practices.

Frustration with insurance companies, especially in the early 1990s. So much paperwork. I was spending more time in the record room than with my patients, and this contributed to leaving hospital work.

In the opinions of several interviewees, things went from bad to worse with the introduction of the electronic medical record (EMR). This further restricted the personal free-form documentation of the patient notes. The EMR necessitated learning new systems for the required documentation of patient encounters. In addition, the lack of standardization meant that physicians who worked in more than one clinic or hospital or those who changed jobs had to learn different systems. The EMR also made records and patient communications continuously accessible. Questions from patients or office staff could demand a physician's attention, even if she were off-duty, asleep, or trying to spend time with family.

You never get away from it. Used to have evenings for myself and my family. Was able to take my children to activities, take care of home and family issues when out of office. Now I am always having to check charts, results, messages, etc. There is no demarcation between work and personal time.

Interviewees of all ages and from all specialties cited documentation and administrative regulations as the principal worst thing about practice. Those in academia were particularly critical of their institutions and felt they carried a double administrative burden, that is, for both clinical work and the academic requirements of teaching, research, and unit management. *I hated all the bureaucratic administration in academia.*

The greatest administrative burden fell on those who ran their own private practices. In addition to regulatory requirements and the demands of payment systems, these women faced the challenges of managing staff and clinical facilities and negotiating local medical politics. A woman who loved her solo small-town practice laughed ironically as she described a continuous black comedy of administrative disasters and frustrations in trying to keep the practice running.

Medicare changed policies in the middle of my practice, and I had no cash flow for three months before it finally was straightened out. I went on vacation, and during that time, my computer system crashed, and I lost all the billing data. Fortunately, we had printed out a backup copy and I was taking an "in town" vacation, so I spent my week's "vacation" trying to get the computer back up and running. Dealing with employees was a big headache. Hiring and firing and getting stable, reliable staff was a nightmare. One bookkeeper decided not to make the bank deposit because she "didn't like my bank." Again, this happened when I had gone on vacation. When I returned, my account was overdrawn because she hadn't deposited the checks. (That was her last day of work.) Another employee had been living with a man who dealt in child pornography. One Thursday afternoon, while I was seeing patients, the sheriff came and arrested her because he thought she was tied up with the situation. It turned out she wasn't, but she was living in a threatening situation with this guy. She was in jail for two or three days because she couldn't make bail. I had to make a decision to let her go. This was one of the hardest decisions I had to make while in practice. The other physician in town suggested that we join practices. He was a wheeler-dealer, and I was skeptical, but I was on the verge of burnout, and I needed relief. We talked about it for a year and had a contract drawn up. I was just about ready to sign it and my accountant called at the 11th hour and said, "Don't sign it. There are too many loopholes. He's a crook." That was the best decision I made. I trudged on until I finally decided to close my practice and proceed with doing a geriatric fellowship.

Changes in Health-Care Systems

Issues in documentation and payment for medical services were among the many consequences of the revolutionary changes in US health-care systems that began in the 1970s. Many physicians transitioned from owning their practices or being directors of physician-owned businesses to being employees of large corporations. Usually, the transition did not go smoothly and brought sweeping changes to practices. The drive for greater efficiency and higher profitability in health systems disproportionately impacted those physicians who spent longer time with each patient and/or provided services that were less well-reimbursed by payment systems. Pediatricians and psychiatrists were most likely to report pressures to *see more patients, work faster, bill higher.* The issues were particularly serious for psychiatrists as health systems curtailed coverage for mental health services, especially for inpatient care. Even in academia, the pressure to generate income changed priorities and undercut cherished values. One interviewee mourned the devaluing of her role as a clinician–teacher–scientist and felt her legacy would be lost in the next generation of her colleagues.

Teaching changed dramatically as faculty added more clinics to make more money. They were not interested in teaching, journal clubs, etc. Couldn't get faculty to come to conferences – everyone was busy seeing patients. Tumor conference used to be sacred: Room would be packed. Everybody was there. Now it's empty, and I'm even looking for people to present. They don't care about academics anymore.

(For additional quotations, see Table 17.2.)

Medical Practice Issues

Bad Patient Outcomes

Of the seven *worst* themes related to medical practice, *bad outcomes* was the most poignant. Throughout the interviews, participants described professional pride in caring for seriously ill or dying patients and supporting families through terrible events. Nevertheless, eight (22%) women specified *the sadness in having to deliver bad diagnoses and prognoses* as one of the worst aspects of their long careers. These women predominantly cared for younger patients as pediatricians, child psychiatrists, or obstetricians. They expressed great empathy for their patients and families, plus their personal grief over the failure of medical expertise to prevent suffering and loss.

Seeing patients die. You used everything to save a life, but they died – that was the hardest part. I felt bad if a family criticized me.

One woman expressed enduring personal grief at the loss of patients, plus resentment and bitterness about the lack of support for young faculty in a prestigious academic unit.

I had a 2-year-old patient with a retroperitoneal tumor who bled to death on the operating table. Then they picked up the body bag like a sack of potatoes to take her to the morgue. Needless to say, I was already upset, and this made me furious – I insisted her body be treated with some respect. I had a pile of papers to fill out for an intraoperative death. I was only a second-year resident. They gave me about 20 minutes to manage all this and then insisted I start the next case. There was no help or support. In comparison, when the pilots landed their plane on the Hudson River – and no one died – they were taken out of work for six months with formal treatment of their PTSD. I got less than 30 minutes. All my close friends there left and went to less-stressful circumstances. We continue to refer to our PTSD from working there.

Self-Doubt, Lack of Confidence

In telling their stories, many interviewees referred to lack of confidence in their professional abilities. Seven (19%) identified it as one of the worst aspects of their careers. For many, this began early but was a recurrent challenge despite career success.

Training was an uphill battle. Long period of self-doubt about being a physician.

Always that impostor syndrome.

As women in a male-dominated profession, they encountered many external challenges to their competence and talked wearily of continuously having to prove themselves and fight for respect.

Always feeling incompetent, unsupported . . . when what I have to give is not respected.

Nevertheless, like many women of their generation, they recognized the equally challenging internal doubts and criticisms. They expressed their struggles in setting realistic goals, establishing boundaries, asking for help, or appropriately articulating their own value.

I don't know how I did it all. I thought I had to. A guy would not have sought approval from male superiors so much. Might have been more confident and, therefore, more independent.

Time Demands

Eight (22%) interviewees prioritized time issues as among the worst aspects of practice. This was the dominant contributor to problems in family life (see later text) but was also identified as an issue by women who were never married and/ or did not have children. In the decades when many of the women were in practice, physicians were commonly on duty or on call for long periods of time, even continuously if they were the only available resource for the community. Some interviewees subjected themselves to *grueling schedules* in order to establish themselves in communities or make practices more financially viable. Some interviewees, mostly anesthesiologists, especially hated night calls or unpredictable schedules.

Interpersonal Issues

The remaining four practice-related themes share a basis in interpersonal problems in the interviewees' professional lives.

Conflicts in Practices

Disagreements among partners or professionals in a practice or clinical unit were not uncommon. For five (14%) of our interviewees, such conflicts were sufficiently distressing to be identified as among the worst aspects of their careers. In at least one case, the conflict over patient safety could not be resolved and resulted in the dissolution of the practice and damage to personal relationships. Distress over conflicts in practice was most commonly reported by anesthesiologists who had to navigate tense situations involving surgeons, nurses, technicians, and others, often in high-stakes emergency situations.

Disrespect

Disrespect and discrimination frequently co-existed, and the distinction was often blurred. Most interviewees used the term *discrimination* to identify negative actions taken against them on the basis of gender, whereas *disrespect* included both active and passive negative comments or actions, predominantly but not necessarily based on gender. An undercurrent of disrespect for female physicians and a perception of being regarded as *second-class citizens* was experienced by almost all our interviewees. Eight (22%) identified disrespect as one of the worst aspects of their careers. For many, it was a pervasive, long-term issue manifest as being patronized or underestimated. Others cited particularly egregious sexism from colleagues or superiors. A more recent phenomenon was verbal abuse from antivaxxers and conspiratory theorists concerning the COVID-19 pandemic.

Discrimination

As described throughout their life stories and addressed in Chapter 19, our interviewees managed or navigated around gender-based discrimination throughout their lives. Five (14%) identified such discrimination as one of the worst aspects of their careers. In each case, the woman qualified the statement by crediting discrimination for making her more resolute in her determination to succeed. The *I'll show you* retort to the high school counselor who told an interviewee she was not good enough for medicine was still evident in the group even after 50+ years in medicine!

Professional Isolation

Despite being intelligent, skillful, and determined, our interviewees found that success as a female physician came at the price of never completely being accepted as *one of the boys* and sometimes subjected to the hostility of colleagues' wives. They were always in the minority or identified as *the woman doctor* in a male profession. They felt the lack of easy camaraderie and the practical support of collegial networks that their male peers took for granted. The lack of patient referrals and coverage for absences was a serious handicap for any woman struggling to establish a practice. Almost all female physicians of this generation, including our group, suffered from professional isolation, and three (8%) identified it as one of the most significant negative aspects of their careers.

(For additional quotations, see Table 17.2.)

Personal and Family Issues

Always Tired, Stressed

The combination of *the grueling schedules* mentioned earlier and the demanding nature of the physician's role resulted in almost all interviewees mentioning stress and exhaustion at some stage of their narratives. Eight (22%) identified feeling tired and stressed as the most significant negative about being a female physician. This factor underlay several other worst entities, especially those related to family life but was not restricted to married women. One unmarried participant described the strain of *always the feeling that you should be somewhere else, doing something else.*

Lack of Personal Time

The time required and/or given by conscientious female physicians to their patients limited opportunities for other activities. While most time-related comments focused on the family and other responsibilities impacted by work demands, eight (22%) interviewees mentioned negative consequences for their personal lives as among the worst aspects of their careers. These women expressed regrets in two areas. The first concerned not being able to invest more time and energy in personal friendships, hobbies, and other interests outside medicine. *The encroachment on my personal life. Work meant giving up a lot of time for fun.* The other area identified was self-care, specifically limited opportunities for exercise and neglecting healthy eating and other lifestyle factors because of work. *Always extremely busy. Sometimes I felt I had no time for myself, to exercise enough and things like that.*

Strain on Family

Reflections on the worst aspects of life as a female physician were dominated by deep concerns about the impact on family life, especially negative effects on children. All interviewees mentioned negative impact of personal and family relationships at some stage of the interview, and 65% identified it as the worst aspect of their careers. They described their perceptions in thoughtful tones that were often sad and tinged with regret. As described in the next chapter, most successfully managed the many challenges to family life and relationships presented by a career in medicine, but doubts and regrets lingered for many women.

The stress and time demands of medicine underlay all family problems. Participants described always feeling *pulled in multiple directions at once.* They were constantly concerned about not providing sufficient attention to either patients or family and of letting down at least some of the many people who depended on them – patients, partners, children, colleagues, and others. *Shortage of TIME – always seems to be cutting corners, then not doing as good a job as you want to do for either family or work.* Such comments were not restricted to wives or mothers; women who had never married and/or were childless also expressed the stress of not being sufficiently attentive to family members, friends, and others because of work-related demands on their time and energy.

Several interviewees spoke about strain on marriages, but the majority of comments concerned the *challenge to be there for my kids.* These challenges were especially severe for single mothers. Most women described regrets about missing activities or being unavailable for their children when they were young, but some pointed out that family responsibilities persist and change as children grow and other family members age, generating *lots of caretaking responsibilities.*

My career has been a mixed blessing. I loved it and feel VERY lucky to have it. I worked VERY hard to get it. The effects on my personal life – some I am not very happy about.

(For additional quotations, see Table 17.3.)

Burnout – When Practice becomes Intolerable

TABLE 17.3

Burnout: Prevalence and Illustrative Quotations

(Number %) Reporting
Never experienced (26: 70%)
<ul><li>*I never felt burned out. I don't give up.*</li><li>*I never once regretted it. I believe I made good choices.*</li><li>*If things didn't go well, something new always turned up.*</li><li>*Never came close to burnout.*</li><li>*Closest was just before change of specialty. I was just tired.*</li><li>*If I ever did feel like leaving, it didn't last long. Even the switch to computers – I stuck it out!*</li><li>*Weirdly not. The people I worked with were lovely. I had been brought up on a farm. If something needed done, you did it and moved on to the next thing. Learned to work through things: Do your best and wait for things to improve.*</li><li>*I don't think so. I worked hard, and in the last few years, the paperwork demands were stressful, but I didn't realize till I quit how tired I was.*</li></ul>
At least one episode of burnout (11: 30%)
<ul><li>*I was gradually becoming bored with my specialty. Feeling it wasn't natural for me. Things fell apart at work and home. Divorce.*</li><li>*Absolutely couldn't continue. It was absolutely horrible. Took years to recover relationships.*</li><li>*I thought about quitting many times. Times when you are so tired you don't know which way is up and ask yourself, "Why am I doing this?"*</li><li>*I wanted to quit often. Sunday nights were terrible, knowing you had to go back to continuous conflict. I did not deal with it very nicely. Nobody likes a woman who gets mad!*</li><li>*I was burned out, exhausted. I kept working but was emotionally drained. Overwhelmed. Seemed like I would catch up one thing, then other things fell apart. Every night carrying the same pain as your patients home with you. You can't refresh. I had to change, to step away. The administration didn't understand. Head of hospital wouldn't speak to me.*</li><li>*The tension. I felt constantly that I could not keep up with all I had to do. All this stress, I believe, culminated in a quadruple bypass at age 58. It was a wake-up call that I couldn't tolerate the lifestyle. We were getting overloaded. I was doing so much synchronously. Looking back, I don't know how I did it all. I thought I had to. Also, I had lots of family caretaking responsibilities.*</li></ul>

"Have you ever felt burned out or thought about quitting medicine?"

When asked this question, 26 (70%) of the interviewees denied ever feeling burned out by their careers or considering giving up medicine. About half of this group provided immediate and emphatic denials: *I have never ONCE felt burned out or wanted to quit.* Several interviewees expressed surprise at the question, and a few found it insulting.

Others who denied burnout or considering leaving the profession described times when they felt vulnerable to overload but described making changes or *powering through* difficult periods to avert burnout and recharge their enthusiasm for medicine.

A couple of real low points, BUT despite working hard and some really tough times, never really wanted to give up.

In several cases, especially during medical school, leaving medicine was described as a transient consideration. *No. Maybe thought about it a couple of times in med school, but not serious.* Later in their careers, several interviewees reported more serious situations when they felt close to burnout but managed to avert the situation.

I came close to burnout several times. The worst was at the end of my career. I retired at 62 in 2003, mainly due to changes in practice.

These women described working determinedly through stressful periods in their careers, typically when periods of excessive workload were coupled with lack of support. These difficult periods frequently coincided with personal issues, such as divorce or increased caretaking responsibilities. As one woman commented, *everything just fell apart at once.*

Never felt burnout or wanted to quit. The closest I came was that time when all the others in my specialty left town – I just could not keep going. I was overloaded.

I worked through some really rough patches, especially around the time of my divorce.

I definitely had periods of vulnerability to burnout. It was especially stressful being the principal caretaker for my mother.

The worst time coincided with my son developing depression: He later died.

Interviewees stressed the importance of lessening the potential for burnout by reducing workload; setting boundaries; enlisting support from colleagues, friends, and family members; maintaining personal health and interests outside medicine; and *taking a break to get things into perspective. Everyone needs to find what works best for her to refresh. Sabbaticals and frequent short vacations worked best for me.*

Several ruefully commented they had not been very good at taking their own advice! *I thought I had to do it all and not ask for help.* If short-term measures were unsuccessful or local solutions could not be found, the most common strategy to avert burnout was relocation to a new community and/or a different medical practice with better working conditions. Four interviewees made significant role changes in mid-career, such as taking administrative positions or entering academia when their original careers became overwhelming or unsatisfactory. Although job-related stress and burnout are usually associated with overwork and overwhelming demands on time and energy, five women described mid-career boredom and made changes as their work was no longer sufficiently demanding and exciting.

No, I never felt burnt out, but positions and activities can become stale. At a couple of points in my life, it's been time for a change – I was losing interest and needed to rediscover – to prevent becoming jaded.

Rather than leave the profession, three women resolved this career ennui by retraining in another specialty, and two volunteered for positions overseas. Two interviewees described regaining their enthusiasm for practice in the course of seriously considering changing specialties.

I came close to burnout in a solo rural practice due to the hard physical work plus all the insurance paperwork, etc. Considered changing to pathology for the hours. I went through all the procedures with getting references and filling out applications. I was offered a position during one interview. When I realized I would have to do anatomical path, I knew I was really an internist at heart. This experience gave me confidence that I was in the right place and I just needed to make it work.

After serving overseas, I didn't want to start over again. Seemed like we had too many changes, but I just needed a little time. I enjoyed my work – loved every moment. Might have considered another specialty, but I absolutely loved what I was doing and was very happy with it.

The 11 (30%) physicians who reported burnout spoke of periods of being *overwhelmed* despite strenuous efforts to fulfill both their professional and personal commitments. Again, they described burnout as occurring during periods of excessive demands or setbacks in more than one area of their lives.

I think I hit burnout a couple of times. I had a terrible time around my divorce. Also, during last year of residency. We separated for a while, and I took my children off for several months while I worked on a Navaho Reservation.

I worked long shifts and frequently covered night shifts because there was nobody else available. Got a lot of bullying from consulting physicians. Held in contempt by the specialists because you're not as knowledgeable as they are about their specialty. Disrespected – not just for being a female. It happens to all ER physicians. I also had serious medical problems and ended up having surgery that left me depressed, in a brain fog. I decided, "This practice is killing me!" It was probably burnout.

Two interviewees specified that they felt burned out at the end of their careers and reluctantly retired feeling *depleted*. One specified the continuous regulation changes and payment disputes as the final straw that precipitated burnout. *My burnout was just at the end over Medicare.*

Burnout was especially prevalent and severe among women whose careers were in academic medicine. They recalled the pressures of the *triple threat* to excel in research, teaching, and other academic activities as well as serving patients in academic units. They described careers of continuous stress with episodes of decompensation and burnout. *Did I have burnout? Oh yeah, repeatedly. Just kept pushing through it.*

All these women spoke of the lack of support from colleagues in the competitive *sink-or-swim, publish-or-perish* academic environment. They were particularly critical of the unsympathetic attitudes of academic institutions. Revealing job-related stress was equated with failure, and asking for help was regarded as counterproductive.

Admitting to burnout changes everything – as if you are a failure.

Rather than finding support, a faculty member admitting to stress was likely to be stigmatized as weak, with consequent serious damage to her career and prospects for advancement.

I was very good at standing up for patients, wasn't so good at standing up for my own career. I felt stigmatized by the burnout. Maybe needed to learn from the daily battles about how to communicate. Men get chosen for administration, and women get ignored. Any indication of burnout or strain in women is perceived as fatal for their careers. I advise women to recognize and take care of themselves regarding burnout, BUT don't tell administration and don't ask for help.

REFERENCES

1. U.S. Department of Health and Human Services. Minorities and women in the health fields. Washington (DC): DHHS;1984.
2. More ES, Greer MJ. American women physicians in 2000: a history in progress. J Am Med Womens Assoc (1972). 2000 Winter;55(1):6–9.
3. McMurray JE, Linzer M, Konrad TR, Douglas J, Shugerman R, Nelson K. The work lives of women physicians; results from the physician work life study: the SGIM career satisfaction study group. J Gen Intern Med. 2000 Jun;15(6):372–80.
4. American Medical Association and AMA Women in Medicine Services. Women in medicine in America: in the mainstream. AMA;1991.
5. Detweiler S, Cartwright L. Women physician pioneers of the 1960s: their lives and profession over half a century. San Francisco (CA): University of California Medical Humanities Press;2022.
6. Martin T. When the personal was political; five women doctors look back. Lincoln (NE): iUniverse;2008.
7. Lo Chin E, editor. This side of doctoring. New York (NY): Oxford University Press;2003.
8. Frank E, Rothenberg R, Brown WV, Maibach H. Basic demographic and professional characteristics of US women physicians. West J Med. 1997 Mar;166(3):179–84.
9. Kletke PR, Mader WD, Silberger AB. The growing proportion of female physicians: implications for US physician supply. Am J Public Health. 1990;80(3):300–4.
10. Jussim J, Muller C. Medical education for women: how good an investment? J Med Educ. 1975 Jun;50(6):571–80.
11. Lopate C. Women in medicine. Baltimore (MD): Johns Hopkins Press;1968.
12. Bowers JZ. Women in medicine: an international study. N Engl J Med. 1966 Aug 18;275(7):362–5.
13. Starr P. The social transformation of American medicine: the rise of a sovereign profession and the making of a vast industry. New York (NY): Basic Books;1982.
14. Frank E, Bhat Schelbert K, Elon L. Exercise counseling and personal exercise habits of US women physicians. J Am Med Womens Assoc (1972). 2003 Summer;58(3):178–84.

15. Frank E, Wright EH, Serdula MK, Elon LK, Baldwin G. Personal and professional nutrition-related practices of US female physicians. Am J Clin Nutr. 2002 Feb;75(2):326–32.
16. Frank E, McMurray JE, Linzer M, Elon L. Career satisfaction of US women physicians: results from the Women Physicians' Health Study: Society of General Internal Medicine career satisfaction study group. Arch Intern Med. 1999 Jul 12; 159(13):1417–26.
17. Frank E, Harvey L, Elon L. Family responsibilities and domestic activities of US women physicians. Arch Fam Med. 2000 Feb;9(2):134–40.

18

Personal Lives

Our interviewees built their personal and professional lives during decades of polarized and often-rancorous controversies over the roles of women in US society.[1] The surging women's movement of the 1960s and the 1970s insisted women could "have it all," paradoxically leaving many women feeling guilty if they did not achieve resounding success in every aspect of their lives.[1] This was nothing new for women in medicine; the constant dilemma of combining careers and personal lives has always haunted female physicians.[2] An 1871 medical journal speculated, "Will the lady continue to practice medicine and her husband follow his own occupation? And if so, and the union should prove prolific, who will train up their offspring in the way they should do?"[3]

Although most female physicians marry and become mothers, they have consistently been taunted with two contrasting caricatures – the hen medic, who is totally devoted to her profession, or the dilettante lady physician, who wastes her medical training to devote herself to family and social pursuits.[4,5] The message has been clear: Be "married to medicine" OR devoted to family. Any attempt to combine roles has consistently been portrayed as deleterious to both and a waste of medical education, with dire consequences, especially for children.[4-10] The powerful impact of this propaganda is illustrated by a 1965 finding that "four out of five college-educated women say that women do not go into medicine because it is too demanding to combine with family responsibilities."[5] As late as 1982, half of male physicians and medical students agreed that "women physicians who spend long hours at work are neglecting their responsibilities to home and family." Women couldn't win either way – in the same study, one-third of the men also believed there was "a significant risk to the optimal functioning of a department that hired a female of childbearing age."[6] The late 1960s and early 1970s were especially difficult for women attempting to build careers and reconcile the many claims on their energies, time, and loyalties. Criticism came from both within and outside the profession. Other women, especially the wives of physicians, were often the most critical of female physicians – and the most vocal about alleged neglect of husbands and children.[4-9] Sadly, some female physicians accepted the criticism as valid. In 1968, a female psychiatrist advised, "A career and children today demand superhuman motivation from a mother which can only include the neglect of children. I would NOT encourage my own daughter to hope for a career involving commitments outside the home."[5]

DOI: 10.1201/9781003539568-18

Partners and Relationships

"The modern woman labors under the handicap of not having a wife."[5]

(The Independent Woman 1920)

Of the 37 interviewees, 33 (89%) married. The timing of first marriage was evenly distributed across training and early practice, with eight marrying before medical school, eight as medical students, nine during graduate training, and eight after entering practice. Most husbands were physicians or fellow trainees. Of the 27 whose first husband's occupation was known, 13 (48%) married physicians or trainees. The others married clergymen (3), businessmen (3), lawyers (2), university faculty members (2), or a teacher, social worker, engineer, or pharmacist. Eleven women (33%) divorced their first husbands. Three of the divorced women remarried.

When interviewed, 16 (43%) were currently married, 9 (24%) widowed, 8 (22%) divorced, and 4 (11%) had never married. Two of the latter group described long-term relationships with women. Several divorced or widowed interviewees revealed current or recent relationships but were wary of remarrying as *a lot of these older guys just want someone to take care of them!* One of the widows described having *several good long-term relationships with very nice men – one lasted 25 years till he died. Currently in good companionable relationship. He's a very nice man, and we're very happy, but what's the point of getting married at our age?* Perhaps this distrust of male romantic motives reflects the exploitative attitudes of male trainees of the 1960s and the 1970s. One 1971 graduate described classmates *seeking a little woman to take care of them. At that time, a lot of men wanting to be doctors looked for a woman to put them through medical school. They would marry nurses or other women who worked, but after they were through medical school, they divorced them.* She added that many men in her age group still held inappropriate attitudes toward women. *Sexist attitudes persist in the e-mail chatter among our former classmates – for example, some of the guys discussing multiple wives, regarding women as expendable, "trading in the old model," etc. I don't think they are joking!*

Several interviewees described how they met their husbands. Those who married prior to medical school described their husbands as college or high school boyfriends. Most were classmates or friends of classmates or brothers. One interviewee married a college faculty member but divorced him just before entering medical school. Couples often met through shared classes or clinical rotations. *I met my husband working in the ER. He was a couple of years ahead of me in the residency program.* Sometimes the initial encounter was not promising. *Four of us married classmates. I was struggling in anatomy to keep up with the group and worried I was letting everyone down. One of the boys did beautiful illustrations and knew what he was doing. I was very shy but asked him to help me. We became friends, and I married him after junior year. I always tell people we met over a cadaver!*

Those women who married fellow medical students or trainees often referred to the typical socializing with classmates, especially hanging out at Jimmy's Jigger – the closest bar to the medical school and a long-standing haunt of medical students. Others met through student parties, outside activities, or mutual friends. *I did date one classmate early on, but most of that time was spent studying together. Most of my socializing was through the church I attended and where I eventually met my husband.*

The women who married after training were more likely to marry non-physicians and older men. One pediatrician married the widowed father of a patient. Another described meeting her husband when working as a divorced mother in a small rural town. *I LOVED that town. I had good friends and lots of group activities – cycling, walking, lunching, etc. My best friend introduced me to "the nicest man in town," who became my second husband.*

Of the 11 divorces, one was immediately prior to medical school, 3 were during residency training, and 7 (64%) occurred while the interviewee was in practice. Most marriages that ended in divorce during practice had lasted a long time – one over 35 years. With both partners in demanding careers, relationships experienced considerable stress. *I was married for seven years, then divorced. It was stressful for both of us. My husband was a fine person and a good physician, but he had issues too. We grew apart.* All but one of the divorced women had children. We did not ask about reasons for divorces, but several women indicated that marriages failed under the demands of sustaining careers and managing family responsibilities. *I divorced in 1975. I had constant concerns about babysitters, especially for overnight, if I was called into the hospital or detained. If I had been a guy, I would not have had two jobs! The men had wives to take care of them, send them out with breakfast, etc. In 1970s, men had not adjusted to women working.*

Several comments echoed the external pressures and internal conflicts of women in the 1970s when both domestic and professional perfection were required of "the modern supermom" and men were not expected to contribute significantly to household or childrearing tasks.[1,4–11]

Residency did cause my divorce. I attribute it to so much time away and always being tired. Have some guilt about it, as the kids were affected. It seemed like I was always not doing anything to the full extent – there were lots of trade-offs.

My husband was a good guy, but he resented doing any of the work at home. Things fell apart, and the divorce was hard on me and my children. I always tried to be home by 5:30 p.m. for my children. I had to learn to set limits. I got pretty good at it but took a lot to get over my upbringing – work was overvalued. I was raised to do it all yourself. The guys had wives at home to take care of stuff! In my upbringing, roles were always pretty rigid – the wife took care of everything at home.

Medical Mothers

"There is pressure on many women practitioners to prove themselves also to be good mothers, devoted wives, and organized homemakers. Considering the multiple responsibilities, it is surprising that women physicians with children are able to practice medicine at all."[10]

Thirty (81%) interviewees were mothers with between one and five children each (average 2.5). Two interviewees adopted one or more children. Three women married older husbands and had stepchildren. All three of these women were very close to their stepchildren, and one adopted her husband's two daughters.

Motherhood during Medical Training

"Throughout the span of training, the problem of marriage and pregnancy is constant."[12]

Four interviewees already had children when they entered medical school. Two were new mothers. One baby was only three weeks old on her mother's first day of medical school. The other new mother divorced her husband, entering medical school as the resolute single parent of a very young infant.

I always had babysitting problems, my vehicle kept breaking down, etc. I just took one day at a time. Money was always a problem. Financed a nickel here and a dime there. Scholarships, beg, borrow, steal (not really, although I sold my blood as often as possible). I did all right but was probably not entirely focused. I had a lot going on as a single mother.

Even in the classes of 1974 and 1975, few female medical students were married, and even fewer were mothers. The mothers felt out of place, more mature than their class-mates, and somewhat overwhelmed by what they had undertaken.

I entered medical school aged 31. I had just had my second baby and was lactating! I was on a different plane from the other students. Faculty, classmates, residents just didn't know how to deal with me. My career was so different from the others. Some classmates were callow boys – silly. Some thought I was exotic, "the old lady with the kids." Most of my friends were men, but nine out of ten classmates were not interested in being friends with me. I think I went to Jimmy's Jigger once.

My kids were three and five when I applied, so I was very surprised to be admitted. There was only one other woman who was married, but she had no children. It was very unusual for a woman with children to be a medical student. Having children and being older made it tough.

The majority of the class were still the traditional White males. My husband was three years ahead and warned me there would be very few women and that I would be the only married woman, but I met another married woman on the very first day. She signed in right after me on the first day at tables arranged alphabetically. I was one of the youngest – only 22 years old – and she was one of the oldest, and the only other married woman. She had a three year old and a three-week-old baby. We became close friends.

Seven interviewees described being pregnant as medical students, and two completed medical school as single mothers – described by a female classmate as *an amazing feat!* Classmates could be very supportive. *One of male classmates told me he would take all my first call – when you had to be in the hospital – because I "need to be at home."* Faced with an unplanned pregnancy, one interviewee was surprised to find supportive individuals both in senior administration and among her classmates.

I was the first unwed mother to graduate from KU Medical School! I was told I couldn't have kids, so when I found out I was pregnant, I was thrilled but scared. The relationship didn't survive, but I wanted the baby. I went to see the dean with great trepidation, terrific anxiety, but he said, "Do what you have to do. If you want to have your baby and graduate, you do it." I had supportive friends – even some non-chauvinistic guys – and had a lovely daughter after third year. There was a group of guys who were surprisingly enlightened, warm, accepting – they even organized a baby shower for me! They helped make life survivable.

Another mother found faculty members less supportive, despite her tremendous efforts to manage medical school and family responsibilities.

It was exhausting. For two years, I drove into Kansas City every day from Leavenworth, dropped the kids off at day care, did classes all day, then drove home. The evenings were for cooking dinner, housework, getting the kids to bed, etc., then I studied from about 9:00 p.m. to 1:00 a.m. and got up again at 6:00 a.m. We moved to Kansas City so I could be close to the Medical Center for the clinical years. My first rotation was radiology. On the very first day, I was told I was on call that night. I said I couldn't do it as I didn't have a babysitter. The professor was not impressed and made it very clear there would be no favors for women with children. I asked for advance notice of the schedule so arrangements could be made and managed to trade that first night with a classmate.

The interviewees described different strategies to manage motherhood during medical school. The most affluent interviewee employed a resident nanny. One arranged for her mother to care for her son and drove back to her hometown whenever possible to see the child. Another spoke of the help from her *wonderful mother-in-law*. Whatever arrangements were made had to be both dependable and flexible, with sufficient backup strategies to ensure care despite students' demanding and unpredictable schedules. *Childcare was a nightmare. Students had crazy schedules and, on some rotations, had to be in by 6:00 a.m. or earlier. I found two lovely people, one to do days and one to do nights. We managed somehow.*

In medical school, neighbor lady took care of my baby during the day, and I can't remember how we managed the call schedule, so someone was always home at night. My husband was a resident, and my parents were not around to help – I wonder, now, how did I do all that?

Most interviewees who had pregnancies during medical school continued their education by arranging clinical rotations to accommodate the expected date of delivery and post-partum leave. *I was not very mature. Fell in love, got married end of second year, and had a baby – thought that was what you did. Took off 6 weeks as the curriculum was in rigid 6-week blocks.* One new mother delivered at the end of the second year and took a year of absence. More commonly, mothers aimed to deliver toward the end of the senior year, when the pressures of coursework had lessened and a break was possible before starting internship or residency. This timing could cause consternation for faculty during the final clinical rotations before delivery.

I was pregnant during senior year. Hugely pregnant during my last rotation, and the attending told me to sit down as I was making him nervous! (He said it in kindness, not adversely. He was a very nice man.)

I was pregnant in third year and absolutely determined to finish the surgery rotation before delivery. I took lots of comments about how unusual it was to see a pregnant physician. On one case, the surgeon joked that I should "belly up to the table" – everyone thought that was pretty funny.

Motherhood during Postgraduate Training

The grueling duty hours and heavy workload made internship and residency the most challenging period for women attempting to combine medicine and motherhood.

"During the internship, the demanding and unyielding 'on twenty-four and off twenty-four-hour schedule' is another major problem. It is frequently impossible for a woman who is a mother to meet such requirements and discharge her responsibilities as a mother."[11]

Residency programs were not always aware of a resident's potential or even impending motherhood. Some programs did not seem to have even considered the possibility.

There was no consideration of accommodations for women in residency. When I asked about maternity leave, I was told, "We don't have a policy. We've never had a pregnant resident." My contract had nothing about maternity leave or pregnancy. I took vacation and sick leave for the delivery and hoped I wouldn't get sick anytime.

Pregnant residents were unusual in the 1970s and cited as a source of major problems for programs, causing resentment and disruptions of workflow.[3–6,12–14] In 1988, a female faculty member declared, "Becoming pregnant is not appropriate during this time period [residency]. If they want to conceive, they should do it on their own time and not inconvenience others."[13] As late as 1998, one expert stated, "It is unacceptable to become pregnant during residency."[14]

Some administrators and faculty member tried to address the situation with understanding and humor; others seem to have been nonplussed.

One of the other residents was also pregnant. This attending said, "What am I to do with you two invalids?" And he thought he was one of the liberated men!

I arrived to start OB/GYN residency visibly pregnant, but nobody said anything directly to me. About six weeks before I was due to deliver, an attending asked, "When are you due?" This was an OB program! I was told that there was great consternation over my pregnancy. Everyone was flabbergasted. It caused a fluster, but this was all behind my back. Nobody would talk about it, and I figured I would not bring it up. I took three weeks off after delivery and used up all my vacation.

In contrast, one interviewee was recruited in the late 1960s by a residency program that was exceptionally supportive. *My second child was born during residency. The chief was excited, like he was the grandfather. He promised the program would "bend like the willows in the wind" to accommodate the pregnancy. I took six weeks off after the birth. There were some comments from the other residents about me "not pulling my weight," but most people were fine.* Similarly, an interviewee completing residency during her husband's military deployment found significant support from those associated with the program during a harrowing experience. *I experienced a miscarriage followed by a stillbirth. It was a terrible experience. We knew for two weeks that the baby was dead. I had lots of support. Wonderful support from nurses, colleagues, and from other Navy wives, but it was a tough time.*

Another interviewee recalled her fellowship program being supportive during a difficult pregnancy. *I was huge, vomiting all the time. People were very nice. Had pre-eclampsia with all three pregnancies but worked till the day each was born. Took two weeks off after first pregnancy, then back to work.*

Postgraduate training was more demanding for mothers than medical school was due to the heavy workload and continuous responsibility for patients. *I could be on for 36 hours then get home and, even then, get called in.* Junior physicians often had no protected hours, and some were expected to live in the hospital. One interviewee recalled starting her married life with a husband who was also a resident. *We lived in the hospital dormitory and ate all our meals in the cafeteria. We were on call continuously for our own clinic patients. I rarely had a full night's sleep for eight months.*

By 1975, conditions for residents had improved somewhat, but agreements for duty hours were not always honored and were regularly overridden by patient urgencies.

I was told in the interview that residents had 1 in 7 overnight call when I was required to be physically in the hospital. Upon arrival, I found it was 1 in 3. It was extremely difficult and stressful to get childcare. I was lucky to find great daytime childcare – a grandmotherly neighbor who was available long hours whenever I needed and was wonderful. For weekends and overnights, I depended on neighbors – stay-at-home mothers where my kids could go.

Mothers had *constant concerns about babysitters, always having to have someone who could stay with the children. I could be away from home day, night, and into next day.* Sometimes, wonderful help was provided by neighbors. *During residency, a lady who lived near the hospital and had children looked after my son and became like a second family to him.*

Backup plans for childcare were essential. Even these sometimes broke down, especially for single mothers, and women resorted to desperate measures. These situations
were recounted with dark humor.

*I had a new baby at the start of residency. Finding good babysitters was essential.
We got names of babysitters from other women at the hospital (students, nurses,
etc.). I was single so had to be prepared for emergencies. One wet winter night, my
overnight sitter had to leave for a family emergency while I was working. I had to
call around frantically to locate another overnight sitter, get someone to cover the
patients while I rushed out to pick up the baby, drive her across town to the new sitter,
and get back as quickly as possible, hoping nothing had gone wrong while I was out.
AND I had to do all this and find the new location without cell phones or GPS – I was
searching for house numbers in strange streets in the rain! I ended up getting stopped
for speeding on my rush back to the hospital. I think I burst into tears, but when the
traffic cop heard this tale, he let me off!*

Sometimes mothers took children with them into the hospital. *At times I took my children with me, and they spent the night in the call rooms (aged about 8 and 10), then
I took them to school and went back to work.*

*It was tough. I had not mastered juggling childcare with being a resident. If I got
called in, I took the baby. There was a room for residents to sleep. I told the staff, "I
got to bring the baby. Help me out. You can hold it together for two hours!"*

None of the interviewees mentioned being reprimanded for sneaking children into
the hospital, but they encountered other risks. *I took my new baby into the wards
during residency while I was breastfeeding. I hid her in a corner of the nursery
until we admitted a baby with TORCH infection, so I had to wean her and leave
her at home.*

Interviewees repeatedly stressed that arrangements to manage family responsibilities were always vulnerable to disruption. Despite careful planning for emergencies,
arrangements often had to be made at short notice. Work requirements for either
or both parents could change, childcare arrangements could fall through, relatives
become unable to assist, or vehicles break down. When children became old enough
for school, finding part-time help was sometimes even more challenging. *It was hard.
It was a big hospital, very busy. We were on call one of three nights and had lots of
sick kids through the ER every night. It was exciting, but hard work. It was especially
difficult with a young child at home after I got divorced. I had a young woman come
to the house to care for the baby. Things got more difficult when my daughter started
preschool, as schools close at regular hours and I needed flexible childcare plus
someone who could pick her up.*

A few interviewees recalled how motherhood had complicated their attempts to complete the national examinations essential for specialist qualifications. They laughed
as they recounted these stories but recalled *being frantic at that time* when facing
potential sabotage of completing this last hurdle in their education.

Oh my! Maybe I have memory loss or repressed things. [Laughing.] I remember things like all three kids had chicken pox just before my oral board exam, and I was sitting on the toilet, studying, while they were all in the bath with colloidal oatmeal to ease the rash!

My daughter was born the year I finished residency. I had to travel to Mayo to take the boards. I remember terrible morning sickness all the way to Minnesota.

I had my first baby two weeks after the end of residency. I took three months off to study for the boards and be with my new baby. I thought he would sleep all the time, so I could study – but I quickly discovered the problems of studying with a newborn and got a babysitter. Then I left the baby with my parents and went to Chicago for the board exam. I was still breastfeeding and developed severe mastitis. I was ill, febrile, and had very inflamed breasts. I asked the examiners if anyone could write a pre-scription, but no local physicians were available – in a huge room full of physicians! There was great consternation and lots of concern about my breasts in the middle of the board exams! Finally, someone persuaded a pharmacist to provide medica-tion. I was so sick. It was difficult to do the questions, especially the microscopy. My breasts were so tender I couldn't bear to bend over to look down the microscope!

Mothers in Practice

Entering practice as full-fledged physicians, most women anticipated more stable working conditions, with predictable schedules and incomes that were adequate to cover childcare and domestic expenses. While generally less hectic than during train-ing, managing both professional and family responsibilities remained challenging throughout their careers.

Some women opted for faculty appointments, believing the hours and working condi-tions would be more compatible with family responsibilities than in private practice. In at least one case, things did not work out as anticipated. Facing budget constraints, academic programs could avoid or delay replacing clinicians, leaving the remaining faculty to carry heavy loads. *There were supposed to be four of us, but I ended up as the only one for the entire excessive workload – seeing clinic patients, doing hospital consults, teaching, and supervising residents. I was running all over the place, not getting home till 11:00 p.m., never seeing my kids. My mother was always available to help, but it was not sustainable. The dean did not seem interested in recruiting or helping me out.*

Even in fully staffed academic units, mothers faced demanding call schedules and frequent emergencies. *Being a single parent, how to constantly juggle job and child? I worried about if she got sick, what would I do? Lots of conflicts, last-minute things. I could get called in for sick babies or bad deliveries anytime.*

I had three children and divorced when the youngest was about 1 year old. For an anesthesiologist, it was challenging if the day care closed and we were still working cases. I often had to pick up my children and brought them back to the medical faculty lounge. The nurses would keep an eye on them for me. Colleagues looked out for one another – someone would watch my patients if I had to dash out to pick up the kids.

As described in earlier chapters, women entering private practice found a variety of situations, ranging from highly supportive to frankly exploitative and abusive colleagues and organizations. Most interviewees worked full-time, with only short breaks around childbirth. Only three women reported working part-time, all while their children were very young. One interviewee made a career change to secure a manageable schedule.

I decided to opt for ER work with 24-hour shifts. My husband learned how to take care of our son. It was really good for both of them. Working ER split up my life into work time and other time. It enabled me to have adult time as well as to be completely with my kids. I used day care and other resources.

As they dealt with multiple challenges in establishing professional credibility and building their careers, mothers worried constantly about not being sufficiently available for their children.

It's hard to be two people at once, doctor-on-call vs. mom. Sometimes I brought it home with me. Difficult to be 100% mom when you are worried about patients. Mostly, I tried not to mix it. I always tried to be there for my own children.

Several spoke of specific regrets. *I missed a lot of my kids growing up, like doing a delivery while my son sang a solo at the church Christmas concert.* Most recognized that their children had done well, despite all the maternal anxiety and the criticism heaped on working mothers. Several interviewees commented on positive outcomes for children of working mothers.

I always worked full-time, even after the divorce. Enough time with kids was always difficult. Made for very independent kids used to doing things for themselves.

My children were very self-sufficient from a young age.

Some even reported affirmation from their grown children. *I didn't do the balancing act very well, but I don't regret what I did. I have great children who don't seem to be too "damaged." My son says I was always there, and he has no memory of me not being present for things. He married an OB-GYN, and they have two children, so he couldn't have had too bad an experience of a physician mother!*

I considered spending more time at home during an especially tough period when the children were teenagers, but things worked out. I found out that the children didn't want me to stay at home! I am very pleased that my children say I have always been there for them, and them for me.

As indicated by the last quotation, women often drew strength and support from their children. One interviewee who was very active in medical politics found her children to be a considerable asset. *I was mostly a single mother with two resilient children. The children were exquisitely fun. They helped a lot. They were very supportive of me and came to meetings, etc., from a young age. The children were often an asset, changing the tone of a welcome or the atmosphere of a meeting and helping me to relax.*

How Did You Manage?

STAMINA! You have to have a good constitution, because it is a LOT of work. Time management – got to be good at it.

When asked about managing both busy personal and professional lives, most interviewees laughed and denied knowing any *secrets.* Several marveled at what their younger selves had undertaken, with comments such as, *I don't know what I was thinking,* or *How did I do it all?* Others revealed a sense of the impostor syndrome, that is, they felt very aware of their shortcomings and were uncomfortable when perceived as having successfully combined family life with demanding careers. As discussed in the introduction, our interviewees and other female physicians of this generation were reluctant to be regarded as heroines or superwomen. While proud of their achievements, they acknowledged their many shortcomings, mistakes, and regrets.

When pushed for practical details on how they managed their working lives, most referred to working hard, being stubborn, and constantly juggling competing demands. Two topics dominated their narratives – sources of help for childcare and housework, and the role of husbands.

Childcare and Household Help

Especially during training, when many were short of money, women described relying on babysitters, neighbors, friends, and family members for support. They often used a combination or network of different individuals to meet changing needs and adjust to the availability of help. During the training years, the absolute priority was reliable, flexible childcare, with plenty of backup arrangements for the inevitable breakdowns in the system. Interviewees rarely mentioned other household tasks, such as cleaning, laundry, or food preparation. They gave the impression of attending to such things themselves as time allowed. *I used my "village" and friends. Also, my mother moved to be close and helped a lot with babysitting.*

Once established in practice, stable, long-term arrangements for childcare and household help became more common, usually involving one or two dedicated individuals, referred to as housekeepers or nannies. Multiple interviewees commented on how *it was hard to find good help,* but several described close relationships and a sense of commitment to their domestic employees.

This was years ago in the rural South, so I had help six days a week. She did everything – cooking, housework, taking care of children.

My mother helped, and I always hired help. Having my own practice, I could set my hours, but I couldn't have done it without help. Always hired someone to clean the house, plus lots of babysitters, friends, etc.

It was difficult to find childcare, then we found this wonderful woman who became family and looked after us for many years, then I took care of her when she retired.

Always had household help – the same lady for 34 years, 90 years old now, and like a grandmother to our kids.

Women who lived in smaller communities perceived they had more support and less difficulty in finding good help.

I practiced in a great little town. Very friendly people, no lack of babysitters, and good help.

Always had someone come to the house for childcare, etc. Help is much easier to find in a small town, where there are hardly any professional women.

Nevertheless, living too far from other people complicated finding support. *Lived in what was then a rural area and commuted into the city. I never had help, mainly because potential employees thought it too far out. The kids and I did everything ourselves – they were pretty capable from an early age. I always worked, did everything at home, and slept 12:00–4:00 a.m.*

Husbands: Helpers or Hindrances?

"'The right husband' is one of the most common requirements set up by women physicians themselves for combining a medical career with marriage."[5]

Most ever-married interviewees commented on the role(s) played by their husbands. These comments covered a broad spectrum, from persisting resentment toward an unsupportive spouse to perceiving their partners as essential to success. Several pointed out that attitudes and expectations about family roles changed dramatically over their lifetimes. Even those who graduated in the 1970s acknowledge that both they and their husbands had been influenced by the norms and values of being raised during a period when the American wife's place was at home.[1] Like most women of their generation, our interviewees felt required to take primary responsibility for childcare and domestic matters, regardless of the willingness of partners to assist. Some felt driven to prove they *could do it ALL.*

The difference is that women are caregivers. You are in charge of the family PLUS working. A job is okay as long as you get all the other things done. Men brought up in the 1950s had a lot of trouble adjusting to women working.

My husband was very good, a very active parent, but the family always felt like my job. I had a second job. At work, I was always looking around anxiously at 4:00 p.m.

to see what needed to be cleared up before you could go home, and praying nothing would come in to prevent you getting home.

Trying to balance career with children was challenging and stressful. Very hard. My husband was a typical male of that time, supportive, but there were assumptions about care of house and children being woman's responsibility. Things were different, and everyone accepted how they were.

Many interviewees recognized their internal drives to do it all based on a sense of obligation, duty, or need to prove themselves. Even at that time, some were aware of feeling like impostors and that the superwoman image they projected was unrealistic.

The guys had wives to support them, to take care of them. I was concerned with the basics – to keep everyone fed and clean. I didn't expect help. 100% I did what I needed to do. I felt a great obligation to future women. I had to show up, work hard to show women could do it. Fortunately, I was very healthy. I was tired, but I had to do it so women in the future could be taken seriously and given a chance.

I felt I had to do so many domestic things. I always projected I can do it whatever it takes. I convinced everybody I could do anything. Even my husband believed it too and went off to medical conferences when I had a new baby and small children.

Some husbands were lovingly described as willing to help but not very effective and somewhat bemused by domestic or childcare necessities. *My husband was pretty good, very good, but the family was "my work." He was not good at initiating things – if I gave him an assignment, he would do things but not think to do them on his own or mess things up. Like rushing to take the kids to day care and leaving the lunch boxes on top of the car!*

One fortunate woman described both an unusually *enlightened* institution and husband. *I had four children and was able to take lengthy maternity leave each time due to generous institutional policies about using sick leave. Also had good child day care. My husband had a flexible schedule and helped a lot – a very egalitarian man!*

The married interviewees were all in dual-career marriages, requiring coordination of schedules and responsibilities. *Very important to choose the right husband! Husband needs to be willing to do 50%. I have a great husband. We managed never to be both on call at the same time and arranged things to share responsibilities. He often got home first. I could get delayed, as pediatrics commonly gets rush of calls in late afternoon, when children return from school with symptoms or mother comes home from work and is concerned about child. I was often not home till after 7:00 p.m. Our evening meal was always after 7:00 p.m. – the children believed that was normal for every family.*

Those not married to physicians perceived themselves at an advantage.

It was always a challenge. My husband was a pharmacist, so we tried to arrange work schedules to stagger hours and be available for family. We were always involved with our kids. I wanted to be there.

I married a schoolteacher, so great for covering holidays, etc. We arranged things – I would get them ready in the morning, and my husband would drop them off at school or day care. Hired once-weekly cleaning help, but mostly we did domestic things on our own. I was very involved with my kids – able to do activities like scouting, teaching Sunday school, etc.

I was really lucky. My husband was a pastor and always had a flexible schedule. We managed to bring the kids up between us with very little use of babysitters.

Verifying this advantage, one interviewee had very strong advice for young women entering medicine.

Have a non-medical husband! My husband worked for himself, so he could be flexible.

More Than Wives and Mothers

"Women are taking their places beside make colleagues as full-fledged professionals determined to demonstrate that leading a fulfilling private life is not incompatible with the competent practice of medicine."[15]

The literature on the family lives of women in medicine focuses on marriage and motherhood, overlooking the experiences of women who were single and/or childless and neglecting all other aspects of the personal lives of female physicians. About three-quarters of our interviewees described being caretakers for adult relatives. *I cared for my husband, then after he died, I started looking after my sister who has dementia.* All the never-married interviewees took responsibility for one or more family members, commitments that often lasted for years and required navigating arrangements even more complex than those for childcare. *I did not marry or have children, but it was always a struggle to balance. Always the feeling that you should be somewhere else, doing something else. It was especially stressful being a caretaker for my mother. My career probably detracted from relationships – I didn't have time to build up social networks.*

I cared for both my mother and sister when they had breast cancer, then eventually retired to care for my mother when she developed Alzheimer's.

All interviewees described constantly navigating competing priorities and time pressures, but they were unwilling to be defined exclusively by their work and managing family responsibilities. They acknowledged that self-care and personal interests always took lower priority than family or career responsibilities, but many described active social lives and interests such as sports, politics, social action, literature, and music. One enthusiastically described playing bagpipes and touring with her pipe band.

I always worked hard but really enjoyed my time off – lots of sports, skiing, hobbies, friends, garden. So blessed in my life.

I had lots of clinical and academic responsibilities but balanced my life with travel-ing, art collecting, gardening, and participating in many sports and activities with friends.

It's really important to lead a well-balanced life. I am VERY grateful for some of the courses I took in college, especially art history, literature, and history. They have given me a lot over the years.

Several described busy retirements, and some had developed new careers after medicine.

I loved medicine, but retirement is SO much fun. I am active in the medical school's geriatric mentoring program and am matched with two freshman medical students whom I follow all four years. After my husband's death, I went to seminary for a year and then have volunteered for many positions in my community. Five years ago, I started an "aging in place" organization in my community that is doing well in pro-viding events and services to allow people comfort in staying in their homes. It has been especially important during the pandemic in supporting older people stuck at home. I am involved in a number of activities – too numerous to discuss!

I retired in 2015. I have now become an interfaith chaplain and am planning after the pandemic to be an interfaith chaplain for retirement communities and establish a chaplain consultancy with a partner, specializing in long-term care facilities.

REFERENCES

1. Douglas SJ. Where the girls are: growing up female with the mass media. New York (NY): Times Books;1994.
2. Williams PA. Women in medicine: some themes and variations. J Med Educ. 1971 Jul;46(7):584–91.
3. Spieler C, editor. Women in medicine. 1976 Report of a Macy Conference. New York (NY): Josiah Macy Jr. Foundation;1977.
4. Walsh MR. Doctors wanted: no women need apply: sexual barriers in the medical profession 1835–1975. New Haven and London: Yale University Press;1977.
5. Lopate C. Women in medicine. Baltimore (MD): Johns Hopkins Press;1968.
6. Martin SC, Parker RM, Arnold RM. Careers of women physicians: choices and constraints. West J Med. 1988 Dec;149(6):758–60.
7. More ES, Fee E, Pary M. Women physicians and the cultures of medicine. Baltimore (MD): Johns Hopkins University Press;2008.
8. Bourne PG, Wikler NJ. Commitment and the cultural mandate: women in medicine. Soc Probl. 1978;25(4):430–40.
9. Morantz RM, Pomerleau CS, Fenichel CH. In her own words: oral histories of women physicians. Westport (CT): Greenwood Press;1982.
10. Anon. Women in pediatric practice. Pediatrics 1983;71(4):S699–705.
11. Bowers JZ. Special problems of women medical students. J Med Educ. 1968 May;43(5):532–7.
12. Finch SJ. Pregnancy during residency: a literature review. Acad Med. 2003;78:418428.

13. Phelan S. Pregnancy during residency. 1: the decision to be or not to be. Obstet Gynecol. 1988;72:425–31.
14. Gold JH, Frechette D, Des Marchais J, Puddester D, Richardson B, Swiggum S. Parental leave: impact on resident education. Ann R Coll Physicians Surg Can. 1998;31:240–3.
15. Morantz-Sanchez R, Sympathy & science: women physicians in American medicine. New York (NY): Oxford University Press;1985.

19

The Gender Thing

An account of the lives of women who entered medicine after WWII would not be complete without addressing gender-based issues, but we tried to avoid emphasizing such issues during the interviews. Participants were encouraged to relate whatever they wished to share about their long careers as women in medicine. Without prompting, interviewees described gender-based issues at all stages of their lives and careers. Recollections ranging from humorous strategies to circumvent dress codes to haunting revelations of sexual abuse were integrated throughout the narratives. Avoiding directly addressing gender-based mistreatment became challenging as the interviews were conducted during the peak of publicity about the *#MeToo* movement and attention to workplace sexual abuse.[1] We therefore added questions about gender-based mistreatment at the end of each interview. To organize the diverse mass of information provided spontaneously or in response to prompt questions, we used the definitions of the National Academies of Sciences, Engineering, and Medicine (NASEM), for gender harassment, unwanted sexual attention, and sexual coercion (Table 19.1).[2] The categories frequently overlapped as disparaging, baiting, teasing, and humiliating behaviors toward women easily transitioned to sexually focused behaviors.

Experiences of Gender Harassment

All interviewees described experiencing at least one form of gender harassment. Ten (27%) denied such experiences when directly questioned, despite voluntarily describing incidents that met NASEM definitions in their narratives. Four of these women believed being female had been an advantage in medical school.

Girls stood out in class. I liked being special. I was never picked on. The small number of women was an advantage. I felt I could be friends with guys without thinking about "dating material." Always liked male company.

Maybe I was treated a bit better because women were still unusual. I didn't feel I was subjected to hardships. Quite the opposite – girls kind of stood out. I think an average girl got more credit than an average guy.

Several interviewees commented that mistreatment was *normal at that time* and was enabled by institutions that took pride in *toughening up* trainees for the rigors of medicine.

DOI: 10.1201/9781003539568-19

TABLE 19.1

Examples of Gender-Based Mistreatment

Sexual Harassment	
Second-class treatment	• *Professors kind of ignored us. They expected us to flunk out.* • *Why are you here? Why are you taking up a guy's place?* • *In hospital and clinic hierarchies, women were not highly regarded. Difficult to be recognized as important.* • *Lots of discrimination in practice – my voice not being heard in committees.* • *We worked harder than the men, had to do more; the environment was NOT friendly.* • *The system was designed for males. Women didn't fit in.* • *Lots of discrimination, especially from nurses.* • *Constantly being underestimated. This angry woman myth if I snapped back too strongly.* • *I had to work twice as hard and know three times as much.* • *People being patriarchal, discounting what I said.*
Recruitment discrimination	• *Finding a job was difficult – lots of discrimination.* • *I was told patients wouldn't like a woman examining them.* • *They acted like it was a HUGE favor to give a job to a woman.* • *I didn't realize there was such discrimination against female doctors; the old boys' network.* • *I was repeatedly turned down, told a female partner would not work.*
Lack of professional support	• *I was expecting to rotate duties and share the work. I ended up doing all the work – taking care of everything. Supervisors did nothing.* • *My partner didn't do what he had agreed. I was on call 24/7, responsible for everything!* • *I assumed partners would share call and assist me getting established, but I ended up always responsible for patients, on call 24/7.* • *I was transferred to the chronic disease hospital – the bottom of the barrel.* • *I was totally unprepared for exclusion, discrimination by my fellow specialists and physicians – even ones I had helped. They would not send me referrals and never reciprocated. A rude awakening.*
Denial/Limitation of resources	• *Uniforms were required. Men could buy them from the bookstore, but women had to make them.* • *Interns were required to live in, but women were not allowed in the interns' quarters. I slept on a couch in the library.* • *Males were always more important. I had to make do – make the best of things.* • *New guys got signing bonuses, referrals, new offices, staff, equipment – everything.*
Financial discrimination	• *I was told, "Get over it, if you want the job."* • *I had been promised a bonus based on earnings, but they wouldn't pay my bonus. They also declined to make me a partner.* • *Some patients were channeled to me, the more lucrative ones to male partners.* • *Definitely underpaid, especially early on.* • *"Honey, don't bother your pretty little head about business."* • *My accountant insisted on coming to the bank to request a line of credit for the practice. The bank was skeptical of a woman.* • *Two women trying to set up a practice – bank wouldn't give us a loan.*

TABLE 19.1 (*Continued*)

Examples of Gender-Based Mistreatment

Sexual Harassment	
Advancement/ Promotion discrimination	• *The guys got more mentoring. Even from a strong female chief.* • *Men rise to power – all the CEOs and chairs are men.* • *Men have the old boys' club; they help one another.* • *I don't think I ever got any mentoring, even from female faculty.* • *They didn't want to promote me. I hired an attorney – was promoted in hours!* • *They didn't want female partners. I was refused after 6 years of successful practice, but a new guy was loaned money for partnership after 6 months.*
Social isolation	• *Lots of discrimination: a departmental party only invited men.* • *Would have been nice to have more camaraderie.* • *A group of students got together to discuss psychological issues, and it just didn't occur to anyone to include women.* • *Career detracted from relationships – didn't have time to build up social networks, etc. I really felt this at retirement.* • *I was used to my father having dinners, social interactions with other doctors, but I wasn't invited to any social gatherings.* • *Men have the "boys' club" – they party and socialize with other physicians and their wives; it is especially difficult for single women physicians.* • *I was always very isolated and am still more comfortable in male company.* • *Morning report was all guy talk – football and things.* • *My invitation to the chair's party was addressed to MISS, but the men were invited as DOCTOR.*
Unwanted sexual attention or coercion	• *A classmate kept asking me out. I refused. He commented, "Female students should all be nuns."* • *Residents were very sexist. Even the married ones flirted heavily.* • *I was married, but a married resident kept coming on to me.* • *Everyone knew which guys were "handsy."* • *Women kept moving away from one man at a departmental dinner. He was all handsy under the table.* • *The neighborhood was not safe when we had to come and go at night. Women could be approached.* • *Multiple things, like professors wanting dates or getting a good letter only if I met the assistant dean at a bar. That never sounded like a date, more like a proposition.* • *I was vulnerable and taken advantage of. Several "#MeToo" experiences that pain me greatly. I bear scars. Way more common than people think.*

Notes:

1. *Gender harassment.* Verbal and nonverbal behaviors that convey hostility, objectification, exclusion, or second-class status about members of one gender.
2. *Unwanted sexual attention.* Verbal or physical unwelcome sexual advances, which can include assault.
3. *Sexual coercion.* When favorable professional or educational treatment is conditioned on sexual activity. Harassing behavior can be either *direct* (targeted at an individual) or *ambient* (a general level of sexual harassment in an environment).

Source: National Academies of Sciences, Engineering, and Medicine.[2]

I thought the approach was like the Marines – to break you down, then build you back up in the expected image. It was derogatory, verbally abusive. Not just to me or the women, but also to the men.

Students were treated pretty badly. Everyone was demeaned, hazed. Faculty members were autocratic.

Even graduates from the 1970s pointed out that mistreatment of women was pervasive throughout American society, and they did not think their experiences were unusual. As a medical trainee, a woman was in double jeopardy of mistreatment.[2-8]

Our interviewees expected challenges to prove themselves *tough enough for medicine.* Some commented that medicine was less misogynistic than other professions at that time.

I was a secretary after college. The only way you were going to work your way up was on your back. I can't watch shows like Mad Men *– I lived it.*

I don't think women were treated as badly in medicine as in some other areas, like business.

Many women accepted mistreatment as an integral part of their acculturation into the profession. Although they recognized that the treatment of trainees was unfair and often cruel, several did not realize the extent of sexual harassment until years later.

I didn't pay attention to harassment from people in power until, years later, a speaker was brought in to talk about it. I thought, "Wow, it had been going on all the time." Maybe I had suppressed the need to understand it.

As females in our time, we thought, "I'm only being prudish, or it's just the way it is." We put up with it. Maybe I wasn't paying attention, or things didn't seem inappropriate at that time.

This perception of the accepted treatment of women at that time may explain the paradox of interviewees denying mistreatment despite clearly describing relevant incidents in their personal narratives.

Types of Gender Harassment

The assumption that women were second-class citizens was pervasive and persistent, but its manifestations changed as careers progressed. As students, women described being routinely ignored, belittled, underestimated, or hazed. As residents, some felt their treatment improved, but a few perceived increased discrimination and disrespect, for example, nurses or trainees who ignored or refused orders and input from women. In practice, interviewees continued to experience discrimination and negative attitudes. Discrimination in recruitment, mentoring, advancement, salary, and resources was a major concern early in practice. Throughout their careers, many reported lacking the professional and social networks that advanced the careers of male colleagues and provided practical support, such as covering call duties, referring patients, and sharing information and resources. Several perceived that they were *not respected or taken seriously* by some colleagues and organizations because, as wives and mothers, they *always had at least two jobs* and were not thought sufficiently committed for important responsibilities or leadership roles. Most interviewees implied that, by the end of their careers, gender harassment was a less-significant issue, due to a combination of their own efforts and changing social and professional environments.

The pervasive gender harassment took two contrasting forms, namely, marginalization and spotlighting.[4] *Marginalization* covers multiple ways of paying too little attention to members of a group. Interviewees described examples of being ignored, overlooked, or underestimated by both individuals and institutions. Marginalization could be active or passive. Interviewees described multiple examples of being denied opportunities, recognition, and advancement or being excessively burdened with unrewarding tasks. The more pervasive and insidious passive marginalization left many women feeling *frustrated and invisible*. The assumption that the careers and professional needs of their male colleagues took priority was so prevalent that some interviewees expected women to have less-prestigious roles and not aspire to stellar careers. Several commented that more mundane work, less recognition, and lower salaries were the price of being tolerated in the profession. *Maybe I should have been more assertive, more confident. I always tried not to make waves. Felt lucky to get into medicine at all.*

In contrast, *spotlighting* refers to excessive unwelcome negative attention, such as being goaded, mocked, baited, or pimped, usually in front of others.[4] Verbal abuse was the principal form of spotlighting. This ranged from inappropriate comments, teasing, and *joking around*, to insults, bullying, baiting, and statements or questions intended to be hurtful, undermine confidence, or sabotage the personal and professional reputation of female trainees or physicians. The perpetrators were predominantly male faculty members, residents, or fellow trainees, but nurses, female staff, and other women could be unsupportive or openly hostile to female physicians. Negative comments from patients were rare. Verbal harassment usually targeted women's sexuality or emotional and physical unsuitability for medicine. A common theme was that they should be raising families rather than usurping male roles in medicine.

My adviser was a bitter man, kept making weird comments, like, "How dare you take up a place here. Go home, get married, and have babies!"

Medical school was like the TV show M*A*S*H: *off-color jokes, lots of prejudice, hazing, sexual stuff at any available woman.*

Verbal harassment later in careers often focused on claims that women generated less income than their male colleagues, were less reliable, and demanded special accommodations as they attempted to meet both family and professional responsibilities.[4–12] Several interviewees reported that their clinical colleagues *made a BIG deal about accepting a woman.* Female physicians felt under continuous scrutiny and pressure to perform well without complaint. Negative attitudes were predominantly encountered from older men, and working environments improved over time.

Some of the older physicians opposed having female colleagues – worried about how to handle pregnancies, and whether I would quit working, etc. I was aware of the negative doctors, the doubts that I could hold up the income. I had to prove myself.

Financial discrimination was routine. *Definitely underpaid, especially early on, BUT we knew what we were signing up for.*

Interviewees recalled first encountering financial discrimination during college and medical school. Although many struggled to pay educational and basic living expenses, some granting agencies only funded male students.

A close friend was depending on a scholarship from her home county, but she was refused, as the widow of the donor would not allow it to be given to a girl.

Locally and nationally, student loan offices had a reputation for hostile treatment and refusing to support women.[4-7]

I was broke. I went to the student financial aid office to request a loan and was told that they did not loan money to female medical students, only single males (that is, wives could support the married guys).

Salary discrimination was prevalent when our interviewees entered practice. Recruiting a woman was perceived to be a risky financial proposition.[9-11] Whereas male recruits were courted with generous salaries, signing bonuses, coverage of moving expenses, and offers of clinical resources, such as new space, staff, and equipment, women were given the impression that they were fortunate to be accepted at all. They felt constantly under scrutiny and pressured to prove their worth, specifically to generate appropriate clinical income.

Initially, I was not paid as well as the men or offered any joining incentives or resources.

My salary was initially lower than they would have offered a man, but I made it up later. I had to prove myself.

Over decades in practice, interviewees benefitted from national progress toward salary equity, but some experienced salary discrimination even late in their careers. One woman resigned from a senior position because of salary inequities.

I left that group after 12 years, when I found out a male associate was being paid more for the same work.

Besides salary, interviewees experienced several forms of financial discrimination. One interviewee described a male colleague who claimed her billings, others knew or suspected they were not being fully credited for their work, and some reported that patients who were unable to pay or likely to generate lower billings were steered toward female physicians.

I did his work, saw his patients, but he billed under his name. The bookkeeper told me, "You see the patients, but he changes the bills to get the credit."

Some partners seemed to think I should just take care of the less-interesting, chronic, low-paying patients.

Another form of financial discrimination was in refusing or restricting resources, thus inhibiting the earning potential of female physicians. Several women described protracted and frustrating negotiations with practices or hospitals over practice facilities, equipment, and staff. These women felt they were unreasonably pressured to justify resources that would have been provided without question to a male colleague.

I was initially assigned ordinary exam rooms and struggled to do procedures. I complained, but the clinic resisted providing more suitable space. I always had to prove my department was important financially.

The hospital didn't have facilities for my specialty, and the CEO said, "We're not looking for someone like you." However, I persisted and got started with a small space in the basement. Not sure if the lack of support was because I was a woman, but a man wouldn't have had to fight so hard to build it up on his own. It was an uphill battle.

Women encountered discrimination in securing financial support from banks to establish practices. Four recounted being treated badly or swindled by financial managers, billing services, or insurance companies, and each of these interviewees speculated that they were targeted because women were perceived to be less competent in financial matters than men.

Our interviewees described a variety of strategies to address financial mistreatment. In a few cases, especially among the older informants, the status quo was begrudgingly accepted as part of generalized second-class treatment. These women described a culture in which women expected to *work twice as hard* but have lower expectations of rewards.

Men are preferred over women, although women work harder. My salary was less than others until fairly recently.

As in other forms of mistreatment, many women tolerated financial discrimination, at least initially, and hesitated to appear aggressive or to gain a reputation as difficult to work with. Some had little scope to negotiate for higher salaries or better conditions, as their families were settled in communities with a limited number of practice opportunities. The option of leaving town was often not available, and setting up an independent practice was a daunting prospect – not just financially, but in negotiating hospital privileges, on-call coverage, and other issues. The situation was especially complicated for those women whose husbands were physicians employed by the dominant hospital or group in the community.

Unwanted Sexual Attention and Coercion

Almost all interviewees reported that women routinely experienced sexual harassment during medical school. Such harassment also occurred, but was less common, later in their careers. Throughout the three decades covered by our interviews, unwanted attention, inappropriate comments, and sexist behaviors were part of a medical culture that would now be characterized as *toxic masculinity*. Sexist attitudes were so deeply ingrained in routine practices that lecture slides including pornographic images and disparaging remarks about female students, colleagues, and patients were daily occurrences and regarded as unremarkable.[3–8]

Was I sexually harassed? Yeah, all the time. Guys would constantly try to do stuff – being grabby, making comments, giving us all the wrong kind of attention.

Men are intimidated by smart women, so they try to put you down, play on your insecurity, say things like "You're not a real woman" if you didn't go along with the sexist remarks and behaviors. It was everywhere, all the time.

There was widespread harassment by faculty. Everyone was targeted.

Sexist comments were encountered on an almost-daily basis during training and ranged from off-color remarks and jokes to obscenities and overt solicitation. Practical jokes were most common during anatomy classes and involved attempts to embarrass women over examination of sexual organs.

Nearly half (48%) of the interviewees were willing to disclose personal experiences of sexual harassment that went beyond the general gender-based bantering, *joking around*, and baiting, to include propositioning, inappropriate physical contact, and even abuse. Fellow trainees were more likely to indulge in crude remarks or practical jokes than physical contact, but several attempted to obtain sexual favors from their female classmates.

One of my classmates was complaining that both his wife and mistress were busy. He offered me a ride home and definitely expected favors. He was surprised and upset when he realized he was not going to be invited in.

The majority of the more serious incidents disclosed occurred during training and involved male faculty members or supervising residents.

The male junior faculty were a problem. One of the instructors in anatomy brushed his hand on girls' bottoms every single time he walked past. Nobody ever called him out for it.

One of the professors was well-known for wanting to have an affair with every single female going through. Nearly everyone was approached. I escaped by the skin of my teeth as I had visitors when he came to my apartment. He was never called out publicly.

A hospital staff physician would find out when female residents were on call for ER and come in late at night to harass them. There was some physical contact.

In the most serious account of sexual abuse, an interviewee described being groomed and abused by a faculty member whom she first encountered as a teenage patient. The abuse continued when she became a medical student.

I have scars. I was groomed and abused for years by a man – a faculty member – who was supposed to be helping me recover from an abusive family situation. It's way more common than people think, and very destructive, especially if it starts at a younger age.

Three participants volunteered examples of sexual coercion when improved grades or a letter of recommendation were offered in return for sexual favors. Several indicated that this was not uncommon, especially in college. The usual perpetrators were junior instructors seeking to exploit the obsession of female premed students with securing excellent grades. Our interviewees were uncertain how serious some of these propositions were. *I think sometimes it was just an ego thing – maybe they were just joking around or trying it on.* Similarly, some residents were reported to imply special treatment or improved grades for a sexually compliant student, but most women did not take such propositions seriously and regarded them as examples of residents being *jerks.*

The few women who did not recall being sexually harassed cited being older, having children, and/or being married as reasons for being left alone – although several married women were harassed. Nine women made self-deprecating remarks to explain not being sexually harassed.

Everyone knew I was married, and I probably projected an image of not to be messed with.

I was never really harassed. Maybe because I was married or not cute!

If I was harassed, I don't remember it – maybe I was too mouthy!

Never happened to me – maybe I was too nerdy!

Addressing Sexual Harassment

Our interviewees stressed that sexist or even misogynistic attitudes and behaviors were *normal for the time*. Several commented, *that's just the way it was.* They had been raised in an era when women were expected to be respectful of male authority. In the masculine and hierarchical medical environment, women often felt tolerated only in sanctioned roles. Medical training was dominated by a few autocratic men who wielded enormous power. Trainees could be penalized or dismissed for any perceived shortcoming or misbehavior. They were completely dependent on the senior faculty for advancement through mentoring and professional recommendations. None dared risk the displeasure of the clinical chiefs or being regarded as a troublemaker.

The attitude was, "Just go away" (more like, "Just be quiet and keep your head down"). We don't want any trouble. There were a lot of dark days.

The options to address inappropriate behavior were severely limited, and the consequences of calling attention to gender-based mistreatment could be devastating. Women did not expect or seek intervention from supervisors or authorities and believed complaining would be counterproductive. Concerns about personal safety or injured feelings were outweighed by the implications of being labeled as difficult to work with, oversensitive, lacking in humor or team spirit, or just not suitable for medicine.

On the wards, there were problems, interactions that probably would end up in court today, but we/I were so intent on school, learning, taking care of patients, so we/I didn't worry a lot about things that might be said. "Mind your elders and go" – that was the way it was. I was fairly liberated, but I didn't do anything to make trouble.

A spirited woman could sometimes handle an interaction or avoid escalation.

There were incidents, but I just got through them. I always got on well with the guys. They would say things that women would find offensive nowadays. We just kidded them back.

It happened to us, but what were we supposed to do? Scream? I think I may have snapped "Cut it out!" one time at that anatomy instructor, but it was just the way it was.

If someone made advances, I walked away or made it clear I was not interested. If they were aware of doing these things, that's their problem. It never did bother me. I do my own thing, and nobody's gonna stop me. I was always independent.

Sometimes, classmates were supportive, and confrontation might eventually be attempted.

I had a couple of "misadventures" with faculty. A physiology professor singled me out. Pointed me out. It was inappropriate and made me angry. The guys in the class came to my rescue. They told me to "just get out of it," "never mind," and helped me push past the incidents. I confronted the professor after graduation. He apologized.

Even during student protests in the 1970s, women did not attempt to improve their situation. The only protests described by our interviewees were modest responses to pornographic material in lectures.

After all this Playboy *stuff, we put up pictures of men from* Playgirl *in the student locker room. This caused great consternation among some of our male colleagues! We had to take them down.*

What Do You Think of the #*MeToo* Movement?

Twenty-eight (76%) interviewees provided positive responses to this question. Several immediately expressed enthusiastic support.

Long overdue. Hell yeah! Some men don't seem to believe or appreciate what goes on. My husband is a nice man, but even he just doesn't get it!

Some supporters had reservations. One believed the initiative would prove futile.

It's long overdue. Will it make a difference? Probably not. Lust for power and money are strong personal urges. People with power feel entitled to do whatever they please, whenever they want.

About 30% of supporters expressed concerns about the movement going too far.

I think they are getting carried away – too much.

Women have been mistreated, and men have to be held accountable, but I think it has gotten out of hand.

Several were cautioned that situations could be misinterpreted, or women overreact.

I am ambivalent about #MeToo. *It's important to be respected, also important not to overread situations.*

A lot of it is justified, but we get too sensitive.

If someone flirts or makes a crack, you don't need to get all defensive and feel maltreated.

Others commented on the difficulties in documenting incidents. Four raised the possibility that accusations could be based on inaccurate or false memories.

I respect the #MeToo *people. Most are probably genuine, but I have encountered individuals who recanted their stories of abuse. . . . Some just need an explanation for their suffering.*

There may be honorable men who have done nothing wrong yet get accused by a vindictive woman, and careers ruined. That bothers me. A female can scream, accuse, and it is just her word against his.

In contrast, another interviewee was less sympathetic. *I realize there may be times when a man may be incorrectly accused, but I am willing for that to happen, as women have dealt with discrimination, sexual harassment for years and years and years. Males need to get up to speed!*

Interviewees were particularly concerned about the potential damage to relationships, communication, and trust among colleagues.

I feel sorry for men now. How can people date, especially if working together? Women are so touchy. Men are falsely accused. I know many men are afraid of complimenting a woman on her appearance, for fear of accusations of harassment.

Four (11%) interviewees had negative opinions about the #*MeToo* movement. These varied from outright dismissal as *ridiculous* to a sense of weariness and frustration. *I have a hard time with it. Women are independent to do what they want to do. I am tired of it.* For these participants, the importance of their work superseded concerns about personal disrespect.

I see dying patients every day and work with anxious patients, people – and yet women are worried if a guy touches a shoulder. They shudder! They believed that a female physician should be able to manage inappropriate behavior without assistance. I don't think much of it. I really don't understand all the fuss.

The opinions expressed about #*MeToo* were unrelated to personal experiences of mistreatment. All the women who were unsupportive or expressed concerns reported unwanted sexual attention in their narratives.

Would Things Have Been Different If You Were a Guy?

Several women provided flippant initial responses to this question. Both flippant and more serious considerations expressed that lives would have been *totally different* and concerned themes of working harder for less recognition, *always having two jobs*, being underestimated or overlooked, and being excluded from *the guys' game.*

Would have made more money, charged more, had a bigger practice!

Whole picture would have been different. Men get more professional support and have wives to care for them.

The men bonded. They were a close-knit community.

I had more hurdles throughout my career. Would have had less trouble getting promoted.

Several reflected that they might have had more confidence, bolder ambitions, or been less anxious to please as males, but only two speculated about specialty choices – all without regrets.

Might have done surgery – would have burned out of medicine sooner, divorced, married my nurse!

Several women believed their experiences made them better physicians and resulted in careers that were more satisfying and fulfilling than those of male colleagues.

All the problems made me more understanding, empathic, able to listen.

I think women physicians are great. We bring compassion and care that the men missed out.

Lots of the men, divorced, died young. Medicine took such a toll.

I suspect women enjoy it more than the men, especially as we get older. Men seem to turn grumpy and complain.

Advice to Young Women

Twenty-three (62%) interviewees enthusiastically encouraged women to become physicians. They conveyed *the joy of interesting, worthwhile work.*

Medicine is a wonderful, wonderful choice. You can change kids' lives, save kids' lives, give children opportunities.

Highly encourage women going into medicine. Wonderful. Certainly satisfying. I really encourage them – it's great.

Several tempered their support with cautions about hard work and overcoming challenges.

Need to be dedicated, work hard, and be persistent. Need to want to take care of people.

It's a wonderful career, but you must be ready to sacrifice. Have a singular purpose, be ready to give things up.

Really wonderful profession, if interested. Don't do it for money. You can make money without getting vomit on your shoes and blood on your clothes.

About half qualified their enthusiasm by stressing personality and motivation.

Fantastic career for women, but a lot are not suited for it. It takes a special kind of woman.

Make sure it is your passion. Do what brings you joy. Need to be smart and devoted.

Go for it if it is your calling. Medicine is a calling. Really need to like people.

About 60% offered advice about behavior, including the necessity of self-care.

Show respect for others, and other people will respect you. How you carry yourself is important. Treat other people well. If you have a chip on your shoulder, people will treat you differently.

Never take on a victim role. For sanity's sake, enjoy your profession. Be calm, not driven by irritability. When at work, give it your all.

Don't be defensive. Laugh things off. Don't get all prickly. Focus on what you want, involve people who can help you succeed. Think about how to care for yourself all the time.

Surround yourself with a community of support. It really does take a village. Learn how to self-promote.

Don't try to do too much. Get lots of outside help. Get the best possible childcare, pay someone to clean your house, make time for your partner.

Summary and Reflections

Our interviewees described multifaceted, gender-based discrimination and mistreatment that changed in focus, intensity, and prevalence as they progressed through their careers. They encountered the most blatant and serious sexual mistreatment as young women in medical school: financial and other forms of discrimination became more dominant later in their careers. The evolution of gender-based problems they described matches the pattern reported by the few available studies.[13] Throughout their lives, they navigated multiple types of both overt mistreatment and the pervasive "micro-inequities" described in the literature.[14] Nevertheless, only one interviewee described her medical school experiences in terms of the unrelenting misogyny portrayed in some writings about female trainees in the early 1970s.[4] The majority of interviewees recalled their training as a complex mixture of experiences – challenging, demanding, and sometimes frustrating or distressing, but also rewarding, fulfilling, and enjoyable times of unprecedented personal growth. Similarly, they acknowledged the many difficulties they had encountered in practice but described their careers with pride and appreciation for their lives as physicians. Above all, they were unwilling for the story of women in medicine to be dominated by the gender-based mistreatment narrative.

The earlier graduates conveyed a generally more benign impression of their experiences as trainees. This may reflect the personalities of the individuals involved, selective recall by elderly interviewees, their interpretations of terminology or events, and/or their unwillingness to share sensitive or personal information. They could, however, have benefited from a more chivalrous environment during the 1950s and the 1960s. When women represented only around 5.0% of the class, they were perceived as a non-threatening minority, or even tolerable and possibly interesting tokens of institutional fairness and modernity.[3–6] By the late 1960s, medical schools felt the impact of student protests and the divisive cultural changes roiling American society. The women's movement was highly critical of the medical profession, especially the pressures on female trainees to conform to masculine values and stereotypes.[4,5,15,16] The influx of female medical students in the early 1970s could have been perceived as threatening to the status quo both in numbers and as bringing in potential troublemakers. Some writers at that time expressed concern about a male backlash to the advancement of women in medicine, especially if the tolerable lady physician evolved into a boisterous feminist.[4] Labeling any assertive women as a "radical feminist" invoked negative images of an ugly, belligerent, and disruptive individual. Several distinguished female physicians have described how the taunt of being a radical feminist was invoked to inhibit their bolder behaviors.[4,8,15–18]

Interviewees used low-key tactics to survive and hopefully progress in medicine. Avoiding confrontation, using humor, or just enduring mistreatment seem incomprehensible to modern readers, yet reports from that time confirm that women used "self-silencing" strategies to navigate difficulties as they worked for credibility in the profession.[4,17,18] When abuse occurred, women commonly attempted to cope by minimizing the event and/or blaming themselves for contributing to the situation or failing to avoid it.[19] Personal distress was suppressed under the priority to meet the demands of robust training programs and attend to the needs of patients.[19]

Given their experiences of mistreatment and powerlessness to respond, we expected our interviewees to overwhelmingly support the *#MeToo* movement.[20,21] Conversely, they expressed a range of opinions, including negative comments. Interviewees were significantly more supportive of *#MeToo* than US women aged 65+ (76% vs. 49%), but many expressed concerns about unsupported accusations and damage to workplace relationships.[1] The interviewees who held negative opinions about *#MeToo* all spoke about ignoring or *powering through* challenges as essential in medicine. Several interviewees voiced concern that *#MeToo* drew too much attention to women's sexuality and vulnerability and undermined the credibility of female physicians, especially in leadership roles. They strongly objected to the characterization of women exclusively as victims.[20]

The female physicians of the generations covered by our interviews worked hard and endured much to establish the credibility of women as colleagues and peers in the profession. Lacking realistic role models, they were expected to be *one of the boys* yet retain certain female characteristics and sensibilities. They cultivated effective behaviors by "carefully constructing one's femininity to strike a balance between appearing too assertive or too weak."[17] Women in medicine nowadays are less likely to face such contradictions and have multiple role models of successful female physicians, including in leadership roles and in traditionally male-dominated specialties. Sadly, studies continue to report high levels of abuse among female medical students, residents, and faculty members – over 80% in a 2020 report – and to document continuing disadvantage in basic issues, including salary, mentoring, promotion, and appointment to leadership positions.[21–24]

REFERENCES

1. Pew Research Center. More than twice as many Americans support than oppose the #MeToo movement. Pew Research Center; 2022 Sep.
2. National Academies of Sciences, Engineering, and Medicine. Sexual harassment of women: climate, culture, and consequences in academic sciences, engineering, and medicine. A Consensus Study Report of the National Academies of Sciences, Engineering, and Medicine. Washington (DC): National Academies Press;2018.
3. Bourne PG, Wikler NJ. Commitment and the cultural mandate: women in medicine. Soc Probl. 1978;25(4):430–40.
4. Campbell MA. Why would a girl go into medicine? Old Westbury (NY): Feminist Press;1973.
5. Walsh MR. Doctors wanted: no women need apply: sexual barriers in the medical profession 1835–1975. New Haven and London: Yale University Press;1977.
6. Lopate C. Women in medicine. Baltimore (MD): Johns Hopkins Press;1968.
7. Bowers JZ. Special problems of women medical students. J Med Educ. 1968;43:532–7.
8. Morantz RM, Pomerleau CS, Fenichel CH. In her own words: oral histories of women physicians. Westport (CT): Greenwood Press;1982.
9. Powers L, Parmelle RD, Wiesenfelder H. Practice patterns of women and men physicians. J Med Educ. 1969 Jun;44(6):481–91.
10. Dykman RA, Stalnaker JM. Survey of women physicians graduating from medical school 1925–1940. J Med Educ. 1957;32:3–28.
11. Bobula JD. Work patterns, practice characteristics, and incomes of male and female physicians. J Med Educ. 1980;55(10):826–33.
12. Spieler C, editor. Women in medicine. 1976 Report of a Macy Conference. New York (NY): Josiah Macy Jr. Foundation;1977.
13. Templeton K, Nilsen KM, Walling A. Issues faced by senior women physicians: a national survey. J Womens Health (Larchmt). 2020 Jul;29(7):980–8.
14. Ludmerer KM. Seeking parity for women in academic medicine: a historical perspective. Acad Med. 2020 Oct;95(10):1485–7.
15. Morantz-Sanchez R. Sympathy & science: women physicians in American medicine. New York (NY): Oxford University Press;1985.
16. More ES. Restoring the balance: women physicians and the profession of medicine 1985–1995. Cambridge (MA): Harvard University Press;1999.
17. Pingleton SK, Jones EV, Rosolowski TA, Zimmerman MK. Silent bias: challenges, obstacles, and strategies for leadership development in academic medicine-lessons from oral histories of women professors at the University of Kansas. Acad Med. 2016 Aug;91(8):1151–7.
18. Pololi LH, Jones SJ. Women faculty: an analysis of their experiences in academic medicine and their coping strategies. Gend Med. 2010;7:438450.
19. Hinze SW. 'Am I being over-sensitive?' Women's experience of sexual harassment during medical training. Health (London). 2004 Jan;8(1):101–27.
20. Walling A, Gillam M, Nilsen K. 'Just the way it was': perspectives on sexual harassment in medical school and #MeToo of women graduating prior to 1975. Kans J Med. 2023 Nov 30;16:280–5.

21. Vargas EA, Brassel ST, Cortina LM, Settles IH, Johnson TRB, Jagsi R. #MedToo: a large-scale examination of the incidence and impact of sexual harassment of physicians and other faculty at an academic medical center. J Womens Health (Larchmt). 2020 Jan;29(1):13–20.

22. Chaudron LH, Harris Toi B, Chatterjee A, Lautenberger DM. Power reimagined: advancing women into emerging leadership positions. Acad Med. 2023 Jan;98:e-pub ahead of print.

23. Richter KP, Clark L, Wick JA, Cruvinel E, Durham D, Shaw P, et al. Women physicians and promotion in academic medicine. N Engl J Med. 2020 Nov 26;383(22):2148–57.

24. Skinner L, Yates M, Auerbach DI, Buerhaus PI, Staiger DO. Marriage, children, and sex-based differences in physician hours and income. JAMA Health Forum. 2023 Mar 3;4(3):e230136.

Index

Note: Page numbers in **bold** indicate a table on the corresponding page.